THE WOMEN'S
HEALTH MOVEMENT

THE WOMEN'S HEALTH MOVEMENT

Feminist Alternatives to Medical Control

Sheryl Burt Ruzek

PRAEGER PUBLISHERS
Praeger Special Studies

New York • London • Sydney • Toronto

RG
14
, U6
R88
1978

Library of Congress Cataloging in Publication Data

Ruzek, Sheryl
    The women's health movement.

    Bibliography: p.
    Includes index.
    1. Women's health services--United States.
2. Women's health services--Political aspects--United
States. 3. Feminism--United States. I. Title.
RG14.U6R88 1978   362.1   78-15483
ISBN 0-03-041436-9

PRAEGER PUBLISHERS
PRAEGER SPECIAL STUDIES
383 Madison Avenue, New York, N.Y. 10017, U.S.A.

Published in the United States of America in 1978
by Praeger Publishers,
A Division of Holt, Rinehart and Winston, CBS, Inc.

89   038   987654321

© 1978 by Praeger Publishers

Printed in the United States of America

For ARLENE KAPLAN DANIELS

I had experienced and heard of widespread mistreatment
of women by doctors. So regular were the tales of abuse
from the first gynecological examination to the last delivery that it began to resemble something more systematic
in character than an occasional lapse we have all been
encouraged to dismiss as phenomenal. It seemed rather
like a rite-de-passage, which, typically of female initia-
tions, is conducted in isolation, without fanfare, and with
brutality.

—Antoinette Groesser, "Is
Gynecology for Women?" 1972

PREFACE AND ACKNOWLEDGMENTS

My interest in the women's health movement comes from a long-standing interest in social reform movements and the role of professionals in society. In the summer of 1971, I was beginning to collect data on the early twentieth-century mental hygiene movement for my doctoral dissertation. My friend and colleague, Rachel Kahn-Hut, returned from the American Sociological Association meeting in Denver that September with a copy of the Boston Women's Health Course Collective pamphlet, Our Bodies, Ourselves. I was expecting a baby in October, and she thought that I might find the pamphlet helpful. It was, and I filed it away for future reference.

During the following year, it became clear that health care was a key feminist issue and that a separate women's health movement was emerging. As a woman, I was personally concerned over issues health activists were raising and interested in discovering how sexism affected women's individual and collective opportunities to live healthy, productive lives. As a sociologist, I was fascinated by some of the similarities and differences between the mental hygiene and women's health movements. Although both movements focused on restructuring beliefs about health and illness and attempted to renegotiate the social control function of professionals, they developed differently. Initially, both were lay movements. But while professionals almost immediately "took over" the campaign for mental hygiene, the women's health movement staunchly resisted professional domination. Both movements reflect their historical social climates. During the early 1900s, Americans believed that science, technology, and professional expertise could and would solve the growing problems of an industrializing nation. It was easy, then, for professionals to use the mental hygiene movement to promote their expertise and solidify their power.[*] By the late 1960s, Americans were wary of professionals' ability to "deliver the goods," and consumer movements sought to reduce what was seen as excessive and dangerous power in the hands of professionals.

By late 1972, I was also working on a research project (studying volunteerism in the lives of women). Arlene Kaplan Daniels, the

---

[*]For various perspectives on the mental hygiene movement, see, for example, Beers 1908; Davis 1938; Deutsch 1938; Meyer 1935; and Ridenour 1961.

principal investigator, encouraged me to follow my growing interest in reproductive health issues by studying volunteer health workers in a family planning clinic.* Eventually, I decided to combine my efforts and study the women's health movement systematically for my doctoral research.

My initial approach was to learn how participants themselves viewed the movement's purpose and structure; a variety of methods were used, including fieldwork, formal interviews, informal interviewing, and review of the growing feminist health literature. I soon discovered that the key feminist issue was who controls women's bodies. I then began studying how different segments of the movement acted to shift control away from professionals and put women themselves in charge of women's health care. Specifically, I focused on feminist approaches to obstetrical and gynecological care, in order to compare them with more conventional approaches. I also sought to compare the development of ideas about women and their bodies in a variety of social arenas. Then, following Glaser and Strauss's (1967) strategies for qualitative research, I collected data to enable me to inductively construct categories of health care worlds and feminist strategies for change. I carried out additional research until I was unable to generate new categories; my research was only yielding additional examples of health care worlds, strategies for change, and views about women and their bodies.

Between 1972 and 1975, I carried out field work and interviewed participants in both conventional and alternative settings (serving women only in California, Washington, and British Columbia). The five traditional settings included a women's clinic in a university-affiliated hospital, a proprietary hospital abortion clinic, two private nonprofit family planning clinics, and one private group practice in obstetrics and gynecology. The 19 alternative health collectives, health centers, and clinics studied were varied. Some were small (fewer than 10 active members); others were large (over 100 active member-workers). Three offered information, education, and referral only, that is, no direct services were provided. Sixteen offered direct services, ranging from routine obstetrical and gynecological care to pediatrics, geriatric services, and abortion.

In addition, I attended many public events related to feminist health concerns: university lectures on women's health issues, abortion rallies, self-help gynecology demonstrations, women's health films, health fairs, and conferences (see Appendix A). At these events, I learned of health projects, chatted informally with health

---

*This study was supported in part by National Institute for Mental Health grant no. MH 26294-01.

activists, and made contacts for interviews and additional fieldwork. I also participated in, obtained printed material from, and/or interviewed members of major feminist organizations involved in health work, including the Boston Women's Health Book Collective, Coalition for the Medical Rights of Women, WEAL (Women's Equity Action League), NOW (National Organization for Women), NARAL (National Association for the Repeal of Abortion Laws), WONAAC (Women's National Abortion Action Coalition), National Women's Health Coalition (NWHC), National Women's Health Network (NWHN), the Women and Health Roundtable, WHAM (Women's Health Action Movement), Women's Health Forum-HealthRight, and the Feminist Women's Health Centers (FWHCs) in Los Angeles, Oakland, and Orange County (see Appendix C for health organizations). Similar information was gathered from non-feminist organizations, including Planned Parenthood Affiliates and Kaiser-Permanente Health Plan, that provide obstetrical and gynecological services.

To round out my data on women's health groups, I obtained information on clinics and collectives in New York, Washington, D.C., Philadelphia, Chicago, Detroit, Ann Arbor, Boston, Denver, Honolulu, and Tallahassee, Florida, by writing to specific groups and individuals and researching the literature. When traveling, I frequented bookstores for local health group material. Friends and colleagues, alerted to my interests, sent me material on other groups and activities.

To keep abreast of new developments, I subscribed to periodicals presenting disparate perspectives—general feminist and health movement periodicals; professional, medical, social service, and social science publications; and women's magazines. (See Appendix B for a list of feminist and health periodicals.) Traditional sources were readily available in the excellent libraries of the University of California at Berkeley and San Francisco. Much of the material I gathered or consulted is organized in a partly annotated bibliography, Women and Health Care (Ruzek 1975), initially prepared for the Research Applied to National Needs section of the National Science Foundation.

When studying a social movement, it is crucial to present oneself so as to maximize opportunities for obtaining data. Although many fieldworkers disagree, I object to participant observation without revealing one's role as a researcher in any but public settings, partly because it impedes asking simple questions outright ("normal" behavior for a researcher but not for everyday participants). I also believe that it is important to explain one's role and specify what is to be investigated, as well as why and how. For presenting an identity other than one's own violates the ethos of many groups and individuals, who are understandably dubious about participating in research unless they see potential benefit to themselves.

As a women concerned with feminist health issues, I had no need for permission to attend public events. Nonetheless, others invariably asked why I happened to be there. While I rarely elaborated all of my research interests, I always discussed what I was working on at that particular moment: studying volunteer health workers, looking for individuals and organizations to include in a roster of women involved in health research, collecting material for a bibliography and resource directory on women's health, and/or analyzing feminist strategies for improving or changing the health care system.

On occasion, I simply presented myself as a person seeking medical care. In a few instances, my role as "patient" remained primary. These were all in traditional settings, where I used the need for service as an opportunity to collect additional data. Rather than make a sharp distinction between data collected in the process of living and data collected exclusively for research, I include both. Much can be learned by using one's self as "subject."

I approached most groups through personal contacts made at public events or on the recommendation of key informants. I wrote to some women's health groups to explain my research interests and asked permission to visit. By revealing in advance my research interests, members of these groups had time to think things over and express their concerns from the beginning. Some groups insisted that the decision to allow observation be approved by the entire collective. Although nearly everyone was cautious at first (and I did encounter occasional skepticism about the value of such research), no one refused to allow observation. Most groups welcomed me back; some invited me to special events; and a lay midwife asked me to attend a home birth with her. Such a movement needs attention and publicity to spread new ideas and approaches; this factor undoubtedly influenced willingness to grant interviews and allow observation.

Initially, I planned to work in several clinics, but I decided that more would be learned by dividing my time over a number of settings. I also decided it was important to maintain a degree of separateness from individual health groups. Because I wanted to discover the array of approaches and perspectives within this farflung movement, I could not possibly become actively involved in many ongoing activities.

My decision not to actively work with or for any particular group was also influenced by concern that "joining" would force me to take sides in schisms and squabbles. By maintaining some distance, I could learn more about all sides of disputes and could maintain a critical stance—difficult when too closely associated with one group.* Overall, the advantages of maintaining some distance seemed

---

*I was reminded of the importance of this after observing a clinic a colleague was studying. When reviewing my observations of

to outweigh the advantages of being a true "insider." As Roth (1963b) points out, researchers who work within organizations eventually develop "management bias."

I should emphasize, however, that I am sympathetic to the women's health movement and now consider myself a participant. The issues raised are serious and important, and the solutions to problems are innovative and exciting.

Many people made this project possible. I extend my gratitude first to the women in the health movement, who inspired me as they generously shared their work, ideas, and time. Some women were particularly helpful. Laura Brown, Carol Downer, Barbara Faltze, Amy Fine, and Lorraine Rothman criticized and commented on my early work, showing me important facets of the movement I had not yet discovered. Diane Carr, Shelley Farber, Lynn Heidelberg, Frances Hornstein, Ann Morehead, and Ellen Peskin all provided information on emerging events and on many occasions took the time to answer specific questions and locate material for me.

Julius Roth's personal encouragement, interest, critical comments, and influence on my sociological perspective—evident throughout—are acknowledged with gratitude. Arthur Lipow taught me to analyze social movements historically and shaped my approach to social stratification. Virginia Olesen's outstanding lecture series on women's roles as providers and receivers of health care at the University of California, San Francisco, beginning in 1973, broadened my perspective. Her interest and encouragement made this project especially rewarding to me. Arlene Kaplan Daniels introduced me as an undergraduate to the study of professions. She has since taught me many things in many ways, offering critical comments, suggestions, and enthusiastic encouragement. This book is dedicated to her in appreciation of her generosity as a teacher, mentor, and friend.

I extend very special thanks to my daughter, Jennifer, who personally introduced me to many conditions in the health care system that I subsequently researched. She also patiently forwent many picnics and trips to the zoo while I completed this book. My former husband, John Ruzek, deserves proper appreciation for the considerable inconvenience he endured while I worked on early parts of the project.

The Committee for Humanizing Health Care of the American Sociological Association Section on Medical Sociology generously provided funds to complete the research. Lucy Ann Geiselman and Velma Parness accommodated my requests for time away from the

---

the clinic's problematic features with her, she bristled; she later told me she was surprised that she felt so defensive over my criticizing "her" health group.

Program for Women in Health Sciences at the University of California, San Francisco, to complete the writing. Ellen Lazer of Praeger Special Studies offered helpful editorial guidance. Mary Alice Hood prepared the index. Carolee Perrett typed and checked references on an early draft; Cassandra Curtiss graciously checked references and typed, retyped, and proofread many subsequent drafts. I thank these women for their technical assistance, encouragement, and personal interest in the project.

My colleagues and friends, Shirley Cartwright, Rachel Kahn-Hut, Patricia Kelly, Nancy Kleiber, Jane Prather, and Barbara Rosenblum, all offered helpful suggestions, information, and encouragement. Belita Cowan, Arlene Kaplan Daniels, Carol Downer, Amy Fine, Lynn Heidelberg, Irwin Kaiser, Ellen Lewin, David Mechanic, John McKinlay, Judy Norsigian, Virginia Olesen, Ellen Peskin, and Julius Roth all criticized various drafts of the manuscript. Their suggestions were invaluable, although I did not always follow them. All errors, omissions, and differences in interpretation are, of course, my sole responsibility.

CONTENTS

LIST OF TABLES AND FIGURES

The Women's Health Movement

1

The Women's Health Movement:
A Challenge to Professional Authority

Recipients of many professional services are no longer accepting whatever they are given with gratitude, especially when they judge
the service to be inadequate or in some way offensive. Increasingly,
clients demand a larger "say" in what they get and how they are
treated in American social welfare, educational, and health care institutions (Haug and Sussman 1969). Disinclined to obey professionals simply on faith, clients openly challenge professionals, arguing
that they can evaluate advice and make crucial decisions about their
own lives. Many of these challenges to professional authority come
from organized consumer groups. This study examines one such
conflict between professionals and clients—the women's health movement.

Addressing the American Psychological Association meeting
in Hawaii in September 1972, feminist health activist Carol Downer
(1972, p. 1) explained why the health care system is deplored:

> In what has been described as "rape of the pelvis," our
> uteri and ovaries are removed often needlessly. Our breasts
> and all supporting muscular tissue are carved out brutally
> in radical mastectomy. Abortion and preventive birth con-
> trol methods are denied us unless we are a certain age,
> or married or perhaps they are denied us completely.
> Hospital committees decide whether or not we can have
> our tubes tied. Unless our uterus has "done its duty,"
> we're often denied. We give birth in hospitals run for the
> convenience of the staff. We're drugged, strapped, cut,
> ignored, enemaed, probed, shaved—all in the name of
> "superior care." How can we rescue ourselves from this
> dilemma that male supremacy has landed us in? The

solution is simple. We women must take women's medicine
back into our own capable hands.

The women's health movement (advocating lay control over
services) is especially important to examine because major social
institutions increasingly are unable to meet clinets' needs for humanistic or affordable treatment. Looking to professionals and other
experts for solutions to such problems has not resulted in widespread
change or improvement. Perhaps it is unreasonable or at least unrealistic to look to these experts for innovative ideas or real commitment to social change, for such persons are too tied into the system,
too dependent upon its continuance, to even have the vision of what
might be.* In contrast, social movements are one of the media through
which new ideas and new practices become part of the social fabric,
providing "valuable clues, articulated in cries of anguish and declara-
tions of hope," about the direction the future will take (Wilson 1973,
p. 4).
    While women's health movement strategies are specifically
intended to alter, improve, or drastically change routine obstetrical
and gynecological care for women, these strategies can also be viewed
as a model of how change might be effected in other fields involving
routine care or treatment. By examining this movement, we discover
how clients as a group can reshape institutions to meet their needs.
That is, in this movement, client power is not limited to individual
efforts to "beat the system" (see Freidson 1961, 1973; Field 1961;
Roth 1963; and Howard et al. 1976). Instead, focus is on group action
to bring about changes on a societal level, on the institutional level,
and in face-to-face interaction between the patient and the physician.
    Health movement strategies also are important to examine be-
cause they demonstrate how the power of the medical profession might
be reduced by altering key features of the health care system: temporal orientation, spacial relationships, distribution of expertise,
etiquette, sex-role expectations, definitions of public and private behavior, assignment of causality, access to curatives, delegation of
tasks, and license to practice. Restructuring routine care along the
dimensions suggested by health movement adherents sharply reduces
the medical profession's ability to insulate itself from public observation and avoid accountability. Finding effective new ways of providing

---

*For discussion of the role of professionals in change, see
especially McKinlay (1973). For perspectives on the importance of
marginality to innovation with particular regard to women, see Daniels 1975b; Lorber 1975; and Millman and Kanter 1975, pp. vii-xvii.

routine care and making professionals accountable for the services they deliver have important consequences for improving the quality of health care for everyone.[*]

Such a movement also reveals some of the intricate interrelationships between change on various levels of society. Studying a social movement that is self-consciously attempting to make changes on several levels of social organization can illuminate how major social institutions structure individuals' interactions. For example, when abortion was largely illegal, patients were powerless to bargain over price or quality. After abortion law reform and repeal, clients' interaction with health care providers changed dramatically, particularly in the now legal feminist abortion clinics. At the same time, one can learn how changes in individual patterns of interaction work their way "up" to change the structure of the larger society. As seen in Chapter 8, women's changing interaction patterns with obstetricians and gynecologists is forcing traditional medical institutions and practitioners to restructure hospital birth procedures, which may have a significant impact on parenting and family relations. In short, we begin to see some important relationships between the structure of social institutions and the more subjective social-psychological aspects of social life and self-identity.

THE PROBLEM OF PROFESSIONAL AUTHORITY

As Hughes (1958) points out, clients don't automatically grant professionals authority and autonomy. Professionals actively seek a mandate to define what is good and right for both the individual and for society at large in some significant aspect of life. Professionals also endeavor to obtain license to carry out their work and prevent others from infringing on their turf (Hughes 1958, pp. 78-87).

Despite professionals' desire for authority over their work, clients are not always eager to give themselves over to experts. In fact, Hughes (1958, pp. 82-83) argues that many lay people hold an aggressive suspicion of all professionals, whether plumbers or physicians. Freidson (1968, p. 27) suggests that given this underlying distrust between clients and professionals, maintaining authority is both difficult and critically important to professionals. In face-to-face

---

[*]For consideration of the importance of accountability systems, see, for example, Daniels 1973; Freidson 1970, 1975; and Freidson and Rhea 1963.

encounters with lay clients, the exercise of professional authority is inherently problematic because lay clients cannot make decisions or accept advice on the same basis as the professional, for they do not share the professional's educational and experiential background. The problem of professional authority is distinctly different, then, from that of scientific authority, which is based on persuasive evidence evaluated by individuals sharing a similar knowledge base.

Professionals who serve clients can maintain their inherently problematic authority because it is institutionalized in ways that minimize reliance on explanation or persuasion (Freidson 1968, pp. 27-29). Certain structural features of medical practice put professionals in a powerful authoritative position vis-a-vis their clients. The professional's quasi-legal monopoly over specific services effectively cuts out competition. Under these conditions, clients must accept professional dictates, since they have nowhere else to turn. In addition, the professional claims exclusive access to related goods and services consumers believe they need to manage problems with or without expert advice. By acting as gatekeeper to what is popularly valued, the professional can make taking his or her advice a prerequisite for obtaining a good or service. Professional authority against client pressure is also buttressed when the profession limits its size (through recruitment or licensing) and the clientele is unorganized. For when the number of practitioners is small relative to demand and the clientele is unorganized, individual practitioners can refuse client requests without risking economic or political ruin (Freidson 1968, p. 29).

The overall consequence of institutionalized medical authority is that lay clients' behavior is limited and channeled, so that when they consult professionals, they have few alternatives for action.* Under these circumstances, it is not necessary to exert influence by persuading the client that the professional advice or service is valid and worth following. Of course, the client can withdraw and refuse to accept what is offered. But when alternatives are scarce, the client may just give in and obey, or clients may happen to agree with what the professional suggests or in the course of the interaction come to believe that what the professional recommends is in fact in their best interests (Freidson 1968, pp. 29-30).

Nonetheless, what the professional really desires or demands is that clients obey out of faith in the practitioner's competence and

---

*See Roth 1977a and Macintyre 1977 for examples of how this process operates in the United Kingdom in a socialized health care system where authority is highly institutionalized.

not on the basis of the clients' evaluation of the advice. Stress is on imputed rather than demonstrated competence. This emphasis reveals the special source of professional authority—encumbency in an expert status (Freidson 1968, pp. 30-31).*

REVOLT OF THE CLIENT

Despite professionals' desire for unquestioning acceptance of their authority, clients no longer obey simply on faith. In fact, conflict between professionals and clients—particularly clients from subordinate or subjugated groups—is a dominant theme of this era. Regardless of the setting where conflicts occur, clients attack the basic legitimacy of professionals to exercise power and authority over key aspects of their lives. Haug and Sussman (1969, p. 156) suggest that clients may question professional authority for any or all of the following reasons:

(1) the expertise of the practitioners is inadequate,
(2) their claims to altruism are unfounded,
(3) the organizational delivery system supporting their authority is defective and insufficient, or
(4) this system is too efficient and exceeds the appropriate bounds of its power.

In the past decade, organized clients have expressed dissatisfaction through varied consumer movements: women, students, minorities, service workers, and some segments of the educated elite who are concerned with "public interest" issues (for example, Nader's "raiders"). Gartner and Riessman (1974) view these groups as a consumer vanguard—a potentially powerful force in transforming society. Since many such groups are relatively disadvantaged in American society, they stand to gain considerably by pushing for social change.

Some suggest that conflicts between clients and professionals in the human services represent the new dialectic. For as the labor force shifts from industrial production to the production of services, control over this segment of the economy increases in importance (Bell 1973; Freidson 1973b; Gartner and Riessman 1974; compare Etzioni 1974). Control over human services necessarily entails conflict with professionals, who dominate major service institutions.

---

*See Schutz 1964 for discussion of the problem of lay persons selecting advice from experts (whose opinions often differ).

CONFLICT IN THE HEALTH CARE SYSTEM

In this age of discontent with social services, the health care system is under constant attack. The young, the poor, minorities, the aged, and feminists all are disenchanted with major aspects of American medicine. It costs too much, is maldistributed, and all too often ranges from ineffective to downright dangerous. Politicians refer to the situation as a "crisis." Physicians do not like the complaints and resent it when patients try to tell them what to do and the government threatens to tell them what to charge. Doomsayers prevail in various camps and even envision "the end of medicine" (see, for example, Carlson 1975; Ehrenreich and Ehrenreich 1971; Illich 1976; Kennedy 1972; and Rushing 1971).

While outside pressure mounts, conflict within the health care system is on the rise. New paraprofessionals and allied health workers, spawned to fill gaps in services, battle over occupational boundaries, laying claim to exclusive control over their turf. They also want bigger roles in decision making and larger shares of the profits (see, for example, Adamson 1971; Bullough 1975; Elling 1971; Freidson 1970; Sadler, Sadler, and Bliss 1972; and Zola and Miller 1973).

Insiders and outsiders alike criticize the helter-skelter way the division of labor is proceeding and decry the class and sex segregation perpetuated by new occupational categories. Nurses and nurse practitioners, for example, fear that physicians' assistants represent a male invasion of medicine at a level inaccessible to female nurses with far more extensive education (Cooper 1970; Reverby 1972a, 1972b). At the lower levels in nursing, race and class lines are reinforced through tracking systems. Working-class women and minority women are channeled into licensed vocational nursing, while white middle-class women become registered nurses in programs requiring little additional training (C. Brown 1975; Navarro 1975).

Physicians, the aristocrats of the health system, must also renegotiate their roles. Some staunchly defend traditional solo practice, while others endorse group practice and large bureaucratically organized health maintenance organizations. While many physicians accept greater specialization and reliance on sophisticated medical technologies, others are moving back toward family centered practice, emphasizing personal contact and empathy rather than space age gadgetry (Cordtz 1971; Howell 1975a; Illich 1976).

Since the mid-1960s, health care consumer and reform movements have grown in several directions. Liberals, radicals, and visionaries all propose to reshape the health care system in keeping with their general values and beliefs about how society is best organized (see, for example, Alford 1975; Bazell 1971; Gossett 1971; Hoffman 1972; Sade 1971; and Wolfe 1971). Liberal reformers, seeking to reduce costs and increase accessibility of services, look to the government to order the chaos they argue arises from a nonsystem of small, uncoordinated providers. Essentially, liberals seek to put regulation into the hands of federal "medicrats," leaving the medical profession's power largely intact and, in some areas, strengthened. The overall strategy is for the government to see to it that it is "good business" for doctors to respond to the needs of the people for health care (Shostak 1974, p. 95).

While liberals believe that medical care can be provided by individual providers on a fee-for-service basis without risking serious abuses, radical reformers do not. Radicals argue that the profit motive is pernicious not only within the health care system but within the entire society. Meaningful change in established health institutions is virtually impossible without concomitant changes in the larger society (Ehrenreich and Ehrenreich 1971; Lichtman 1971). Some suggest that a major obstacle to change is the presence of professionals. Geiger (1971, p. 25), for example, argues that the health care system is run for the benefit of professionals, who ignore, accept, or profit from a social order that creates poverty, racism, inequity, oppression, and indignity. Professionals' roles in these institutions are, then, by nature, reactionary and oppressive.

For both practical and ideological reasons, radicals focus on the contributions of paraprofessionals in a national health system. Midwives and Chinese barefoot doctors are idealized as desirable models of "peoples' healers." Free or low-cost health care for everyone in community-controlled clinics is seen as a crucial link in the process of the people taking control over the entire society.

Others take issue with both liberal and radical reform schemes. Shostak (1974) identifies these reformers as visionaries, because they conceptualize health and illness in a completely different way. Health is regarded as a state of being, a heightened sense of self-realization, self-liberation, and self-actualization, whereas illness reflects a breakdown in individuals' normally harmonious balance of mind and body in relation to the social world in which they live. Central to visionary reform is cooperative care based on self-help and patient participation—a rejection of all that is currently authoritarian in our health care system (Shostak 1974, p. 117).

Visionaries also reject the notion of health care as a product—something to be purchased or delivered—preferring to regard themselves as participants rather than as consumers in health. Visionaries (Costanza 1972, p. xxviii) thus pose very fundamental and startling questions: Should not people be active participants in decision making concerning their health? Should not the patient be regarded primarily as a thinking, responsible person?

Health care professionals are understandably threatened by visionaries, for they imply that health professionals have no instrinsic expertise about the moral, social, and political wisdom of the health care system. Visionaries, in fact, suggest that given the facts, the American public can decide what a reasonable national health care system should be. They also imply that patients can actively decide about their medical treatment, just as they decide whether or not to accept the advice of counsel (Costanza 1972, p. xxviii).

When such visionary views are called "utopian," "cultish," "antitechnological," or "apolitical," proponents argue that the profound political ramifications of their proposals are misunderstood or ignored. In fact, Marieskind and Ehrenreich (1975, p. 41) suggest that the crucial political aspects of the women's health movement are incorrectly dismissed as "only palliative." They argue that in medicine, the present organization of production, which concentrates knowledge and control in a professional elite, is not the inevitable outcome of a rational science and technology but, rather, is generated by the need to preserve prevailing patterns of class, race, and sex domination. By reversing or altering the hierarchical, scholastical, and antiempirical relationships in the health system, women can pave the way for a socialist transformation of society. Illich (1976, pp. 8-9) similarly suggests that medicine is a key area for political action by groups wishing to halt the industrial mode of production. Only people who have the ability for mutual self-care (combined with the application of contemporary technology) will be ready to limit the industrial mode of production in other major areas.

SOCIAL PROBLEMS AND SOCIAL MOVEMENTS

How has the health care system come to be regarded as a major social problem by organized client groups? As Fuller and Myers (1941, p. 320) point out, social problems are conditions defined by a considerable number of persons as deviating from some cherished social norm. Although objective conditions are necessary, they are not in themselves sufficient to constitute a social problem, unless people involved in them regard them as such.

Cultural values play a causal role in what objective conditions are defined as problems (Fuller and Myers 1941, pp. 320-21). Theoretically, social problems could develop as a result of (1) changing objective conditions that conflict with established cultural values, (2) changing values that conflict with pre-existing objective conditions, or (3) a shift in both values and objective conditions. A significant social movement can emerge when a substantial group of people define a condition as an intolerable injustice rather than as a misfortune warranting charitable consideration (Turner 1969, p. 391).

The appearance of social movements is a sign that part of the existing social order is being challenged, having lost its sacredness in the process of becoming irrelevant or detrimental to peoples' needs. The rise of social movements also indicates that new social worlds have been conceived, new hopes have arisen, and faith has been renewed in the idea that humanity can improve the human condition through its own efforts (Wilson 1973, p. 4).

Social movements are situated at a nexus between the institutionalized and noninstitutionalized aspects of life, where they can function as agents of social change. In contrast to mere aggregate action, social movements are conscious, collective, and organized attempts to bring about or resist social change—often through the use of noninstitutional means (Wilson 1973, pp. 8-11).

Movements are often complex, consisting of various levels that should be clearly distinguished. A general social movement has no firm sense of direction and neither organization nor formal leadership. General social movements are expressed in a variety of ways—through trends in literature, art, the popular press, and novel life-styles (Blumer 1946, pp. 200-202; Wilson 1973, p. 11). General movements involve cultural drifts, which in turn act as seedbeds of many specific social movements—movements that possess leaders and have a more definite direction and "we-consciousness." Within these specific social movements, numerous movement organizations plan, organize, and carry out specific actions (Wilson 1973, p. 11; Zald and Ash 1966, p. 327). It is crucial not to confuse formally constituted movement organizations with social movements themselves, although these groups may function as the active components of a movement (Ash 1972, pp. 1-2).

The contemporary feminist movement is a general movement that has changed opinions, attitudes, and self-conceptions and has produced ideas arousing new consciousness and new basic cultural values about women. It has also spawned numerous specific social movements and movement organizations. The women's health movement is a specific social movement, distinguished from the general movement by its emphasis on health and body issues. It emerged as a result of changes both in women's values and in the objective conditions of health care during the late 1960s and early 1970s.

During the late 1960s, women's values and self-concepts began to change as they participated in the feminist movement. As feminists became more assertive and self-sufficient, they rejected the stereotypical passive feminine role supporting the traditional authoritarian medical-professional model, particularly in obstetrics and gynecology. As we shall see in subsequent chapters, dissatisfaction with conventional obstetrical and gynecological services is now widespread, even among women not actively involved in either the women's health movement or the larger feminist movement. While many of the objective conditions feminists decried existed prior to the emergence of the contemporary feminist movement, feminism aroused awareness of these conditions in ways that led to their being defined as problems. Investigating objective conditions, activists identified and interpreted existing practices as manifestations of male domination of medicine. Finally, certain objective conditions of women's health care worsened: the abortion mills and the medical community's discovery of iatrogenic (physician-induced) disorders related to reproductive technology (publicized in the early 1970s) shaped feminists' view that health care is hazardous to women's health.

2

Health and Body Issues:
The Feminist Imperative

WOMEN AND THE HEALTH SYSTEM

While critics argue that the health system is oppressive and unresponsive to the needs of both men and women, feminists find it particularly problematic for women. First, the very organization of the health care system reflects and perpetuates the social ideology of women as sex objects and reproductive organs. In the promotion of the specialty of obstetrics and gynecology, women are encouraged to enter the health system through their reproductive organs. Marieskind (1975b, p. 48) suggests that

> we would think it very humorous to have men entering the health system through their penises, reproductive systems, and urologists; why do we not find it equally ludicrous that women's health care is principally organized around her uterus and her reproductive potential?

Gynecological Imperialism

Women do more than "enter" the health system through their reproductive organs; they often organize their health care around gynecological care. From puberty until well past menopause, many women see no other physician on a regular periodic basis (Burkons and Willson 1974).

With sharply declining birth rates, obstetricians and gynecologists must look for ways to expand their roles (Gibson 1976). One plan recently advocated by the American Medical Association (AMA) is to have obstetrician-gynecologists formally recognized as women's

11

primary health providers, since many already function in this role
(Pearson 1975). Feminist health activists strongly oppose this desig-
nation, for they seek to limit, rather than expand, gynecologists' influence and authority (see, for example, Howell 1975b; Marieskind
1975b; Marieskind and Ehrenreich 1975). They are especially adamant
that surgical specialists should not provide routine care (Cowan 1978).

Much of the desire to restrict physicians' roles grows out of
feminists' deep distrust of the male-dominated medical system and
its reflection, in microcosm, of the larger sexist society. Medical
sexism is especially pernicious, for it is veiled in the medical mystique of science and rationality. Because women have been largely
excluded from acquiring scientific knowledge, they have had little
opportunity to question medical practices in this culturally sanctioned
manner. Thus, their complaints have been disregarded as emotionalism or neuroticism. Nonetheless, although medicine purports to
be grounded in science, many medical practices have neither been
systematically examined nor scientifically validated. They are simply
practices grounded in untested assumptions, beliefs, and stereotypes
that have been embedded in the general culture and incorporated into
clinical practice (Ruzek 1974).*

The medical profession has shown itself capable of treating
women in ways that uphold the beliefs, values, and needs of men. As
subsequent chapters will show, male lawmakers and physicians are
accused by feminists of restricting access to contraception and abortion without regard for women's welfare or rights to control their own
fertility. With equal disregard for women's health and safety, profiteering inventors and drug companies and ineffective regulatory agencies promote widespread use of hazardous drugs and devices primarily
affecting women. Physicians also perform a disproportionate amount
of unnecessary reproductive tract surgery. Childbirth practices are
tailored to the convenience of physicians rather than patients—often
to the serious detriment of both mother and child. Many psychological
therapies are specifically designed to make women's behavior conform to traditional sex-role behavior. In short, many feminists view
obstetrics and gynecology as a devastating form of sexual politics,
putting men's interests ahead of women's health.

----

*For example, physicians often declare without any systematic
appraisal of actual patient preferences or reactions that patients prefer being addressed in certain ways, cannot handle medical information, and will develop psychosomatic symptoms if informed of drug
side effects.

Utilization Patterns

The health care system is also more problematic for women than men because they use it more often and under different circumstances, especially during their reproductive years. Women's greater dependence on the medical system is reflected in their utilization rates. National studies of health services utilization reveal that in a given year in the United States, approximately 71 percent of all women visit a physician, compared with 65 percent of all men. In addition, women report more visits each year—an average of 4.5 visits, compared with 3.6 for men. A similar pattern is found in hospital admissions. Each year, 16 out of every 100 women are admitted to hospitals, compared with 11 out of every 100 men. However, despite common stereotypes, women are not necessarily "sicker" than men, for when physician visits and hospitalization for pregnancy and delivery are subtracted, the differences in utilization rates between men and women disappear. Women simply have much more contact with the medical profession than do men. If one also adds visits to pediatricians, women have nearly 100 percent more physician contact than do men (Kravits 1976; Anderson, Kravits, and Anderson 1975; Lipman-Blumen 1975).

Many of women's contacts with the health care system occur when they are "well" rather than "sick." Feminists complain that they are denied the right to participate fully in making decisions when they visit physicians during pregnancy, or when they seek routine gynecological examinations, contraceptives, or abortions, or when they accompany their children to pediatricians. These women say that they are not in need—either psychologically or technically—of a powerful authority figure in these situations. Yet, typically, women must seek care in institutions organized around a health care delivery model based largely on the assumption of acute illness, where such authority on the part of the physician has been considered justified. Women feel strongly that this inappropriate role relationship perpetuates the stereotypical sex-role relationship, where the female must be passive and dependent, while the male is active, instrumental, and authoritative. When women attempt to break out of these traditional sex roles, they meet with anger and hostility and face labeling as "mentally disturbed."

The Medicalization of Female Culture

Despite inaccurate stereotypes of women as inherently "sicker" than men and as "weak" or neurotic overusers of health services, their greater dependence on the health system stems largely from the medicalization of crucial biological life events—menarche, pregnancy, childbirth, and menopause. All of these events are important rites of passage for females and have significant consequences for their sense of self and feminine identity (Hammer 1975). In American society, these crucial status-passages are presided over by men— medical men—who claim to know best how to steer women through these important events (Glaser and Strauss 1967, p. 10).

With the revival of feminism in the mid-1960s, women began to question whether or not medical men are in fact best qualified to assist them either technically or symbolically. Feminists seriously question physicians' technical expertise in many areas related to female sexuality and reproduction. In addition, they doubt physicians' altruism and ethics and suspect that profit, rather than professional judgment, motivates many physicians to practice as they do. Finally, some feminists believe that women's routine health needs cannot and should not be met by male professionals, regardless of their competence or humaneness. Instead, routine care should be deinstitution- alized, deprofessionalized, and reintegrated into female culture, as it was historically in Western countries and as it remains in primitive societies.

In primitive societies, male and female worlds are typically separate and distinct. In women's worlds, female healers instruct young girls in the beliefs and practices surrounding their reproductive functions. Older lay women and midwives guide girls through their first and subsequent menstruation and assume responsibility for per- forming female initiation ceremonies (Brown 1963; Young 1962; Young and Bacdayen 1965; Shandall 1967). Pregnancy and childbirth, of course, are the traditional domain of female midwives and kin (Haire 1972; Mead and Newton 1967; McArthur 1973).

Feminist historians argue that prior to the early twentieth cen- tury, American women's reproductive functions (from menarche to menopause) were firmly enmeshed in a female culture, which offered sympathetic personal support and guidance (Smith 1970; Smith-Rosen- berg 1973, 1975). The biological realities of frequent pregnancies, childbirth, nursing, and menopause bound women together in physical and emotional intimacy, so that mother and daughter roles shaded imperceptibly into each other (Smith-Rosenberg 1975, p. 9).

In the twentieth century, female culture disintegrated, or was diminished, by declining birth rates, increases in geographical mo- bility, and the superficial entry of women into male culture. But the demise of female culture began earlier, during the early 1800s in the United States, as males assumed obstetrical and gynecological tasks.

Ehrenreich and English (1972) argue that American women's traditional roles as healers were deliberately usurped by white upper- class males as part of their struggle to gain ascendency. During the early 1800s, there were few restrictions on practice, so medicine was open to anyone who professed or demonstrated healing skills (Ehrenreich and English 1972, p. 20; Shryock 1966, pp. 156-58). At this time, women functioned autonomously as midwives and general healers and frequently practiced jointly with their husbands. Some entered practice after caring extensively for family members or serving an apprenticeship with an established healer (Ehrenreich and English 1972, pp. 20-21). Although there was a growing number of formally trained white male doctors, or "regulars," their education varied tremendously in length and scope and sorely lacked a scientific base (Ehrenreich and English 1972, pp. 21-22; Shryock 1966, pp. 71-89, 152-54; Wood 1973, pp. 32-33). Nonetheless, by 1830, 13 states had passed medical licensing laws establishing the regulars as the only legal practitioners (Ehrenreich and English 1972, p. 22).

Despite the early nineteenth-century efforts of medical regulars to establish themselves as the official doctors, they were accepted only by certain segments of the middle and upper classes; their expertise and authority were doubted and openly challenged by others. Between 1830 and 1870, reaction against the medical regulars erupted into a popular health movement, supported heavily by feminists and working-class radicals, who assailed the regulars for their ineffective and hazardous "cures" and for elitism. Gradually, the popular health and feminist movements merged and became indistinguishable (Ehrenreich and English 1972, p. 24; Shryock 1966, pp. 111-25; Wood 1973, pp. 40-52).

Shryock (1966, pp. 120-22) argues that the attacks on the medical profession were far more successful than is generally recognized. The principles for which these early health reformers fought—recognizing the dangers of drugs, the importance of hygiene, and the soundness of the philosophy of prevention—were ultimately accepted by the regular profession. In addition, all American laws against irregular practice passed during the early 1800s were repealed or nullified by midcentury. Thus, virtually anyone could be a "doctor" (Shryock 1966, pp. 120-22).

During the latter half of the nineteenth century, feminists viewed the admittance of women to medicine as a test case for their whole movement for equal rights and campaigned for women to take their rightful place in medicine (Shryock 1966, p. 179; Wood 1973, pp. 43-52). In fact, some challenged the propriety of men's involvement in medicine. For example, in 1852, Sara Josepha Hale, editor of Goday's Ladies Book, remarked: "Talk about this (medicine) being the appropriate sphere for men, and his alone! With tenfold more plausibility and reason, we say it is the appropriate sphere for women, and hers alone" (Shryock 1966, p. 179). Apparently, many women patients agreed. As early as 1853, the Boston Medical Journal reported that competition was becoming serious; women were already cutting in on the profits in obstetric cases. In Boston, a Dr. Gregory directly accused the doctors of desiring a male monopoly of the market. In the following years, there was open suspicion that doctors opposed medical women (both regular and sectarian) out of fear of economic competition (Shryock 1966, p. 187).

By the turn of the century, the regular medical profession was able to reconsolidate its power through the patronage of foundations, whose benefactors shared the same class background and interests as did the elite of the regulars. In 1903, with the intention of creating a respectable, scientific American medical profession, the foundations began pouring funds for training and scientific research into the elite schools (Ehrenreich and English 1972, pp. 29-30).

Impressed that university affiliation and scientific research would indeed improve medical training, many women physicians, such as Emily Blackwell and Mary Putnam Jacobi, strove to have women admitted to regular schools. By 1900, women were technically accepted at major university medical schools, and all of the regular women's medical colleges except the Women's Medical College of Pennsylvania merged with other schools or closed. However, many women continued to train in sectarian schools, which were more open to female students (Shryock 1966, p. 190).*

Concerned over the discrepancies in training between university and proprietary medical schools after the turn of the century, the Carnegie Foundation sent Abraham Flexner on a national tour of medical schools. Flexner evaluated programs against the scientific model of Johns Hopkins, and in 1910 published his recommendations on which schools should and should not survive. Flexner's report resulted in the closing of scores of medical schools, including six of the eight black medical schools and the majority of the sectarian or irregular colleges, which had been a haven for female students (Ehrenreich and English 1972, pp. 29-30; Shryock 1966, p. 188).

As medical knowledge grew, better training was surely needed. However, Ehrenreich and English (1972, pp. 30-31) argue that the foundations had no intention of making better training available to the great mass of healers. Instead, the foundations ensured that medicine became an almost exclusively white male profession. Professionalizing medicine in this way did not immediately improve the quality of care, however, for the run-of-the-mill regular doctor did not suddenly acquire a knowledge of medical science but rather the mystique of medical science (Ehrenreich and English 1972, p. 31).

---

*For a detailed history of women in medicine, see Walsh 1977.

With increased power and prestige, organized medicine sought to improve its monopoly position further by driving out the last hold-outs of irregular practice—midwives. In this endeavor, regular female physicians were as adamant as men that anyone practicing obstetrics should have a full medical education. Thus, the few attempts to revive midwifery through better training were submerged by the cry for more women medical practitioners (Ehrenreich and English 1972; Kobrin 1966, pp. 350-59; Sablosky 1976; Shryock 1966, p. 182).

Beginning in 1910, licensing laws enacted throughout the United States created a medical monopoly over obstetrical and gynecological care (Ehrenreich and English 1972, p. 31; Kobrin 1966, pp. 350-51). Outlawing midwifery hurt women in several ways. Despite physicians' attempts to convince the public that midwives were dirty, ignorant, and incompetent, it is far from certain that physicians offered superior care. A study conducted by Dr. J. Whitridge Williams at Johns Hopkins in 1912 indicated that most American doctors were less competent than the midwives; quick to blame uterine infections and neonatal blindness on midwives, doctors themselves were unreliable at preventing these complications. Furthermore, the new medical specialists were sometimes eager to use surgical techniques not fully mastered and thus lost more patients from ineptness than midwives did from infection (Ehrenreich and English 1972, pp. 31-32; Kobrin 1966, pp. 351-53). In some areas, infant mortality rates actually rose in the years immediately following the bans on midwifery (Kobrin 1966, p. 362).

Outlawing midwifery also undermined and diminished women's culture. As Millet (1970, p. 35) points out, by declaring reproduction the proper domain of male physicians, childbirth was taken out of the home—the only area where female authority was permitted. Thus, as childbirth was transformed into a medical event, women were robbed of the core of their female world. Without the shared experience of childbirth, where they were heroines and healers, no sphere of life remained to hold roles actually and symbolically more important and prestigious than those of men.

As women became less interdependent upon each other and as childbirth became a medical procedure, women's culture—and with it, women's traditional source of strength and pride—began to diminish. As women were treated like helpless children by the medical profession in childbirth, they became less competent. The more women were "helped," the more they needed assistance. Indeed, Millet (1970, p. 47) argues that patriarchal circumstances and beliefs seem to poison women's sense of physical self until it often truly becomes the burden it is said to be.

ABORTION: THE KEY ISSUE

With the resurgence of feminism in the late 1960s and early 1970s, female culture was rediscovered. As women met in large and small groups, they soon discovered many common concerns over their health and their reproductive lives. Along with their growing criticism of women's subordinate role in every social institution, feminists voiced particular dissatisfaction with the medical care they received. They were outraged at the demeaning manner in which they were treated and critical of the quality of care available regardless of how much they paid. Above all else, they rebelled at the control men had over their bodies and reproductive functions. From the Supreme Court to the examining room, men were making fateful decisions about women's bodies and their reproductive lives.

As women discussed their problems, attempts to gain equal rights in education, politics, employment, and the family were soon seen as impossible unless women could control their own reproduction. For as Cisler (1970, p. 246) points out, without the capacity to limit reproduction, a woman's other "freedoms" are illusory. This was not a new feminist issue. Margaret Sanger, heroine of the earlier twentieth-century feminist agitation, spent her life campaigning for birth control, arguing that no woman is free unless she owns and controls her own body and can choose consciously whether she will or will not be a mother (Sanger 1920, p. 94).

Contemporary feminists (like Sanger in earlier years) recognized that the abortion issue goes beyond terminating unwanted pregnancies. Frankfort (1972, pp. xxxiii-v) argues the real reason that moralists in the church, state, and medical profession oppose abortion so strongly is that they recognize the revolutionary impact of fertility control. They fear that if women are free to end unwanted pregnancies, they might choose not to have children at all, to remain unmarried, or even to love women rather than men. In fact, all the traditional role expectations that subordinate women for the convenience of men might be destroyed.

While abortion was controversial, even within the growing women's movement, it was a powerful issue because it was clear and concrete. It also created personal conflict, for while unwanted pregnancies have been a major source of women's oppression, women have been socialized to equate their sense of self with motherhood. Abrogating motherhood for anything but life-threatening reasons counters the expectation that women wholeheartedly embrace the maternal role.

The abortion campaign proved to be the one issue that aroused mass participation. While some women were drawn into battle out of feminist consciousness, others developed a greater awareness of their subjugation in society through active participation in the abortion campaign. This campaign, then, was crucial not only to women's freedom but, also, to the growth of the women's movement itself. Fighting for a concrete issue with both real and symbolic importance provided the cohesion, sense of group strength, and recognition of powerlessness vis-a-vis established institutions needed to build and sustain a broad-based movement.

Moves Toward Abortion Reform

The women's movement was not the only organized attack on the abortion laws in the United States. In 1959, the American Law Institute (ALI) recommended that abortion should be available under the following circumstances:

1. When continuation of pregnancy would gravely impair the physical or mental health of the mother,
2. When the child might be born with a grave physical or mental defect,
3. When pregnancy resulted from rape, incest, or other felonious intercourse, including illicit intercourse with a girl below the age of sixteen (Lader 1967, pp. 145-146).

While some regarded the ALI code as a step in the right direction, critics argued that anything but complete legalization compromised women's freedom. The ALI reforms were also seen as unmanageable, leaving physicians to determine what constituted "health" (Lader 1967, pp. 168-69).

The public entered the debate in 1962 when it came to light that the tranquilizer thalidomide caused severe birth defects. Sherri Finkbine, who used the tranquilizer during early pregnancy, was unable to obtain an abortion in the United States. Widespread publicity followed when she obtained an abortion in Sweden. Public discussion of abortion resurfaced in 1964 when a German measles epidemic resulted in the birth of over 20,000 seriously deformed children—many to mothers who would have had abortions if permitted (Hole and Levine 1971, pp. 283-84; Lader 1967, pp. 10-16).

Despite restrictions on abortion during the early 1960s, an estimated 1 million women each year obtained abortions—most of them illegal (Lee 1969, pp. 5-6). By 1970, feminist sources estimated one-fourth of all American women had had illegal abortions (Morgan 1970, p. 559). Illegal abortions were sought not only by single women but by married women who had all the children they wished or could support (Lee 1969, p. 6). Nor was illegal abortion the exclusive province of any single social class or ethnic group. However, poor and minority women suffered most from illegal abortions, with death and complication rates far higher than for white middle-class women (Morgan 1970, p. 559; Polgar and Fried 1976).

Although many women sought abortions during the 1960s, public opinion was largely unfavorable. Blake's (1971) analysis of data from five Gallup polls (taken between 1962 and 1969) and the National Fertility Study conducted by Ryder and Westoff (1965) reveals that during this period, women were particularly opposed to abortion. In fact, abortion was most acceptable to non-Catholic well-educated "establishment"-oriented men. Although disapproval of abortion declined somewhat during this decade, Americans were generally against abortion, except to preserve the mother's health or prevent deformed births. Purely elective abortion was disapproved of by 80 percent of the population (Ryder and Westoff 1965, p. 540).

Blake's analysis of these data is interesting—particularly in light of later developments in the feminist movement. Blake (1971, p. 544) argues that upper-class men, who were most open to abortion, had much to gain and little to lose by legalizing it. They were satisfied with small families and were particularly vulnerable to financial and social responsibility for accidental pregnancies—in or outside marriage. In addition, it is women, not men, who undergo the procedure.

Upper-class women were more opposed than men, according to Blake (1971, pp. 544-45), because motherhood was the principal career for such women. Legalized abortion would not only remove much of the "mystique" of motherhood but might also undercut a woman's opportunity to create a respected occupational niche "simply by being careless." Inconvenience notwithstanding, pregnancy could provide a woman with a source of income, social status, and sense of achievement.

Blake (1971, p. 545) also argues that resistance to abortion is greatest in the lower classes—especially among females—because the norms supporting reproductive behavior are central to many noneconomic goals of most of the population. Despite the economic advantage of having fewer children, the majority of women (and less-advantaged persons) derive most of their lifetime rewards from the family and tend to support it unconditionally. The legal restriction on abortion indicates the state's recognition and support of their life's work. Lifting these restrictions would suggest the state's indifference to this work.

Despite negative public opinion, a growing number of Americans were calling for liberalization of restrictive laws by the middle 1960s. As might be expected from Blake's analysis, upper-middle-class men were active in organizing the early abortion reform movement. In 1964, the Association for the Study of Abortion was founded by doctors, theologians, social workers, and lawyers to compile data on abortion and to make it a public issue. The same year, birth control advocate Bill Baird established the Parents' Aid Society in New York to help women locate qualified (albeit illegal) abortionists—the first such "aboveground" abortion service (Hole and Levine 1971, p. 284).

Legislative reform was first enacted in Colorado in 1967 along the lines suggested by the ALI code. By 1970, 11 other states (Arkansas, California, Delaware, Georgia, Kansas, Maryland, New Mexico, North Carolina, Oregon, South Carolina, and Virginia) had passed similar reform laws. As the laws were about to be liberalized, abortion referral services appeared (Hole and Levine 1971, pp. 284-85).

Reform Versus Repeal

The first "official" involvement of the women's movement in the abortion issue came in November 1967 at the second National Organization for Women (NOW) convention. The NOW bill of rights, adopted after lengthy emotional debate, demanded that laws limiting access to contraceptive information and devices be removed from the penal code and that laws governing abortion be repealed (Morgan 1970, pp. 512-14).

By 1970, three states—Hawaii, Alaska, and New York—repealed their restrictive laws (Hole and Levine 1971, p. 285). The shift from reform to repeal was crucial to feminists. Abortion reform was totally unacceptable because it took the decision making out of the hands of women and turned it over to men. In addition, reform ignored the underlying basic feminist goal—to guarantee women the right to limit their reproduction. All the other reasons for repealing the laws, ranging from lowering welfare expenditures to making happier families, were simply embroidery on the real feminist issue (Cisler 1970; Hole and Levine 1971, pp. 294-302).

Nonetheless, even feminists were divided over just what constituted repeal. The three first abortion repeal laws, in fact, specified some qualifications, including one or more of the following:

...the woman must be a resident of the state.
...a married woman needs the permission of her husband; a minor, as with any medical procedure, needs the permission of a parent or guardian.
...the operation may be performed only in a licensed hospital.
...the operation may be performed only by a licensed physician.

> ...the operation may not be performed beyond a certain
> date in the pregnancy (Hole and Levine 1971, p. 286).

Liberal reformers generally accepted these qualifications, except the husband's permission clause. Radical feminists objected to other seemingly "reasonable" restrictions, noting that residency is not a qualification for any other medical procedure. Whether or not the procedure should be performed in a hospital by a physician created some of the most heated debate. Many feminists (including a number of physicians) argued that abortion is an extremely safe medical procedure, which is easily performed in a clinic or doctor's office by trained paramedics. (Legalizing nonhospital abortion makes abortion more available to poor women—an important feminist goal.)

The "time limit" argument, involving legal, medical, moral, and theological considerations, created even greater furor. Total repealers argued that any woman who had religious or moral scruples about late abortion would not seek one. Nonetheless, feminists often disagreed over this issue, partly because maternal death and complication rates increase with late abortions.[*]

Early feminist abortion action took several directions. A number of groups were founded to work for abortion law repeal by lobbying through established legislative channels. NOW's Task Force on Reproduction and Its Control was the first such organization. New Yorkers for Abortion Law Repeal (NALR) and the Women's National Abortion Action Coalition (WONAAC) were subsequently formed.[†] While national organizations provided a sense of cohesion and served as a communications network for abortion repeal groups, most abortion action occurred on the state level, where many feminist groups constituted for broader concerns became involved in abortion repeal (Hole and Levine 1971, p. 295). Ad hoc actions designed to raise consciousness became common. For example, in the spring of 1969,

---

[*]For extended discussion, see Cisler 1970; Hole and Levine 1971, pp. 286-90; Lader 1973; and Sarvis and Rodman 1973, pp. 15-27.

[†]Although differing somewhat in approach, both the Association to Repeal Abortion Laws (ARAL) and the National Association for Repeal of Abortion Laws (NARAL)—two older general abortion rights groups—worked cooperatively on many issues with the feminist abortion groups. For details on these groups, see Freeman 1975, pp. 129-32; Hole and Levine 1971, pp. 295-96; and Jenness et al. 1973, pp. 2, 13-14.

the Redstockings, a radical New York group, disrupted a state legislative hearing on abortion reform, demanding that the meeting be turned over to them on the grounds that women are the only "real experts" on abortion. In addition to calling for abortion repeal, the Redstockings questioned why of the 14 official speakers on the platform, only one was a women and she was a nun. The hearing was moved and closed to the public; a month later, the Redstockings held alternative "public hearings," attended by over 300. In January 1970, a small group of radical women invaded an antiabortion law rally in the state of Washington. Carrying picket signs depicting the instruments and methods of illegal abortionists, the women argued for complete abortion law repeal rather than reform. While the Michigan legislature debated an abortion reform bill in 1970, the Detroit Women's Liberation Coalition staged a funeral march, mourning women's deaths from illegal abortions. Dressed in black and veiled, 50 women and 5 men marched to the city morgue to protest the thousands of unnecessary deaths, wailing and displaying coat hangers, safety pins, and other self-abortion instruments. During the 1970 American Medical Association (AMA) convention in Chicago, local feminists staged several skits about medical treatment and the AMA position on abortion.[*] In a unified show of support, on August 26, 1970, abortion demonstrations were held throughout the country (Hole and Levine 1971, pp. 298-99).

Abortion Referral

While ultimately, repeal of laws was desired, some groups also sought to make abortion immediately available by organizing both legal and underground abortion referral services. Hole and Levine (1971, p. 299) estimate that a referral service existed in every area where a women's liberation group had appeared. Most services were independent, but many local chapters of NOW and other national organizations also offered referral services. Feminist groups in some areas worked closely with the referral groups established before the existence of the movement in 1967: ARAL, Parents' Aid Society, and Clergy Consultation Service.[†]

---

[*]Hole and Levine (1971, pp. 296-98) provide detailed accounts of these actions.

[†]Antagonism developed in some areas, however, with the clergy group. Feminists accused the clergy of operating with a

The purpose of all the referral services was to keep an up-to-date list of doctors who performed medically sound abortions at a reasonable fee. When and where abortion was legal, the services tried to find the safest and cheapest care performed by sympathetic, humane abortionists. In Southern California, for example, the Women's Abortion Referral Service (WARS) and the Feminist Women's Health Centers (FWHCs) scheduled hospital abortions, provided counseling and education, and accompanied women throughout the abortion procedure in the hospital (Heidelberg 1978). In some areas, the services developed a degree of bargaining power over fees, forcing doctors to lower costs considerably (Hole and Levine 1971, p. 299).

Many early abortion services operated publicly to test restrictive laws, but others functioned quietly to avoid legal difficulties. Where harassment was likely, referrals to out-of-state doctors were preferred in order to minimize the risk of arrest and prosecution. However, such a strategy was expensive, and women without resources had to risk seeking local abortionists (Hole and Levine 1971, p. 301; Lee 1969; Maxtone-Graham 1973).

While referral services run by feminists and nonprofit agencies, such as Planned Parenthood, rarely charged referral fees, profit-making referral services sprang up in the early years of abortion law change. Some of the most blatant abuses occurred between 1970 and 1972 in New York, the abortion capital of the United States. By simply booking a woman for an abortion, some agencies collected from $100 to $150, plus kickbacks from "package deals," covering hotel rooms, deluxe hospital accommodations, and other frills (Lader 1973, pp. 163-64; Frankfort 1972, pp. 57-71).

After considerable public outcry, the New York State attorney general and the New York State Senate Committee on Health held hearings on commercial referral services (Frankfort 1972, pp. 63-71). A number of the profiteers were investigated, and in February 1971, the attorney general closed Abortion Information Agency, a notorious offender. By July 1971, the New York State Legislature outlawed all profit-making referral services (Lader 1973, p. 164).

The Feminist Abortion Underground

Some referral agencies "branched out" to fill gaps in needed services. For example, The Service, a group of 40 women from the

---

self-righteous, patronizing attitude, and in turn, the clergy criticized some feminist services of haphazard management (Hole and Levine 1971, pp. 298-99).

Chicago Women's Liberation Union, organized in 1969 to provide referral only. As the group (informally known as "Jane") developed
close relations with several abortionists, the price dropped from
$500 to $200, and the quality of care improved. When the group discovered that its primary abortionist was not a physician but a skilled
health worker, several members decided to learn to perform abortions themselves. By 1973, Jane was providing over 50 abortions a
week for an average fee of $50. In four years, over 11,000 abortions
were performed. No one was denied an abortion for lack of funds
and no one died (Bart 1973, p. 28; Bart 1977; Chicago Women with
HealthRight 1975, p. 3).*

The Court Acts

While debate continued over the qualifications for abortion and
over specific techniques and technicians, abortion laws were challenged through the courts on the grounds that women's civil rights,
rights to equal protection, and rights to privacy were violated by
restrictive laws. By 1971, 70 civil and criminal cases were pending
(Hole and Levine 1971, p. 285; Lader 1973).
On January 22, 1973, the U.S. Supreme Court handed down a
decision in Roe v. Wade and Doe v. Bolton that went beyond what anyone had predicted. In a vote of seven to two, the Court decreed that
during the first three months of pregnancy, abortion was to be a free
choice to be negotiated between a woman and a physician.[†] It also
prohibited any state intervention in the second three months except to
protect maternal health. The decision exceeded in scope any of the
18 state laws enacted since 1967 with the exception of the New York
law (Lader 1973, p. 221-22).

Abortion: Catalyst for Health Reform

While women were divided over many aspects of abortion,
abortion action brought together otherwise hostile factions of the

---

*Similar feminist lay abortionists are still operating in Italy
(Bart 1977, p. 11).
[†]Kaiser and Kaiser (1974) point out that, in fact, this leaves
women in a very vulnerable position, since patients' ability to negotiate with physicians is severely limited.

women's movement, serving as a catalyst for wider health reform in a number of ways. Frankfort points out that following the July 1970 liberalization of abortion laws, women's experiences in the New York abortion mills—both as patients and as paraprofessionals—were profoundly radicalizing. While some clinics offered good care at moderate cost, others were shyster operations. For example, a woman fortunate enough to be referred to the Women's Medical Center in New York City by a nonprofit agency, such as the New York Abortion Project or Planned Parenthood, could have a vacuum aspiration abortion for $75; the same procedure cost from $300 to $1,500 in many other facilities, many of which were poorly equipped and staffed by inadequately trained personnel (Frankfort 1972, pp. 57-71).

Women also faced humiliating encounters with medical personnel. Women were forced to sign fetal "death certificates," had machines to record fetal heart beats set next to them, were given bags with a picture of a fetus to return to the hospital after aborting at home, or were aborted on the same ward with women giving birth (Frankfort 1972, p. 40). Such practices were constantly reported in the feminist press (see, for example, Alper, Hoffnung, and Solomon 1972; Fruchter 1970; "Funeral for a Fetus" 1974; "Harassing Jane Doe" 1974; and Leinfelder 1974). Control over quality of care quickly became as serious a matter as access to abortion. The situation was shocking to middle- and upper-class women, who usually believed they fared well in the health care system but found themselves subjected to these conditions (Frankfort 1972, p. 93).

Frankfort (1972, p. 93) emphasizes that the abortion struggle gave women both a sense of enormous leverage with a powerful social institution and fostered the view that there was something radically wrong with the health care system. Even after abortion law repeal, women were pitted against an unresponsive health system.*

The abortion struggle provided the initial impetus for a broader women's health movement by creating widespread awareness of how medical and legal systems obstruct women's right to control their own fertility. It also exposed women to objective conditions in the health care system that demanded correction. Some of these conditions (for example, the attitude of medical personnel, high costs, and insurance exclusions) predated the abortion movement, but others, such as excessive profiteering, inadequate facilities, and poorly

---

*For discussion of the slowness of health institutions to make abortion available following the Supreme Court decision, see especially the 1975 Alan Guttmacher Institute study.

trained personnel, were unintended consequences of abortion reform. With abortion more socially and psychologically acceptable, demand for services rapidly exceeded supply. Profit-oriented providers, stepping in to fill the gap between supply and demand, created objective conditions far worse than had existed previously in "legitimate" operations.

FEMINIST BODY CONSCIOUSNESS

At first glance, it seems paradoxical that later developments in the women's health movement grew directly out of the larger feminist movement, since many feminists minimize or disregard biological differences between the sexes entirely. Occasionally, this disregard is carried to the extreme of denying nearly all biological differences between men and women. In their attempt to overthrow the dictum "Biology is destiny," very real and important differences between the sexes are sometimes ignored (Hole and Levine 1971, pp. 171-93).

Women's needs related to reproductive functions have also stirred controversy. Some feminists deny that women have any special physical or social-psychological needs, arguing that menstrual cramps, nausea during pregnancy, postpartum depression, and menopausal symptoms are culturally induced problems best treated with consciousness raising; others disagree. Some believe childbirth to be so dangerous and degrading that test tube babies are preferable; others see childbirth as a woman's peak experience. Ehrenreich and English (1973, pp. 87-88) note that the real trouble is that whatever women say about these bodily events can and will be used against them. If women argue menstruation is painful and distressing, women will be barred from certain occupations; if it is believed to be unnoticeable, women may be required to work the same hours and lift the same weights as men, regardless of the discomfort. If pregnancy is viewed as an illness, women may be fired early; if defined as a perfectly "healthy" state, women may be held to overly rigorous work schedules.

As feminist interest in health and body issues grew, confusion over the propriety of such concerns increased. Many health movement developments—for example, women's clinics, body courses, and pregnancy counseling—were puzzling, even to basically "sympathetic" observers. The editors of Health/PAC Bulletin, for example, observed that while the women's movement struggled to debunk the definition of "woman-as-reproductive-beast," women's clinics and the health issues reinforced the image, for the only health problems that pertain to women and women alone focus on the female reproductive system, making it easy to focus on women as users of contraceptives, seekers of abortions, bearers of children, victims of venereal disease and vaginitis, that is, as a collection of ovaries, uteri, vaginas, and other sexual appurtenances ("Women's Clinics" 1971).

Despite the image problem, health movement activists attend to body issues for many reasons. But basically and most fundamentally, feminist focus on health and body issues is a strategy to subvert the ideology of sexism at its base: the social interpretation of biological sex differences (Marieskind and Ehrenreich 1975, p. 38). The social interpretation of sex differences is crucial to attack, for traditionally, biological differences have been used to denigrate women and justify their subjugation and oppression. In scientific circles and the political arena, as in every patriarchal institution, women's bodies have been belittled. Freud, for example, argued that "Anatomy is destiny," while Mussolini put it more starkly, "Genius is genitals" (Seaman 1975, p. 43).

To counter biological determinism, feminists argue that their subservient position is socially conditioned and, therefore, can be socially redefined (Hole and Levine 1971, p. 171). From this perspective, it is only necessary to alter the social value of women's biological characteristics in order to alter their overall social position; there is no need to change or apologize for female anatomy. Thus, rather than minimizing or ignoring their biology, health movement participants seek to re-examine and redefine health and body issues from an exclusively and uniquely feminist viewpoint. This requires putting aside preconceived notions of the value, beauty, and importance of the female body, for such taken-for-granted notions are inextricably part of the patriarchal culture and value systems. Once these values, beliefs, and practices are laid aside, the value of female biology can be discovered, explored, and integrated into the social self.

This redefinition also requires fostering considerable body consciousness. Women learned that the way they related to their bodies and allowed others to relate to their bodies was central to their conception of self and their liberation. Restructuring social definitions of the body-self, then, became central tasks to liberate women from all forms of oppression (the Boston Women's Health Book Collective 1973, 1976; Dodson 1974; Rush 1973; Salomon 1974).

That health activists did view their bodies as their primary essential selves through which they related to the world was reflected in the final decision of the Boston Women's Health Book Collective (1973, p. 1) to call their enormously popular health manual Our Bodies, Ourselves instead of Women and Their Bodies—a title they initially used. This perspective and approach toward social change is consonant with certain traditional psychodynamic views of the importance of the body in establishing a social self. Significantly, such psychological approaches have gained considerable attention during the past decade. The phenomena of women reasserting control over their bodies and health care and establishing female worlds largely excluding men and male authority also mirrors the behavior of racial and ethnic minorities, who become exclusionary in order to establish a positive sense of self and to gain strength to renegotiate their position in the larger society.

Body Imagery in Art and Literature

Feminist artists, novelists, and poets suggest that female body experiences profoundly affect women's sense of self. However, until recently, women's sense of self has been distorted. Female body experiences that contradict cherished male perspectives have been discouraged from expression as either trivial or taboo (Millet 1970; Nochlin 1971; Showalter 1973; Tuchman 1975).

In some feminist circles, painting and sculpture is explicitly sensual and sexual. "Vaginal art" particularly explores female perspectives on women's bodies; breasts, vulvas, vaginas, clitorises, abortion, childbirth, and all types of sexual intercourse are graphically portrayed (Prescott 1976a). Art critic Maryse Holder suggests that in these works, women artists as a group were for the first time not copying from men.

> A record of female experience, it offered a completely different view of reality. And it was imaginative, often brilliant work about an area of human experience that had not been dealt with before, or even now, by men. "Sexualism," then, to use a more accurate term than "eroticism," is exciting. It is new and it is a movement (Holder 1973, p. 17).

Betty Dodson, a prominent feminist artist, was one of the first women to present this new perspective on female sexuality.* In a series of photographs, drawings, and paintings of women's genitalia, her intent was to help women become what she termed "cunt

---

*Initially, Dodson's work went beyond the bounds of acceptability, even in liberal New York artistic circles; several portraits of women masturbating were removed from a show in 1972.

positive"; her artwork is now used in "body-sex workshops" for this purpose (Dodson 1974, pp. 23-55; Salomon 1974).

In Los Angeles, 26 women artists transformed an old mansion into "Woman House." In the "Womb Room," fibers drooped "like an exhausted uterus," according to Judy Chicago, co-founder of the feminist art program at the California Institute of the Arts, which sponsored the 1972 show. In the flesh-colored kitchen, sponges fashioned into fried eggs transmuted into human breasts adorned the walls and ceiling ("Bad-Dream House" 1972). In Michigan, Kathe Roger's "cunt sculptures"—boxes of wire mesh concealing deep red slits—were described as "shocking, assertive and liberating" (Prescott 1976a). Feminist artists Chicago and Miriam Schapiro caution, however, that the visual symbolism in works such as these should not be taken as "vaginal art" in a simplistic sense. What these artists have done is to have taken the central feature that defines them as women and to have then developed from it an imagery to reverse cultural views of women (Haas 1977).

While feminists are enthusiastic that women are no longer exclusively exposed to male portrayals and images of female sexuality, thus far, women's sexual or erotic art has had limited showing in art galleries and museums. Feminist sexual art is perhaps making a greater impact in other areas. Sexologists and therapists who seek to demystify the body find it useful; Helen Singer Kaplan's (1974) widely acclaimed sex therapy manual is noted for Dodson's outstanding illustrations ("The New Sex Therapy" 1976). Integration of feminist artistic portrayals of female sexuality into conventional mental health literature will probably affect cultural attitudes toward women's bodies and sexuality.

Women's redefinition of their body-selves is also evident in feminist literature. In some authors' works, body themes have become progressively more prominent. Erica Jong's first volume of poems, Fruits and Vegetables (1971a), reflects a fundamental body consciousness. Her second, Half-Lives (1971b), directly addresses childbirth and sexuality. And in Fear of Flying (1973), she writes explicitly about menstruation and sexual arousal and response.

Sylvia Plath's work, written a decade before female topics were "acceptable," reveals a similar line of development. Her first volume of poetry, Colossus (1960), only hints at sex-role conflict (Rapone 1973, p. 408). In The Bell Jar (1963), Plath began exploring contraception, abortion, sexuality, and childbirth. Her two last volumes of poetry, Crossing the Water: Transitional Poems (1971) and Ariel (1961), focus on alienating aspects of the female body-self experience. Worth and fertility are often connected, and the body is portrayed as a means through which woman is controlled by others. A frequent image is the patient whose body is reduced to an object for tending (Rapone 1973, p. 410-11).

Medicalized body events are particularly noticeable in small feminist anthologies, where such topics as childbirth (for example, Miles n.d.a, b; Alta 1971), abortion (for example, Joyce 1972; Zahler 1973-74), menstruation (for example, Regal 1972; Alta 1971), and miscarriage (for example, Alta 1971) are featured. Female biology and sexuality appear also in the popular fiction of Doris Lessing, Joan Didion, Margaret Atwood, Marge Piercy, Cynthia Buchanan, and Joyce Carol Oates (Duffy 1972, pp. 98-99) and in Nora Ephron's Crazy Salad (1975) essays. Prior to the resurgence of feminism in the 1960s, all of these "women's topics" were regarded as too trivial to be taken seriously (Showalter 1973).

In art and literature, then, women's social-psychological-physical reality is presented differently than in the past. Despite the fears of some, who assume body consciousness necessarily leads to objectification or degradation of women, it need not. As Gould (1975) points out, there are worlds of difference between the male fantasy-oriented world of pornography and the exploration of female erotisicm and sexuality within feminist circles. In women's health groups, for example, sexuality is treated seriously. Joking and telling "off-color stories," so common in all-male or mixed groups, are noticeably absent.

Toward a Women's Health Movement

Initially, feminist body issues were the right to contraception and abortion. Feminists gradually expanded these concerns, arguing that far more was involved in women taking control over their bodies. Ehrenreich and English (1973, p. 5), acknowledged movement spokespersons, emphasized that the whole medical system is strategic for women's liberation; it is the "keeper of the keys."

With increasing vehemence, feminists directed their attack toward male gynecologists, who came to be seen as perpetrating some of the cruder forms of patriarchal domination. In fact, the gynecological examination and gynecological surgery are often called "socially sanctioned forms of rape" (see, for example, Downer 1972; Frankfort 1972; Barry 1972; Edmonds 1975). Similarly, throughout Vaginal Politics, Frankfort (1972) uses sexual exploitation as a metaphor to describe various aspects of the health system that oppress women. Feminists also saw the significance of science in defining and enforcing male perspectives of female reality and began to attack existing theories and practices for perpetuating patriarchal dominance. How did the sexual politics of health attract such widespread attention and grow into a separate social movement?

3

The Rise of the Women's
Health Movement

With the growth of feminism, women discussed health and body
issues in small consciousness-raising groups and larger public forums.
There were numerous concerns over contraception, abortion, and
gynecological care that men did not seem to understand but which
troubled feminists. In the spring of 1969, several women who had
participated in a "women and their bodies" discussion at a large
women's conference in Boston decided to meet to explore health issues. They had all experienced frustration and anger toward specific
doctors and the health system. To do something about doctors who
were condescending, paternalistic, judgmental, and noninformative,
they decided they would have to learn more about their own bodies.

The following summer, the Boston women researched and
wrote papers on anatomy and physiology, sexuality, venereal disease,
birth control, abortion, pregnancy and childbirth, medical institutions, and the health care system in the context of a capitalist society.
Using these papers, the women began organizing health courses in
day schools, nursery schools, churches, and women's homes. The
course was an immediate success, and the mimeographed notes and
papers were bound together into the first printed edition of the enormously popular health manual, Our Bodies, Ourselves (The Boston
Women's Health Book Collective 1973, p. 1).[*]

---

[*]Early editions of the pamphlet were distributed by the small
left-oriented New England Free Press in Boston. By January 1973,
Our Bodies, Ourselves had gone through 11 printings; 225,000 copies
were in circulation. The growing volume of requests strained the

Word of the Boston course spread quickly to New York, where health issues were already a major feminist issue. By 1971, feminist groups across the country were meeting specifically to discuss health issues. That a full-blown feminist health movement was emerging became clear in March 1971, when over 800 women assembled in New York for the first Women's Health Conference. Some came from as far away as San Francisco and Seattle. The topics included everything from a practical exchange of ideas on health matters to the planning of future health movement policy. A significant aspect of this conference was that women discussed "technical matters" (for example, abortion techniques and drug safety), formerly regarded as the sole property of male professionals (Frankfort 1972, p. 235).

ROUTINE CARE—AN AFFRONT TO SELF-DETERMINATION

From the earliest days of women's health discussion groups, women voiced complaints over the treatment they received during routine gynecological examinations. Overall, early health activists were offended by the way most gynecologists treated them, as well as by gynecologists' denial of their right to participate fully in decisions about abortion, sterilization, contraception, and treatment of routine problems.

The women perceived that when attempting to make their own decisions about standard medical procedures, they faced deeply ingrained attitudes of what women are like and what is "appropriate" for them to do or say. Physicians, like many men in American society, treat women as children—persons to be sheltered and protected from unpleasant facts and relieved of responsibility for decision making, ostensibly for their own good. Thus, when women seek medical care, physicians often fail or openly refuse to give women enough information to discuss procedures or make decisions in a reasoned, competent manner.

Feminists were and are bitter that they are often ignorant not out of choice or inability to understand but because doctors make it

---

small press, and the Health Book Collective turned distribution rights over to Simon and Schuster but retained copyright and other controls (Boston Women's Health Course Collective 1971, pp. 137-38). By 1976, when a second, revised edition was issued, the first Simon and Schuster edition had sold over 1 million copies. A Spanish language edition was released in 1977.

difficult to acquire the information they need to make competent decisions for themselves. In waiting rooms, there is little health education material to help patients understand their bodies or aid them in communicating with doctors. In the examining room, they feel demeaned when called "honey" or "dear." Most wonder why they must address physicians as "Doctor X" when they are addressed so familiarly by pseudo-intimate terms or by their first names. Women also complain that when they are stripped and draped and lying on their backs with feet in stirrups, it is difficult to interact with physicians. In such an awkward position, women can neither see what is being done nor ask questions easily.

Women's basic complaints all reflect serious disagreement over appropriate style of patient-physician interaction, access to information, and right to decision making in health matters. These were and are especially burning issues, because many standard medical practices and procedures were found to be ineffective or hazardous in the late 1960s and early 1970s. Unless women can interact with physicians in a style allowing full exploration of risks and hazards associated with routine treatment modalities (including contraception, abortion, treatment for routine vaginal disorders, and childbirth), they are unable to make informed decisions. In Seaman's opinion (1969, 1972), patient passivity, whether enforced or willing, contributes significantly to many inappropriate and hazardous medical practices.

Feminist analyses of physician-patient interaction focus on how typical role relationships between women and physicians are related to women's general social status. Groesser (1972), discussing the work of Szasz and Hollender (1956), notes that the most common interaction style mirrors the parent-infant relationship. Termed the activity-passivity model, it is the traditional clinical relationship. A second interaction style, the guidance-cooperation model, fits the parent-adolescent paradigm. This mode is more common in situations where there is little urgency and the patient's active cooperation in the treatment is needed. The third model, mutual participation, is an adult-to-adult form and is exceedingly rare. Groesser (1972, p. 14) observes that patients with power and money are more likely to be treated as adults, whereas those without it are more liable to be treated as children. Women and members of lower economic groups typically are treated as children.

Because feminists seek equality and individual self-determination in every aspect of life, typical interaction with gynecologists was galling. Women who attempted to interact in gynecological examinations in the mutual participation, or adult, mode were met with everything ranging from astonishment to outright hostility. For example, Monty (1973) reports how several physicians reacted when she revealed that she examined herself:

> Telling him that I had been examining myself for some
> time with a plastic speculum, I explained that that was
> why I wanted to watch. Incredulous, he then looked at me
> as if I were a rare species of caterpillar. Like a little
> boy whose toy had been taken away, he said, "You have
> no business doing that!" It really was scary to see what
> happened when his "omnipotence" was threatened.
>
> On another occasion, I read that some women have
> a friend come into the doctor's office with them as a
> "patient advocate." ... On my next visit, Deb came with
> me. When I introduced her and told the doctor that she
> wanted to watch the examination, he said that it was against
> his ethics. When we questioned him further as to what he
> meant, he said, "Look, dear, I just won't do it." I was
> stunned.

An often repeated story in self-help groups concerns a woman who
went for an exam and asked the doctor a lot of questions about why
the drape was necessary. Finally, the doctor replied that the drape
was to avoid embarrassment. The woman replied, "Oh, doctor, I
didn't know you were embarrassed!" At this, the doctor tossed away
the drape, and the examination continued without it.

Some physicians seemed to understand the importance of style
to feminists. For example, at ob-gyn rounds at the University of
California at San Francisco in July 1973, gynecologist Sadja Goldsmith told her colleagues:

> Overall it's the attitude of the physician women are com-
> plaining about. Women want to be treated as equals. They
> don't want to be talked down to. They want doctors to an-
> swer questions and explain what's going on. Women feel
> they can't talk to their doctors. They want more honest
> discussion. They want to be brought in as decision makers
> (Stephen 1973b).

She also told the group that women don't want to be called "girls,"
which

> is a putdown, it connotes immaturity. Some women want
> to watch their pelvic exams. You should either offer with
> a sign or by just asking. This may seem funny to men but
> your genitals are exposed ... whereas women have been
> told not to look or touch (Stephen 1973b).

Nonetheless, most physicians were not eager to include women
in decision making. A year later, at a public forum on women's roles

in health care decision making at the University of California, San Francisco, Maureen Murphy of the School of Nursing faculty opened the session, stating that when the notion of discussing the role of women in decision making about their own care was first suggested to her, her first reaction was to have two hours of silence and then go home. That would sum up women's role in decision making. The following two hours of discussion were anything but silent. Participants pointed out that as women were becoming more familiar with their bodies and gaining medical knowledge, they were demanding a greater voice in all aspects of their care. At first, the demand for choice revolved around routine matters—what contraceptive to use or which drugs or anesthetics to accept during childbirth. Now some women argued they had exclusive right to make decisions regarding abortion and sterilization. Even more threatening to physicians was the growing demand that women ought to be fully involved in decisions regarding major surgery, particularly for breast cancer. One surgeon on the panel complained bitterly that women were insisting that he perform lumpectomies rather than radical mastectomies on the basis of things they had read in women's magazines. Although he acknowledged that medical practice in the previous 30 to 50 years was perhaps overly authoritarian and lacking in consideration of humane factors, swinging into a phase where women make decisions about their own surgery was going "too far."

It is important to understand that women demand a greater role in decision making for an array of overlapping reasons. As already noted, feminists believe it is necessary for women to make all decisions regarding their reproductive lives. They are willing to take risks based on their own assessment of the situation because they no longer have faith in either the goodwill or technical competence of the medical profession. Much of their distrust stems from growing revelations of hazardous medical practices and technologies.

DRUGS AND DEVICES

Oral Contraceptives

Barbara Seaman opened Pandora's box when she published The Doctor's Case Against the Pill in 1969. At the time, an estimated 12 to 15 million women throughout the world (including 8 million American women) were taking oral contraceptives (Seaman 1969, p. 12). For several years, rumors had spread among physicians that there were major complications associated with pill usage. However, the evidence—scattered in the international medical literature— was difficult to interpret.

NC.

..n, whose husband is a physician, was alarmed over
..orts of pill hazards. After combing the international
..ls, Seaman analyzed the growing evidence that oral
..vere neither as safe nor as effective as physicians
..believe. Particularly alarming was that as women
..ong periods of time, the effects of synthetic estro-
..pronounced. Combining a review of the research
lit ..tic clinical narratives, Seaman presented to the
la) ..g evidence of links between the pill and blood
clott..g, su.. .., sterility, decreased sexual responsiveness, cancer, heart disease, diabetes, genetic changes, jaundice, thyroid
malfunction, weight gain, urinary tract infections, arthritis, skin
and gum problems, depression, and other medical conditions.

It was also clear that physicians prescribed the pill to many
women without considering their family medical histories or informing
them of the risks. Women who expressed concern were routinely
reassured of pill safety. Dr. Hugh Davis of the Johns Hopkins University School of Medicine pointed out that doctors who pushed the
pill's safety were now in a bind; they were embarrassed to admit that
they were wrong. Physicians who strove to be infallible were particularly uncertain about how to backtrack on the pill and still maintain their patients' respect (Seaman 1969, p. 10).

It also became clear that the Food and Drug Administration
(FDA) approval was no guaranty of safety or efficacy. Oral contraceptives had passed through the FDA without being subjected to recognized standards of scientific experimentation for safety. The Puerto
Rican study on which the original FDA approval was based had included only 132 subjects—a sample so small it was later described
as a "scientific scandal." In addition, at least two or three deaths
among these women had never been explained or even reported to the
FDA (Mintz 1967; Silverman and Lee 1974, pp. 99-100; Seaman and
Seaman 1977, pp. 61-149].

Hearings and investigations were held in Washington, D.C.,
in 1970 over pill safety. Midway through Senate hearings, Newsweek
published the results of a Gallup poll revealing that two-thirds of the
women taking the pill had never been warned by their physicians of
any hazards. The FDA shortly announced that a warning label should
be inserted into pill packages, a move vehemently opposed by the
AMA and the drug companies. A watered-down form was finally adopted in June 1970 (Silverman and Lee 1974, p. 102). However, late
in 1977, the Pharmaceutical Manufacturers Association together with
the ACOG filed a lawsuit against the FDA, claiming that the drug
companies did not have to insert labels for patients in drugs containing estrogen. The National Women's Health Network, Consumers
Union, Consumer Federation of America, and WEAL joined in the

lawsuit (as intervenors on behalf of the FDA) to represent the interests of women patients. The judge upheld the FDA's requirement that labels be included in all estrogen drugs, including those used for estrogen replacement therapy during menopause (Cowan 1978).

At the San Francisco forum in 1974 on women's roles in decision making, a panelist who had been involved in the pill issue in the Department of Health, Education and Welfare at the time of the insert controversy reflected that

> the amount of attention devoted to the question at the highest levels of government, it seems to me, was much less than would have been the case if the secretary of HEW had been a woman taking that pill and the assistant secretaries advising her had been women. That isn't to say that everybody who was there was a male chauvinist or anything. It's a question of what attracts your attention. If you're blind, you tend to be concerned with the problems of blind people if that issue comes up as a matter of public policy. And if you're female, you would, I assume, tend to be concerned with this problem.

In feminist circles, no amount of fancy footwork could restore physicians' or government agencies' respectability. The controversy Seaman's work engendered ranged far beyond immediate concern with the pill. The pill fiasco simply pulled out the cornerstone in women's belief that the FDA fully tested drugs prior to marketing or that physicians were truly concerned with safety.

As new pill hazards were discovered, they were reported in the feminist press (see, for example, "British Pill Study" 1974; Cowan 1974d; Dawson 1975; and "Liver Tumors and the Pill" 1974). Feminist health material, articles, and pamphlets clearly stated known risks (see, for example, The Boston Women's Health Course Collective 1971; Gray and Gray 1971; and Hansen, Reskin, and Gray 1972).

The DES Tragedy

Women soon learned the horrors of other iatrogenic disorders. Reports of a rare form of vaginal cancer in young girls began appearing in the medical literature in 1970 (Herbst and Scully 1970). Prior to this time, vaginal adenocarcinoma in adolescent girls was unknown and was unusual even in older women. Cancer experts quickly traced the cause to exposure to synthetic estrogens in utero; most of the mothers of the young cancer victims had been given a synthetic estrogen

drug, diethylstilbestrol, commonly known as DES, during their pregnancies (Cowan 1977, p. 26-29; Frankfort 1972, pp. 112-15; Greenwald et al. 1971; Seaman and Seaman 1977, pp. 1-37; Weiss n.d.,
1972, 1974, 1975a).

Between 1945 and 1970, approximately 3 million women were
given DES to prevent miscarriage, although the medical literature
contained six scientific reports that DES was ineffective in preventing
spontaneous abortions (Weiss 1972; Meyer 1974).* At puberty, DES
daughters tend to develop vaginal adenosis, or precancerous lesions.
One million more DES daughters will reach puberty in the next two
decades. Unfortunately, the prognosis for vaginal adenocarcinoma
is poor. One-quarter who have developed it have died within 18
months of diagnosis.† Treatment of both adenosis and adenocarcinoma
has involved progesterone therapy (believed now to be ineffective),
surgical extirpation, and cauterization and radiation (Seaman and Seaman 1977, pp. 30-31; Weiss 1972, 1974, n.d.). Tentative calcula-
tions suggest that 1 out of every 250 DES daughters may suffer adenocarcinoma by the age of 30; the low estimate is 1 in 1,000. One out
of every 25 DES daughters may develop carcinoma in situ—a less
virulent form of cancer. Overall, up to half of all DES daughters may
need at least minor surgery in their twenties (Seaman and Seaman
1977, pp. 29-30).

To make matters worse, none of the public health agencies
(FDA, National Institutes of Health [NIH], National Center for Disease
Control, American Cancer Society, National Cancer Institute) were
willing to initiate a national effort to contact women who had been exposed to DES in utero. In addition, many hospitals and doctors refused to give individual women information on whether or not they had
been given estrogens during their pregnancies (Seaman and Seaman
1977, pp. 17-19; Weiss 1974).

As if the history of this drug was not sufficiently distressing,
NIH awarded ten universities research grants in the early 1970s to
test DES as a "morning-after" pill. The FDA-approved experimental
dosage as a postcoital contraceptive was massive: 250 milligrams
for five days (Weiss 1974).

By 1972, an NIH official announced that the morning-after pill
was being given by most university health services. The rapid adoption

---

*Daniels (1976) suggests it would be interesting to know how
many articles during this period reported the opposite to be the case.
†For accounts of the personal tragedy of these women, see,
for example, Seaman and Seaman 1977; Spake 1978.

of DES as a postcoital contraceptive was stimulated in part by an article by Lucile Kuchera in the October 26, 1971, issue of the Journal of the American Medical Association (JAMA). The author claimed that in a study of 1,000 Ann Arbor, Michigan, women, there were no pregnancies and no serious adverse reactions. To the embarrassment of the JAMA, patients from the University of Michigan health service read the report and started an investigation, because the report did not fit the facts. Some women had discontinued the full five-day treatment because of severe nausea. Others who took the medication properly had remained pregnant. A subsequent investigation revealed that out of a sample of 69 DES patients, only 1 in 4 had ever been contacted by the health service after being given the pills. Local women who continued to monitor the effects of DES repeatedly found facts that contradicted the JAMA report (Seaman and Seaman 1977, pp. 40-41).

Belita Cowan's survey of over 200 women aged 18 to 31 who had taken DES for this purpose between 1968 and 1974 at the University of Michigan showed that over 29 percent had taken the morning-after pill at least twice within one year. The study also revealed that DES was prescribed carelessly and casually, sometimes to women for whom estrogens were contraindicated. Six percent of the women were DES daughters (Seaman and Seaman 1977, pp. 41-42).

After the JAMA's study had been severely challenged, Lilly, the prime maker of DES, made a concerted effort to inform doctors that since the drug's safety and efficacy had not been proven, it should not be used as a postcoital contraceptive. (Lilly continued to supply DES to Tablicaps, the company that marketed morning-after pills as an ideal contraceptive.) The FDA took no action, however, to limit the use of DES for nonapproved uses or to warn doctors and women to stop using it (Seaman and Seaman 1977, p. 43).

In May 1973, the FDA mailed a bulletin to physicians approving DES for use in preventing pregnancy under restricted conditions; in September, reporters received a similar press release. In July 1973, the Medical Letter, a scrupulously careful non-profit consumer-oriented prescription drug publication, reported that DES had recently been approved as a "morning-after" contraceptive. Nonetheless, at Senator Edward Kennedy's hearings in 1975, FDA Commissioner Alexander Schmidt revealed that the FDA was just about to approve DES as a postcoital contraceptive so that it could be better regulated. Senator Richard Schweiker and others at the hearing were confused; the bulletins on DES had been issued two years earlier. Marvin Seife, an FDA physician, testified that the FDA had issued a statement published in the September 26, 1973 Federal Register that 25 milligrams of DES could be used as a post-coital contraceptive (Cowan 1978). Commissioner Schmidt testified that the drug bulletins only specified the conditions under which DES would be marketed. "None of this has taken place yet" (Seaman and Seaman 1977, p. 44).

In fact, hundreds of thousands of women, including many DES daughters, were receiving DES. And because the treatment was not always effective, a whole new generation of children was being born that had been exposed to massive doses of the drug in utero.[*] Seife and another physician, Vincent Karusaitus, testified that they were shocked that the FDA (their employer) had allowed the Federal Register to publish a new use for a drug without any study or investigation (Seaman and Seaman 1977, pp. 43-45). Frankfort (1972, p. 115) had earlier speculated that the male authorities might not have delayed action on stopping the drug's use if DES had been shown to cause cancer of the penis in young male adolescents and the standard treatment was removal of the penis.[†]

Incensed over the DES tragedy, the feminist press widely publicized DES issues as they developed. Kay Weiss's fact sheets (1972, 1974b) on vaginal cancer and review of the scientific literature (n.d.) were circulated through health centers and feminist literature outlets. Her-Self editor Belita Cowan published a series of articles on various aspects of the DES problem, including Lilly's decision not to sell the clearly hazardous drug (1974c). (For additional coverage, see, for example, Cowan 1977, 1974c, 1974g; Dejanikus 1974; Greene 1974; Goodman 1974; and Jones 1974).

By 1974, the growing incidence of vaginal cancer was well known in medical circles, yet many physicians were ignorant of the appropriate screening measures. Even among those who were knowledgeable, few had the proper diagnostic equipment in their offices (Goodman 1974; Weiss 1974).[‡] The San Francisco-based Coalition

---

[*]Vicki Jones' 1976 retrospective analysis of rape victims' medical records at Grady Memorial Hospital in Atlanta, Georgia, revealed that women given DES had the same rate of pregnancy as the group not given DES, shedding serious doubt on the claims of DES' efficacy as a post-coital contraceptive. The study was conducted at the Center for Disease Control, Atlanta, Georgia (Cowan 1977, p. 27).

[†]Recent studies indicate high rates of reproductive tract abnormalities and undersized penises in DES sons (Seaman and Seaman 1977, pp. 36-37). There is now growing evidence that the mothers who took DES during pregnancy may have an increased rate of breast cancer (Wolfe 1977).

[‡]There is some controversy over whether a colposcope, which costs $1,520,000 is really necessary to carry out adequate screening.

for the Medical Rights of Women (founded in 1974) mounted an educational campaign to alert DES daughters, physicians, and public health officials to the need for screening and limiting these women's exposure to other synthetic estrogens (Coalition for the Medical Rights of Women 1975; "DES Groups Plan Summer Programs" 1976). The mass media gradually followed suit.*

The Growing Concern over Dangerous Drugs

Alarmed over the DES tragedy, feminists kept a watchful eye on medical research reports to keep abreast of newly discovered hazards. Feminist papers, including Her-Self, Off Our Backs, The Monthly Extract, and The Spokeswoman, all publicized potential problems, including the FDA approval of Depo-Provera as a contraceptive after only limited testing, dangerous levels of mercury discovered in Koromex contraceptive jelly (this has now been removed), side effects of vaginal sprays, powerful prostaglandins as contraceptives, and carcinogenic properties of Flagyl (routinely prescribed for trichamonis, a common vaginal infection) and Tinidazole (a new rival to Flagyl). These papers also carried articles on the problems related misuse of tranquilizers, drugs, anesthesia, and medical devices in childbirth. Concern increased over oral contraceptives and estrogen-replacement therapy for menopausal women.[†]

Some experts believe that this is another example of how expensive medical technology gets "pushed" on the public (Kaiser 1978).

*For example, early in 1976, Newsweek presented the plight of DES families and described screening procedures.

[†]Most major feminist newspapers and newsletters reported on these issues. The following examples illustrate the type of coverage afforded; often in-depth coverage followed initial news items. See, for example, with respect to Depo-Provera: "FDA Approves Depo-Provera" 1974; with respect to Koromex jelly: "Mercurial Jelly" 1973; with respect to prostaglandins: Chapman 1973a; with respect to Flagyl: Dejanikus 1974; with respect to Tinidazole: "Tinidazole: Another Carcinogen for Women" 1974; with respect to tranquilizers: Castleman 1974; with respect to vaginal sprays: "Vaginal Sprays" 1973; with respect to childbirth hazards: Cowan 1974k and "Machine May Cause Many Birth Defects" 1974; with respect to oral contraceptives: "British Pill Study" 1974 and "Liver Tumors and the Pill" 1974; and with respect to estrogen-replacement therapy: Fruchter 1976. See Cowan 1977 for additional references.

Intrauterine Devices—Hidden Hazards

Although a shock to many, more radical health activists saw
the FDA's laxness at screening drugs as to be expected in a capitalistic society. Nonetheless, they were amazed to learn that medical
devices, such as the widely prescribed intrauterine devices (IUDs)
were not even under the purview of a regulatory body. From the
FDA's perspective, IUDs were no more subject to regulation than
sun lamps or exercise equipment. In essence, just about anyone
could invent and market an IUD or other medical device without any
testing (Butler 1974). And they were invented! During the 1960s and
early 1970s, at least 3 million American women and 7 million women
in other countries received IUDs—none ever tested by a government
agency.

At a House subcommittee hearing in 1973 on device safety,
army physician Russell Thomsen testified that several hundred gynecologists had carved and twisted various metals, plastics, and fibers
into objects to insert into the depths of trusting patients; nearly every
month one read about another new and improved IUD (Butler 1974,
p. 11). Some devices were wiggly coils; others were shaped like
bows; still others appeared as insect antennae. One—the Dalkon
Shield—was shaped like a small fish, with sharp "teeth" all around
the body.* Touted as the most effective device for women who had
never borne children, Dalkon Shields were inserted in the uteri of 2
million women (Butler 1974, p. 7).

Critical reports on IUDs began circulating informally in the
medical community and within the FDA between 1968 and 1970.
Physicians and bureaucrats were aware of deaths, sterility, hemor-
rhage leading to anemia, disabling pain, unwanted pregnancy, miscarriage, ruptured tubal pregnancy, massive infection, and other
disorders. Many of the complications resulted in hospitalization,
major surgery, blood transfusions, and exposure to pelvic X rays.
Although systematic reporting on IUD complications is not available,
by 1974, at least 36 women had died, 3,500 women had been hospitalized, and over 200 women had suffered infected miscarriages while
using the Dalkon Shield (Butler 1974; Dejanikus 1974; Katz 1975; see
Seaman and Seaman 1977, pp. 153-74 for recent data on IUD hazards).

---

*For discussion and illustration of the most widely prescribed
IUDs—the Lippes Loop, Dalkon Shield, Saf-T-Coil, Ypsilon-Y, Cop-
per "T," Copper "7," and Progesterone "T"—see The Boston Women's
Health Book Collective 1976, pp. 196-200.

Despite calls for investigation and regulation, the FDA claimed that the IUD was a "device" over which it had no authority. However, two 1968 Supreme Court decisions gave the FDA legal authority to classify IUDs as "new drugs," subject to premarket testing. Nonetheless, the FDA bureaucracy ignored chief counsel William W. Goodrich's recommendation to treat IUDs as new devices. Finally, in May 1973—three days before Congress opened hearings on IUD safety—the FDA seized 12,000 Majzlin springs from the manufacturer—devices known to be extremely hazardous (Butler 1974, p. 7).

After lengthy hearings, the FDA began serious attempts to remove other dangerous devices from the market. In 1974, the FDA recalled 200,000 Copper "7" IUDs after physicians complained of defectively sealed sterile packages. About the same time, the Planned Parenthood Federation asked 183 affiliated clinics to stop prescribing Dalkon Shields ("Dalkon Shield Recall" 1974). Shortly thereafter, the FDA convinced Dalkon Shield manufacturer, A. H. Robins Company, to stop producing the device. The Department of Health, Education and Welfare subsequently banned the Shield in 3,000 public birth control clinics and instructed physicians to remove previously inserted devices when patients came in for routine checkups.

However, as feminists and the Health Research Group in Washington, D.C., complained, the FDA still refused to classify all IUDs as drugs, an action that would subject them to premarket testing on both laboratory animals and clinical populations. Finally, on May 28, 1976, President Gerald Ford signed legislation mandating the FDA to regulate medical devices—including IUDs and clips, rings, and bands used for sterilization—products over which the agency previously had no clear statutory jurisdiction. Devices already on the market are now required to apply for approval and submit evidence of safety and effectiveness ("Device Legislation Empowers the FDA to Regulate IUDs as Well as Clips, Rings, and Bands Used in Sterilization" 1976).

EXPERIMENTATION

While women demanded safer drugs and devices, they decried the way women were used as guinea pigs in medical research (see, for example, Brown 1973; Farber 1973; and Johnson 1975). The original testing of oral contraceptives in Puerto Rico on unsuspecting women—several of whom may have died because of the experiment—was viewed as an example of the blatant disregard for women, particularly nonwhite women.

Subsequent attempts to study side effects of the pill raised serious doubts in the minds of many that the medical profession could or should be trusted. In March 1971, Joseph Goldzieher, a gynecologist at the Southwest Foundation for Research and Education in San Antonio, presented a paper at a meeting of the American Fertility Society in New Orleans. The well-received paper described a double-blind study he had conducted comparing the incidence of headache, nervousness, nausea, vomiting, depression, and breast tenderness in women taking the birth control pill as opposed to a placebo.

The subjects, mostly poor Mexican-American women, were enrolled in the experiment when they came to the clinic for contraceptives. They were neither told of the experiment nor informed that some of them would receive a dummy pill rather than a contraceptive. The women were given a contraceptive cream and advised to use it along with the pill. At the end of four months, 10 of the 76 women given placebos were pregnant. When questioned about his procedures, Goldzieher replied, "If you think you can explain a placebo test to women like these, you never met Mrs. Gomez from the West Side" (Seaman 1972, pp. 180-81).

Goldzieher's experiment was clearly irresponsible if not unethical. The noted Christoper Tietze of the Population Council had declared in 1968 that no responsible investigator could take it upon himself to study oral contraceptives by means of an ordinary double-blind trial involving a placebo that would expose women seeking protection to the risk of pregnancy (Tietze 1968). Nonetheless, the medical community largely ignored Goldzieher's experiment. One gynecologist who did speak out against the San Antonio physician anonymously told Medical World News that he considered the experiment "totally unethical." George Langmyhr, medical director of Planned Parenthood International, suggested that Goldzieher should have had a fund to abort the pregnant women. While Langmyhr also expressed concern over whether informed consent was properly obtained, neither he nor Planned Parenthood had any plans to censure or repudiate the study or even to stop referring clients to Goldzieher (Seaman 1972, pp. 181-82).

While ignored by the medical community, the Goldzieher experiment caused a furor among feminists. The Third World Woman's Caucus, a women's liberation group, attempted to bring legal action against him. Robert Veatch of the Institute of Society Ethics and the Life Sciences criticized Goldzieher at length. Veatch's criticism, including his questioning of the relationship between Goldzieher, Syntex Laboratories, and the United States Agency for International Development (USAID) were widely discussed in the women's health movement (see, for example, Bart 1973 and Brown 1973).

Members of the Feminist Women's Health Centers (FWHCs), in particular, spoke out against experimental procedures. At a meeting of the American Public Health Association in San Francisco in 1973,

Laura Brown, co-director of the Oakland FWHC, explained that she and her associates spend a lot of time and energy in exposing and criticizing experimentation and research methods because they feel that much of the inaccurate, invalid, and incomplete research controlled by men is dangerous to women's health. Brown (1973, p. 4) elaborated on some of the fallacies in releasing products to the general public on the basis of "favorable" results obtained in premarket research studies. She pointed out that in these studies of IUDs, for example, women with any previous difficulties with IUDs are excluded, as are women with a history of pelvic inflammatory disease (PID) or recent abortions or births. In and of itself, this exclusion is reasonable, except that such research is used to justify widespread use of the devices. When the devices are prescribed for women with these conditions, the effectiveness rate begins to drop and the complication rate rises.

At the same meeting, Shelley Farber (1973) of the Los Angeles FWHC expressed concern that population controllers were experimenting on women in underdeveloped countries—the most blatant experiments being performed on people least able to defend themselves. In New Zealand, women were given Copper "7" IUDs and Depo-Provera injections without being informed that these contraceptives were experimental.

STERILIZATION

Surgical sterilization is a form of contraception that can only rarely be reversed by subsequent surgery. Women have typically found it difficult or impossible to be sterilized unless they meet stringent age and parity criteria set by the American College of Obstetricians and Gynecologists (ACOG). Often a spouse's consent has been required (Agate 1973; Lader 1972). Arguing that these requirements were violations of women's right to control their own bodies, feminists began pressing for the right to sterilization on demand regardless of age or parity (Agate 1973; Boston Women's Health Book Collective 1976).

While feminists were demanding the right to be sterilized voluntarily, black women in the South were concerned over "Mississippi appendectomies," in which their fallopian tubes were tied or their uteri were removed without their knowledge or consent. Medical services in ghettos also sterilized poor black and non-English speaking women without obtaining consent (Boston Women's Health Book Collective 1976, p. 212; Caress 1975; "Sterilization Abuse of Women: The Facts" 1975).

In 1973, two black girls aged 12 and 14 in Montgomery, Alabama, were sterilized in a federally funded family planning program without their informed consent. Their mother had been persuaded to give consent by signing an X on a form she could not read. She was not told the operation was permanent. The same year, it was revealed that a South Carolina obstetrician routinely refused to deliver a third child to a welfare mother unless she consented to sterilization. In a six-month period, he performed 28 sterilizations, mostly on black women (Herman 1976).

The Alabama case received national attention, and a $1 million lawsuit was filed in the girls' behalf ("Alabama: Sterilization of Minors Leads to Controversy" 1973; "$1-Million Sterilization Suit Filed" 1973; Rosoff 1973). In response to public outcry, the Department of Health, Education and Welfare began to develop guidelines to prevent such occurrences (Coburn 1974; Rosoff n.d.; "Sterilization Guidelines Criticized by ACLU" 1973).

Nonetheless, since 1970, female sterilization has increased rapidly, particularly among poor women and ethnic minorities. In the United States, 20 percent of the black married women and 14 percent of the Native American women, compared with 7 percent of the white married women, have been sterilized. A recent survey of gynecologists in four major cities revealed that 94 percent favored compulsory sterilization of welfare mothers with three or more illegitimate children (Herman 1976).

Feminist reaction to forced sterilization was slow to develop until recently, in part because it did not directly threaten white middle-class feminists. In addition, the population control organizations that promoted sterilization were needed allies in abortion repeal (Caress 1975; Herman 1976; "Sterilization Abuse of Women: The Facts" 1975).

CHILDBIRTH PRACTICES

Even before the women's health movement gained momentum, American childbirth practices were questioned by such groups as the International Childbirth Education Association (ICEA) and other "natural childbirth" proponents. And there were indicators that public dissatisfaction might be extensive. For example, in August 1956, the Ladies Home Journal (a conventional women's magazine) published a letter to the editor from a nurse who wanted an investigation into the common maternity ward practices of leaving women unattended, holding women's legs to delay birth, pulling babies out with forceps, unnecessary strapping and drugging, and unwarranted withholding

of drugs. The Journal editors cautiously suggested that an investigation into what they termed "undoubtedly rare cases" might be useful.
They were deluged with horror stories corroborating the assertions
of cruel maternity ward practices. In response to this flood of reader
concern, the Journal advocated midwifery training, admission of
husbands to delivery rooms, and increased sensitivity of maternity
personnel in its September 1956 issue. Considerable weight was
given to indignant letters from health professionals, however, and
the Journal absolved the medical profession from responsibility or
even complicity in reported abuses (Marieskind 1976, pp. 144-45).

In 1972, Doris Haire, then co-president of the prestigious
ICEA, published "The Cultural Warping of Childbirth," a low-key
scholarly assault on high-technology childbirth. Haire had visited
maternity care facilities in North and South America, Western Europe,
Russia, Asia, Oceania, and Africa, and as a result of her investigation discovered that many commonly accepted or enforced American
childbirth practices, which often disregard human physiological and
psychological needs, are not supported by scientific research but are
rooted in hospital and medical tradition.

Haire pointed out that 14 other developed countries have lower
infant mortality rates than the United States. Drawing on international
research on the use of various types of medication and anesthesia,
Haire revealed that many American hospital practices inhibit spontaneous birth and increase the need for all types of medical-surgical
intervention—themes elaborated later by other feminists, including
Nancy Shaw (1972, 1974) and Suzanne Arms (1975). In short, many
"modern" practices create problems, in turn requiring more medical
tinkering—to the detriment of both mother and child.

The dehumanizing aspects of labor and delivery were frequently discussed among feminists, who argued that women must regain
control over this important life-event (see, for example, The Boston
Women's Health Course Collective 1971; Cagan 1970; Groesser 1972;
Ostrum 1975; Pollard 1969; Shaw 1972; Treseder 1970). Haire's
documentation of specific medical hazards was followed by feminist
exposes of other problems related to childbirth, including discrimination against pregnant women in education, employment, and credit
(see, for example, Cowan 1974i; Dejanikus 1973a; "Federal Court
Rules in Favor of Pregnant Women in Unemployment Benefits Case"
1973; Hayden 1973; and "Pregnancy Ruled a Disability" 1974).

As with many other health problems, objection to male domination of obstetrics previously had been raised in the social scientific
and medical literature. Ostrum (1975) points out that in 1949, Margaret Mead described American birth procedures as designed primarily for the benefit of obstetricians, and Helene Deutsch (1945)
argued that modern, efficient masculine obstetrics deprived women

of their active monopoly of this area of life. The isolation of women in impersonal obstetrical wards was written about extensively. Nonetheless, this literature was largely ignored until the contemporary feminist movement brought public attention to the male domination of obstetrics and how it has worked against the best interests of women.

SURGERY—THE AMERICAN WAY TO CURE

Researchers have long recognized that where medicine is practiced on a fee-for-service basis, surgery rates are higher than in prepaid health plans or in countries with socialized medical schemes. Surgical intervention is also higher for patients with surgical insurance than for those without such coverage.

Pelvic surgery, in particular, has been cited in the medical literature as excessively performed; perfectly healthy uteri, ovaries, and fallopian tubes are too frequently excised (see, for example, Carter 1961; Lembcke 1956; Miller 1947; and Morehead and Trussell 1962). Although this information has been available for several decades, these facts attracted widespread attention only with the advent of a social movement that defined health care for women as a problem.

Early editions of Our Bodies, Ourselves reported that in a study at the Columbia University School of Public Health, one-third of the 6,248 hysterectomies reviewed were judged as having been done without medical justification; the percentage of unnecessary hysterectomies in some hospitals has been as high as 66 percent. Appalachian doctors were alleged to have removed healthy organs from 11- and 12-year-old girls to collect the $250 fee. The Boston women wondered how often unnecessary testectomies are done (Boston Women's Health Course Collective 1971, p. 125).

Seaman's expose of unnecessary surgery rested heavily on existing studies of pelvic surgery abuse. Particularly alarming were her reports on audits performed in New York by the Columbia School of Public Health during the late 1950s and early 1960s for the Teamsters Union. The investigators (including the late Alan Guttmacher) noted that there were two causes for care to be judged inferior. One type was surgery performed on essentially normal organs (for example, removal of the uterus) where patient exploitation was suspected. The other type of inferior care resulted from poor clinical judgment (Seaman 1972, pp. 185–86).

The auditors raised the issue of gynecological exploitation in several ways. While most poor ratings were given for inferior clinical management or operative technique in general surgical cases, gynecological cases rated as poor typically were so rated because the surgery was suspected to be unnecessary. Of the hysterectomy cases audited, a review of all records, including the operative report and pathology findings, led the auditors to judge that one-third of the women were operated on unnecessarily; another 10 percent of the operations were of dubious necessity. The reviewers added that these women should have had a dilation and curettage (scraping of the uterus), followed by an observation period, prior to hysterectomy. In many instances, dilation and curettage would probably have allevi-ated symptoms (Seaman 1972, p. 187).

Guttmacher and his associated also indicated that 7 out of 13 Caesarean sections reviewed may have been unnecessary. In many of these cases, various practices consistent with good obstetrical care were omitted, including failure to get a consultation, failure to rup-ture membranes, and failure to stimulate labor with Pitocin—any of which might have obviated the need for surgery (Seaman 1972, pp. 187-90).

Citing the work of John Bunker (1970), Seaman noted that in the United States, 516 hysterectomies are performed each year for every 100,000 women, whereas in England and Wales, the number is less than half—only 213. Breast operations show a similar pattern: in the United States, the rate is 278 per 100,000, compared with 171 per 100,000 in Great Britain. Seaman also reported that when a plan for reimbursement of surgical fees was offered to the United Mine Workers, an excessive number of surgical bills were submitted. Concerned over the increasing rate of gynecological surgery, the Mine Workers required preoperative consultation; hysterectomies decreased by as much as 75 percent (Seaman 1972, pp. 190-93). (See Carter 1961 for a detailed account of the United Mine Workers medical audits.)

Seaman (1972, p. 191) gingerly raised the issue of mastectomy abuse in a footnote, referring to an October 6, 1961, Medical Tribune article stating that the English, who approach breast surgery more cautiously than Americans, get just as good results physically and better results psychologically. Seaman cited John Hayward's London study, which showed that after 90 months, there was no significant difference between the percentage of patients who survived after having a radical mastectomy compared with those who had a "wide excision" of the tumor. With the radical mastectomy (removing the breast, the entire pectoral muscle, and the armpit nodes, often leaving the arm swollen and useless), 64 percent of the women were still alive. With the excision (only removing the tumor—a procedure barely no-ticeable in women with large breasts), 67 percent were still alive after 90 months (Seaman 1972, p. 191).

Frankfort (1972, pp. 127-40, 1973a) took a stronger stand against radical mastectomies. Citing research conducted at St. Bar-tholomew's Hospital in London; the University of Iowa; the Radiation

Center in Copenhagen; Rockford, Illinois; Cambridge, England; and Scotland, Frankfort argued that most women with evidence of breast malignancy undergo extensive surgery (radical or modified radical mastectomies), although numerous studies have shown that simple surgery (removal of only the breast or the tumor itself), followed by radiation treatment, is as effective; many physicians actually believe that radiation treatment alone is as effective as surgery. Despite growing evidence, surgeons continue to perform the most extensive operations.* Although the controversy over treatment for breast cancer is not "settled," Frankfort has argued that women at least ought to be informed there are no clear advantages in choosing radical surgery (1972, p. 135).

Frankfort added that the sole researcher to study the differences between operating at the time of breast biopsy and waiting until after a patient learns the biopsy results (so a choice of treatment can be discussed) was Houston physician Vera Peters. Peters found no difference in outcome based on waiting or cutting immediately. The advantage, of course, is that women need not undergo anesthesia for a biopsy without knowing whether they will have a breast upon awakening.

Part of the problem in Frankfort's view is that medical students learn to disregard the breast in anatomy classes. Recalling her early days in medical school, she wondered what it would be like if breasts were not introduced as greasy masses to be cut off as quickly as possible in order to make way for the study of the axilla. Perhaps if that part of the anatomy, a symbol of womanhood, were to be treated with more respect, doctors would extend their respect to women by giving them a choice when it came to cutting up their bodies (Frankfort 1972, p. 137).

While the surgical approach to breast cancer may be due in part to doctors' desire to behave as if they know the answers even when the evidence is unclear, they may have other motives to perform extensive surgery. Radical mastectomies are more costly operations than simple excisions. Frankfort (1972, p. 137) adds that it is not by accident that the most thorough studies on breast cancer have been done in England and Scandinavia, where doctors are not encouraged by money to mutilate a woman's body unnecessarily.

---

*For discussion of the controversy, see especially Cope 1977, 1971; Cope et al. 1967; Crile 1974; Eagan 1976; Kushner 1975; and Switzer 1976. In the film Taking Our Bodies Back (Lazarus 1974), Cope takes a firm stand against radical mastectomy and suggests that local excision, radiation, and chemotherapy are preferable for many women. See also Cope's statement in Cowan 1977, pp. 30-32.

Shocked by these exposes, feminists sought to investigate and analyze other surgical abuses. For example, in October of 1972, Boston women organized Speakoutrage, a public hearing for women to testify about their experiences with abortion, forced sterilization, unnecessary surgery, and other forms of exploitation and mistreatment. Conditions at the Boston City Hospital Ob-Gyn Clinic were particularly decried. One Boston City Hospital medical student reported that a common joke was that the only prerequisite for a hysterectomy was to not speak English. Another student reported on the practice of choosing operations for teaching reasons rather than because women needed them. A 17-year-old black woman, for example, was given a hysterotomy abortion in her 12th to 13th week of pregnancy instead of a saline induction, which meant that all her future children would have to be delivered by Caesarean section—major surgery. The physician in charge implied it was done largely for the "experience." Another woman was given a complete hysterectomy during surgery intended only to remove her left tube and ovary; again, the only indication was to provide the resident with experience (de Maehl and Thurston 1973, p. 17).

The choice of hysterectomy as a sterilization procedure at Boston City Hospital was particularly disturbing, since it carries far greater risk than tubal ligation—the usual method. (For comparison of risks, see Hibbard 1973.) When the student asked the teaching physician why hysterectomy was chosen over a tubal ligation for a 32-year-old black welfare woman, he was told quite simply that a hysterectomy was more of a challenge, that it was good experience for the junior resident—good training (de Maehl and Thurston 1973, p. 18).

Another student reported that a physician became angry when he saw pamphlets on vasectomies in the birth control counseling office and ordered the pamphlets removed immediately for fear their presence would decrease his female surgery. The Boston women added that the litany goes on and on: sterilization and experimentation without women's knowledge and consent, other unnecessary operations performed for teaching experience or for profit—and throughout, an attitude of contempt for women. But what most surprised these investigators was not the stories themselves but the realization that they had not heard them before (de Maehl and Thurston 1973, p. 20). During the following few years, feminists were determined to learn all they could. Ferreting out further evidence of medical abuses in city after city and hospital after hospital generated a broader-based women's health movement.

SELF-HELP GYNECOLOGY

The "invention" of self-help gynecology more than any other event transformed health and body issues into a separate social movement. Self-help gynecology was born on April 7, 1971, at the Everywoman's Bookstore in Los Angeles. For some time, feminists had met there to discuss health and abortion issues. After exhausting "book learning," Carol Downer, a member of the group, urged empirical observation. That evening, Downer inserted a speculum into her vagina and invited the other women present to observe her cervix. In September that year, a similar demonstration of self-examination was presented at the national meeting of NOW in Los Angeles (The West Coast Sisters 1971).

Self-examination and self-help gynecology (developing in its wake) were revolutionary concepts. For self-help provided women the opportunity to reclaim parts of themselves controlled by male professionals. What seemed an "accident of anatomy" no longer prevented women from becoming acquainted with parts of their anatomy usually reserved for male observation. As Price (1972) points out, men have had more intimate contact with, and far greater access to, the vagina than women have ever had. The male organ, on the other hand, has always been exposed, and seeing it reinforces its reality. Women now have this possibility.

Most women first view their own cervixes with awe and excitement (Reynard 1973, p. 99). Not uncommonly, women experience their first viewing as a mystical or even spiritual event.* The concept of self-examination spread rapidly through the feminist movement. Members of the Los Angeles FWHC (including Carol Downer, Lorraine Rothman, and Coleen Wilson) traveled throughout the country demonstrating cervical self-examination. On the East Coast, Lolly and Jeanne Hirsch, a mother-daughter team, coordinated self-examination activities. In addition to giving self-help demonstrations and classes, the Hirsches, along with Millie Alleyn, founded a newsletter in August 1972.

---

*Women often express their experiences poetically. For a good example of the common themes in these experiences, see the poem written by a member of the Mother Lode Collective 1972, p. 6. See also L. Hirsch 1972, p. 22.

The Monthly Extract—An Irregular Periodical was billed as the communications network of the global self-help movement. Its purpose—stated on the cover of each issue—was "to fire the Revolution by which WOMEN WILL RIGHTFULLY RECLAIM OUR OWN BODIES." The Monthly Extract was the crucial first health movement communications network through which women learned of each other's activities. The informal newsletter format—short articles, letters from readers, reprints of newspaper clippings, and announcements of conferences and other events—encouraged women to share ideas and exchange information.

Within a year after Downer began publicizing self-examination, over 2,000 women had attended clinics and demonstrations. By 1975, self-examination had been demonstrated not only throughout the United States but also in Canada, Mexico, England, France, Germany, Italy, Northern Ireland, Belgium, Denmark, West Berlin, and New Zealand. In the United States, self-help groups and women's gynecology clinics now operate in most major metropolitan areas and in many smaller communities as well. (See Appendix C for a list of self-help clinics.)

Of course, women did more than simply "look" at themselves. With regular self-examination, women could detect signs of common gynecological disorders. Using a simple hand mirror, a lamp, and a plastic speculum, women learned to recognize early signs of vaginal infections, syphilis, and pregnancy. They also discovered how to check the placement of IUDs and perform breast examinations. In addition to comparing notes on what types of drugs were commonly prescribed for certain disorders, the women found a number of simple home remedies very effective. The most famous remedy, which attracted worldwide attention, was yogurt, applied directly to the cervix to relieve monilia—commonly referred to as yeast infection. (Monilia is actually a fungus infestation rather than an infection.)

Had self-help advocates simply stuck to yogurt in the privacy of their own homes, the medical and legal authorities might have ignored the matter. Instead, women publicized what they learned, sharing their new-found knowledge with laywomen and professionals alike. At the September 1972 American Psychological Association meeting in Hawaii, Downer told conferees: "Abortions are so simple, they are downright dull; vaginal infections are diagnosed with a microscope; pap smears are easier to do than setting our hair; fitting a diaphragm is less complicated than stuffing a turkey. We can do these things" (1972, p. 4).

"What they could do" that most upset the medical establishment was to remove the contents of the uterus. Early in 1971—even before publicly demonstrating self-examination—Downer and Rothman developed a procedure termed menstrual extraction (The Feminist Women's Health Center n.d.). The technology making menstrual

FIGURE 3.1
Del-Em: Self-Help Clinic Menstrual Extractor

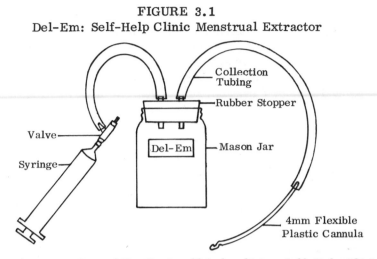

Source: As a member of the first self-help clinic, Self-Help Clinic One, Lorraine Rothman invented and patented the Del-Em menstrual extractor. The illustration of the Del-Em is by Suzann Gage. Lorraine Rothman and Suzann Gage are health activists at the Feminist Women's Health Center in Los Angeles. Material is being reprinted with permission.

extraction possible was Rothman's ingenious Del-'Em jar—a syringe connected to an airtight vacuum-controlled bottle, which provides the suction needed to draw out the uterine contents in about five minutes through a small-diameter cannula inserted into the cervical os (Price 1972; The West Coast Sisters 1971). Essentially, the Del-'Em jar is a simpler version of the more cumbersome and expensive vacuum aspiration equipment that was being used by physicians for early abortions in the late 1960s.*

At the same time Rothman was developing menstrual extraction technique and technology, physicians in San Francisco, Los Angeles, Washington, D.C., and New York were experimenting with similar procedures for very early termination of pregnancy. Referred to

---

*Women trained in self-help do not use the device as frequently as medically trained personnel use regular endometrial aspiration equipment. To compensate for possible risk related to infrequency of use, the Del-Em is equipped with an extra by pass valve to prevent the possibility of air entering the uterine cavity.

euphemistically as <u>menstrual induction</u>, <u>menstrual regulation</u>, or
<u>endometrial aspiration</u>, physicians were inserting a narrow-diameter
cannula through the os of the cervix and using suction to remove uterine
contents in the legally "gray area" between the time a woman missed
her period and the time pregnancy could be confirmed. In 1970,
Downer and Rothman had visited abortion facilities throughout the
country and investigated these abortion techniques thoroughly (Price
1972). (For medical details on these procedures, see, for example,
"Atraumatic Termination of Pregnancy" 1973; Goldsmith and Margolis
1971; "Population Report" 1973; and Stim 1973.)

As late as 1972, there had been no court cases testing the legality of physician-performed menstrual induction, nor had state legis-
latures debated whether or not it should be classified as an abortion.
The states where it was performed, however, had liberalized abortion
laws before the procedure was publicized (Dejanikus 1972, pp. 4-5).
For obvious political and legal reasons, menstrual extraction was
never publicly presented by Downer and Rothman as an abortion technique. Instead, it was touted as a means for women to reduce the
length and discomfort of their menstrual periods (Downer 1972; Price
1972; The West Coast Sisters 1971). However, no one denied that if
the uterine contents contained a fertilized egg, it would be gone after
performing the simple procedure. Furthermore, if one could extract
a normal period, one could also extract a "late" period—up to five
weeks late (Price 1972, p. 4).

Menstrual extraction performed by laywomen was roundly denounced by professionals as a dangerous "do-it-yourself" abortion
technique (see, for example, Blair 1972; "<u>Hospital Tribune</u> Report"
1973; and Naismith 1973). At the other extreme, popularizers spread
the view that women ought to have "period extraction jars" in their
bathroom medicine cabinets—just like a toothbrush or bottle of aspirin
(Grau 1971).

Neither of these portrayals were what the inventors had intended.
Self-help advocates emphasized that the procedure was only intended
to be performed in a group of thoroughly screened and trained women—
never alone. In such groups, women could avail themselves of collective knowledge, collective expertise, and sisterly concern for one
another. Outside the context of the group, menstrual extraction was
both unsafe and in violation of feminist principles (The West Coast
Sisters 1971; Dejanikus 1972, p. 5). Furthermore, as Lolly Hirsch
explained, unless women were "gymnastic geniuses," it was absurd to
believe women could even do menstrual extractions on themselves
(Dejanikus 1972, p. 5).

Some of the initial confusion stemmed from an article written
by Peggy Grau in October 1971 in <u>Everywoman,</u> a West Coast feminist
newspaper. Harvey Karman, who sometimes claims to have invented

menstrual extraction, has been accused of responsibility for this article ("Feminist Women's Health Center Report" 1973). In response
to Grau's article, Downer and Rothman disclaimed anything to do with
self-abortion (Price 1972, p. 5; The West Coast Sisters 1971).

Despite self-help proponents' public attempts to differentiate
between menstrual extraction and abortion, no one took the disclaim-
ers too seriously. Feminists themselves were divided over the issue
of menstrual extraction. While proponents saw it as a means for wom-
en to gain greater control over their bodies, others argued that there
were too many risks (Dejanikus 1972; Price 1972; Frankfort 1972).
Some feminists even questioned whether or not such a procedure
should be performed as a standard abortion technique by physicians.

"The other side" was certain, however, that laywomen should
not be doing menstrual extractions, regulations, inductions (or whatever one might call the procedure), or any other procedures that
could conceivably fall under medical authority. By the summer of 1972,
the FWHC in Los Angeles had been subject to undercover surveillance
for six months. On September 20, eight plainclothesmen and two uni-
formed Los Angeles police officers entered the center with a search
warrant. During the three-hour search, officers confiscated plastic
tablecloths, a 50-foot extension cord, books, health records, plastic
specula, curettes used in educational programs describing hospital
abortion procedures, birth control devices, and cannulas. Yogurt,
used in the vagina to treat monilia, was taken from the refrigerator.
Carol Downer and Coleen Wilson were arrested on assorted charges
of practicing medicine without a license.

Wilson, charged with 11 counts, pleaded guilty to the charge
of fitting a diaphragm and was fined $250 and placed on two years'
probation.* Downer, charged with the misdemeanor of practicing
medicine without a license (for helping a woman insert a speculum
and apply yogurt), chose to stand trial. The Monthly Extract, in the
November-December 1972 issue, sent out a special appeal for financial support to defray the legal fees and publicize the case. Other
feminist newspapers and newsletters followed suit (see, for example,
The Spokeswoman 1972).

Downer's trial became a cause celebre. Comparisons were
made between the Los Angeles women and the suffragettes, who had

---

*In June 1973, Wilson applied for a teaching credential in Cal-
ifornia. After many delays, the state denied the credential on the
grounds of "moral turpitude." See Feminist Women's Health Center
Newsletter 1976, p. 2.

risked going to jail to promote their causes. The similarities were also drawn between Downer and early birth control crusaders Margaret Sanger and her sister, Ethel Byre, both of whom were jailed for opening the first American birth control clinic in Brownsville, New York. Sanger had gone to jail eight times, and Downer seemed willing to follow in her footsteps (The Monthly Extract 1973, p. 1).

Money and support flowed into the FWHC from disparate groups and individuals. New York Congresswoman Bella Abzug proclaimed the trial of Downer to be an enormously important test case, and feminist periodicals and newsletters from Ms. to The Monthly Extract openly supported Downer, repeating the plea for defense funds (Reynard 1973, p. 96). Margaret Mead observed that "men began taking over obstetrics and they invented a tool that allowed them to look inside women. You could call this progress, except that when women tried to look inside themselves, this was called practicing medicine without a license" (Los Angeles Times, February 5, 1974, pt. IV:1, p. 6).

On December 5, 1972, Downer was acquitted after two days of deliberation by a jury of eight men and four women in the Los Angeles courtroom of Judge Mary Waters. After the ordeal was over, Jeanne Hirsch wondered:

> WHAT MAN WOULD BE PUT UNDER POLICE SUR-
> VEILLANCE FOR SIX MONTHS FOR LOOKING AT HIS
> PENIS? What man would have to spend $20,000 and two
> months in court for looking at the penis of his brother?
> This case is a clear cut version of the position of women
> in America—the lengths to which we must go and obstacles
> which must be overcome to be FREE (J. Hirsch 1974,
> p. 2).

FEMINISM AND NATURAL CHILDBIRTH ADVOCATES

Interest in self-help gynecology was paralleled by a growing interest among feminists in childbirth (see, for example, Alexander 1974; Cagan 1970; Marguerite 1973; Olds 1973; and Pollard 1969). Of course, childbirth was also of concern to counterculture people leading "natural" life-styles that included home-birthing, natural or prepared childbirth proponents (often affiliated with the ICEA) and breast-feeding advocates (whose interests were furthered by La Leche League, a traditional self-help and mutual aid organization).

Feminists, "hippies," home-birth and prepared childbirth proponents, and breast-feeding advocates all recognized their common interests and sought to work toward common goals despite their many differences in life-style and political orientation. This coalition, which made the movement broad based, was fostered in part by women's overlapping involvements in various reform movements. Feminists Norma Swensen, a member of the Boston Women's Health Book Collective, and Doris Haire, a prominent health writer and educator, for example, were both active in the ICEA.

Many of the demands health movement activists make are remarkably similar to those made by the ICEA (strongly supported by many prominent physicians over the past two decades). Haire's work in particular (1972, 1973) encouraged women's groups to demand changes in maternity practices and has been used to support both nurse-midwifery and lay midwifery.

Lay midwifery became a feminist cause celebre in March 1974 when three key members of the Santa Cruz, California, Birth Center were arrested on charges of practicing medicine without a license after a year of undercover surveillance. Linda Bennett and Donna Walker, a physician's wife, were arrested after arriving at a private home to deliver a baby for an undercover agent. Kate Bowland, the third midwife, was arrested at the Birth Center by eight armed officers, who entered with a search warrant (Goldberg 1974; Von B. 1974; Butler 1974; Christeve 1974).

Feminist newspapers and newsletters reported the "bust," and calls for volunteers to work on the legal defense went out immediately.* Pretrial motions delayed hearing of the case. On August 20, 1974 the Berkeley-Oakland (California) Women's Union (including several local women's health clinics) sponsored a benefit for the Santa Cruz midwives, featuring Bennett, a defendant, along with Barbara Ehrenreich and Deirdre English as speakers. Over 200 people, mostly women and small children, attended.

English argued that the midwives' trial was political because it concerned who would be allowed to provide health care. The medical establishment felt threatened and responded to women organizing by trying to keep medical secrets and technology out of their hands. The arrest of the midwives was thus a direct assault on women's right to control their own bodies and health care.

English emphasized the affinity and solidarity between the self-help movement and the lay midwives and likened the midwives' situation

---

*See, for example, the call for financial support, letters of protest over the arrests, and information on the legal position and accomplishments of midwives in other states printed in The Monthly Extract 1974, p. 7.

to the arrest of Downer and Wilson in Los Angeles for their self-help activities, repeating the importance of winning this legal battle many times. The lay midwives and their clients, with all their traditional values, came to be viewed as warriors in the feminist battle for freedom of choice.

After many delays and prosecution attempts to "drop the case," the midwives finally came to trial in the summer of 1976. The appellate court ruled that because pregnancy was not a disease, midwives could not be practicing medicine without a license; they were declared merely assisting in a normal physiological process. However, the California attorney general requested a rehearing of the case. Media observers suggested that the state was concerned that the ruling would be interpreted to mean that anyone could participate in home delivery without fear of state interference ("Santa Cruz Center Victory" 1976).

In August 1976, the state supreme court reconsidered the charges and ruled that the midwives could indeed be formally charged with violation of the Medical Practice Act. Subsequently, however, the charges were dropped, so the women never stood trial.

A conviction of the midwives would have reinforced health activists' belief that the male-dominated legal and medical professions collude to maintain vested class interests, power, and authority over women. An acquittal would have legitimated feminists' claim that childbirth is the appropriate province of women and would have been a clear victory for women's right to choose who will assist them in crucial life-events, typically presided over by medical men. Either outcome would have had serious repercussions for established medicine.

FEMINISM AND RADICAL HEALTH POLITICS

Feminism exerted an influence on many social movements flourishing in the late 1960s, altering the direction of some movements and leading women in others to break away from the older, male-dominated movements. Women involved in the free clinic and radical health movements formed crucial initial constituencies of the women's health movement.

Free Clinic Movement

A prominent feature of health activism during the 1960s was the growth of alternative institutions—particularly free clinics. Like alternative services in many fields (ranging from educational institutions to runaway houses), free clinics were intended to provide services that were less expensive, less dominated by professionals, less hierarchical, and more open to advocacy and social change than traditional ones (Gartner and Riessman 1974, pp. 83-84).* Free clinic advocates, in particular, aimed to offer services in a humane, nonjudgmental setting where any and all life-styles would be accepted (Glasscote et al. 1975; Harding, Harrington, and Manor 1973; Health/PAC Bulletin 1971).

But there was considerable sexism in the otherwise humanistic free clinic movement. A member of a large women's health collective (an outgrowth of a major free clinic) explained that although the doctors had learned not to be racist or antihippie, they were still sexist; neither women staff nor patients were treated with respect. Some women in free clinics publicly complained about doctors who said they were tired of looking at vaginas, who performed crude pelvic examinations, and who made insensitive and moralistic comments to women ("Women's Clinics" 1971, p. 14). Women clinic workers reported that patients were often subjected to sexual advances by both the staff and other clinic patients.

In response to sexist treatment, women organized their own free clinics in Berkeley, Seattle, and Baltimore early in 1971. Groups in New York also responded, and by the end of the year, at least half a dozen more clinics were opened. In establishing them, women extended the feminist ethos into direct health services and broadened the base of the women's movement. While the women's clinics served to recruit women health workers and patients into the women's movement, the reverse was also true. Already committed feminists were attracted to clinic work, and many ultimately pursued further training in health occupations and professions ("Women's Clinics" 1971, p. 15). This segment of the women's health movement involved in direct service has had the greatest commitment to, concern over, and difficulty with, operating organizations collectively.†

---

*The Haight-Ashbury Free Clinic, founded in 1967 to serve San Francisco's "flower children," set the style for an estimated 400 clinics that subsequently opened (Glasscote et al. 1975, pp. 28-29).

†See especially Kleiber and Light's 1978 extensive study of the organizational aspects of the Vancouver Women's Health Collective. For another perspective on the difficulties of collective organizations in the social services, see Galper and Washburne 1976.

Medical Committee for Human Rights

Between 1964 and 1974, the Medical Committee for Human Rights (MCHR) was by far the most active and best-known new left health group. Primarily an organization of physicians and nurses, MCHR activists provided medical services during civil rights protests, urban riots, and other political confrontations and supported anti-abortion repeal, welfare rights, food programs, the prisoners' rebellions at Attica, free clinics, and occupational health and safety programs (Kotelchuck and Levy 1975).

During the civil rights movement, women nurses and a few women physicians did much of the nitty-gritty work but received stingy wages and none of the glory.* Male doctors were flown South to put in brief appearances and then antagonized women by paternalistic references to the "grand work being done by our little maids in Mississippi" (Kotelchuck and Levy 1975, p. 6). Tensions over this treatment did not surface until April 1971, when the MCHR national convention met at the University of Pennsylvania.

Organized around the theme "The Consumer and Health Care," the MCHR convention attracted large numbers of women, Third World people, nonprofessional health workers, and consumers for the first time. Under substantial pressure from militant women, the MCHR considered its internal racism, sexism, elitism, professionalism, and organizational hierarchy and opened its leadership to its new constituencies. In the process, the MCHR developed a disdain for organizing doctors or medical students, because of the developing ideology that such individuals could ultimately act only in their own, already privileged counterrevolutionary self-interest. As a result, the MCHR was transformed into a mass organization without a clearly identifiable constituency or strategic thrust. By 1974, the organization had virtually disintegrated (Kotelchuck and Levy 1975, pp. 16-29).

Health: Just Another Commodity?

A major force in radical health care during the past decade was the Health Policy Advisory Center (Health/PAC), which sees

---

*Many of these women were active in several reform movements. For example, Phyllis Cunningham, a nurse, had worked formerly with the Student Nonviolent Coordinating Committee (SNCC), and June Finer, a physician, was later active in antiabortion repeal and activities.

itself as part of a larger movement for radical social change in America.* Two of the original ten Health/PAC staff members, Barbara and John Ehrenreich, wrote major critical analyses of the health system, describing it as an industry organized for profit—not for peoples' health (1971). Under capitalism, they argued, health care is transformed into a commodity, but a commodity difficult to "purchase" wisely, for although patients are "consumers," they have none of the rights or protections that consumers of other goods and services expect (1971, p. 12). What health radicals essentially demanded was more product for less money with some assurance of quality control.

At the Berkeley benefit for the Santa Cruz lay midwives (who had been arrested for practicing medicine without a license) on August 20, 1974, Barbara Ehrenreich declared that in retrospect, the health radical vision was rather limited and that feminism had dramatically changed her goals. Previously, she and other health activists had let the medical profession tell people what they needed without looking at what was "inside the wrapping." Whereas previously, she and others had been interested in quantity, they were now quality conscious and concerned with deprofessionalizing and demedicalizing the health care system (ultimately creating the basis for a new feminist-socialist alliance).

Feminist theorists like Ehrenreich expanded the narrow economic outlook limiting earlier radical critiques of the health system. They argued that while health care is a capitalist commodity, this analysis fails to address the health care experience adequately. Because feminists take an experiential perspective, the actual production of health care must be analyzed in terms of its total effect on the participants (Marieskind and Ehrenreich 1975, p. 39).

In the typical health care relationship (which mirrors larger social relationships), women feel humiliated and powerless vis-a-vis condescending and contemptuous physicians. Because professionals have a monopoly over the production and application of medical knowledge, physicians can dominate their less-privileged, less-knowledgeable patients. Socialist-feminist health activists see self-help activities as a means to alter this by giving patients access to the knowledge

---

*Organized in 1967 by Robb Burlage, Health/PAC's primary mission was to provide information and analysis of immediate usefulness to health activists. Gradually, Health/PAC's activities expanded to include educational projects and direct technical assistance to the student, worker, and community groups involved in health activities (Ehrenreich and Ehrenreich 1971, p. vii).

and skills required for medical production (Marieskind and Ehren-reich 1975, pp. 39-40). Thus, radicals see self-help as offering a necessary condition for building a nonauthoritarian collectivist or socialist (rather than simply socialized) medical system; the Chinese system is the model (Marieskind and Ehrenreich 1975, pp. 41-42).

4

Women, Medicine and
the Moral Order

In health groups, women's clinics, public demonstrations, and in the feminist press, women responded to revelations of medical outrages with anger and surprise. Some felt betrayed—a good indication of their previous faith and trust in the medical mystique. Members of the Mother Lode Collective (1972, p. 1) commented:

> When women come together to talk about their experiences in doctors' offices, everyone has a story to tell, or many stories, of humiliation, of bullying, callousness or outright carelessness on the doctor's part. Why is this so? Given that we are thought of in this society as inferior creatures whose role is confined to sexual/procreative functions, who are unable to comprehend or control our own lives, it is not surprising that doctors reflect the general attitude in their treatment of us. The doctor is paternalistic and uses his professional mask to make us feel stupid, clumsy, unsure and ignorant. His religious/cultural orientation influences how he sees our physical condition, especially if that condition has to do with sex or reproduction, and his attitude is often more "moral" than it is medical.

Arguing that medicine is embedded in, and an embodiment of, patriarchal society, women began clarifying the role of science and sexism in American medicine. Significantly, the inquiry quickly spread from the underground feminist press to academe. Although the tone and style of ideologists, commentators, and academic researchers is different, their concerns and contentions are strikingly similar. Allegations of medical sexism in the feminist press are

65

impressionistic and rhetorical. Nearly identical claims have appeared in the medical and social scientific literature which are written in neutral language and buttressed by statistical measures of significance. Such claims are considered more "legitimate" to the annoyance of many lay health activists who equate professionalism with patriarchal elitism.* As more than one health activist has complained, "Academics are just proving what we women already know."

The rush to validate and verify feminist perspectives actually indicates widespread adoption of a new paradigm, which assumes male-female relations to be a crucial dimension in understanding and improving the social and behavioral sciences, medical science, and clinical practice. As such a paradigm is put forth and gains credence in established disciplines, efforts are made to verify basic concepts and to consider their ramifications—the tasks of "normal science" (Kuhn 1962).

Barbara Seaman has been credited by the Library of Congress as the first author to raise sexism in health care as a worldwide issue. Others rapidly used existing data to elaborate on this theme. Ehrenreich and English's pamphlets, Witches, Midwives and Nurses: A History of Women Healers (1972) and Complaints and Disorders: The Sexual Politics of Sickness (1973), were early efforts to develop a theory of the sexual politics of health. The enormously popular pamphlets generated tremendous interest in medical sexism and medical history and motivated academic scholars and laywomen alike to document the moral—or, as sometimes stated, immoral—features of medical science and practice.

Although there is no single document offering a unified critique of the health care system—nor could there be given the movement's diversity—certain issues and themes appear regularly in feminist health literature and in discussion groups, as well as in the academic literature. Some of these themes appeared earlier but were largely ignored before the movement gained momentum. The lay movement's ability to generate academic inquiry and draw attention to little-known early studies suggests how far the direction of medical, as well as the social and behavioral sciences, can be altered by extrascientific factors.

---

*I have included references to material from a wide variety of sources to emphasize the distribution of ideas throughout society. That similar statements are made in The New England Journal of Medicine and Off Our Backs indicates how widespread the issues are.

Beginning with an historical analysis of the social control function of physicians, the feminist critique (culled from many sources) focuses on the transformation of the medical-scientific establishment's assumption of biological inferiority into psychological terms detrimental to women. Feminists also speculate on, and offer empirical evidence to explain, the sources and supports of sexism in society and in medical institutions.[*]

THE SOCIAL CONTROL FUNCTION OF THE PHYSICIAN IN HISTORICAL PERSPECTIVE

Historically, physicians have served the interests of those in power, not only offering technical medical skills but also serving as arbiters of morality and agents of social control.[†] In patriarchal societies, where men claim proprietary rights to women as husbands, fathers, and lovers, men have relied on physicians to assist them in maintaining prestige, status, purity of lineage, and property rights by managing female sexuality (Bullough 1974; Millet 1970; Smith 1970, p. 6). As McLaren (1975) points out, by the early 1800s, French physicians had taught men forms of contraception (for example, the rhythm method), which put all control in their hands. Women were not instructed in these techniques by physicians, for: "all forms of birth control would presumably provide the woman with some dangerous insights into the workings of her own body" (McLaren 1975, p. 50).

The Victorian Era—Upper-Class Confinement

In Victorian America, physicians acted as watchmen of morals, authorities on fashion, and staunch defenders of the status quo. Haller and Haller (1974) report that the medical profession actively reinforced societal attempts to keep women dependent and subordinate to men by using a mixture of anthropometric studies, biblical references,

---

[*]The purpose of this section is to present the world view of feminist health activists, not to critique the historical approach taken by specific authors. For critiques of feminist perspectives on medical history, see especially Fruchtbaum 1976; Morantz 1974; Ozonoff and Ozonoff 1975; and Verbrugge 1975.

[†]See Zola 1972 for discussion of medicine as an institution of social control.

medical evidence, and evolutionary law to explain women's proper role and place in nature. Roles other than those that assured the stability of the home circle were thoroughly denigrated by medical science (Haller and Haller 1974, p. 47).

In late nineteenth-century America, keeping middle- and upper-class women in the home was regarded by many as essential to the survival of the nation, and physicians joined the effort to convince, cajole, or coerce women into fulfilling traditional roles. Fearful of militant upper-class feminists, physicians directly attacked the emancipiation of women (Haller and Haller 1974, pp. 47-48). Despite considerable research which indicated that higher education was not detrimental to women's ability to bear children, many physicians continued to assert that thinking would stunt the growth of the ovaries, breasts, and future fetuses. In addition, physicians claimed that the nervous stimulation accompanying social, political, and educational emancipiation was hazardous, for nervous stimulation was said to trigger menstruation—a condition regarded as pathological (Bullough and Voght 1973).

Indeed, all female reproductive functions were defined as pathological to upper-class women. Puberty was regarded as a period of crisis, turning the entire female organism into a state of frailty and turmoil. Menstruation was a state of ill health, to be treated with rest. Pregnancy was defined as a disease requiring the care of a physician, and childbirth was transformed into a surgical event. Menopause was regarded as the final illness—the "death of the woman in the woman" (Ehrenreich and English 1973, pp. 6, 20-21; Wood 1973).

Constricted by social conventions, upper-class women had few options but to be "sick." Indeed, some made lifelong careers of the cult of invalidism. Admired as romantic heroines, tubercular women exemplified the prevailing standard of frail feminine beauty (Ehrenreich and English 1973, pp. 19-22). Many women suffered from neurasthenia—a catch-all category used by physicians to describe the female syndrome attributed to nervousness and overexertion. The typical treatment—rest and isolation—often exacerbated women's problems and brought on additional symptoms and increasing lethargy (Ehrenreich and English 1973, pp. 17-22; Haller 1971; Haller and Haller 1974, pp. 5-43; Smith 1970, pp. 131-39; Wood 1973).

Physicians soothed many women into lifelong alcohol and opiate addiction (Haller and Haller 1974, pp. 273-303). Some fought back or escaped temporarily through hysteria (Ehrenreich and English 1973; Smith-Rosenberg 1972; Wood 1973). According to Smith (1970, pp. 138-39), ill health was also a birth control measure and an attempt on the part of women to gain some measure of control of their own bodies.

Gynecological Surgery

Some have argued that medical control over middle- and upper-class women reached its heights in the late nineteenth century in the form of gynecological surgery. Barker-Benfield (1972, p. 59), for example, argues that gynecologists' underlying aims were inseparable from those of the dominant society. These aims were retaliation against, and control of, women and the assumption of as much of their reproductive power as possible.

Surgical control took several forms. Clitoridectomy was performed in the United States beginning in the late 1860s, and along with female circumcision (removal of the clitoral hood), was advocated to stem the allegedly growing tide of masturbation.* However, female castration (ovariotomy) was a more common surgical treatment than either circumcision or clitoridectomy. Invented in 1872 by Robert Battey, "normal ovariotomy," or excision of the ovaries for nonovarian conditions, was indicated by a number of conditions, including

> neurosis, insanity, abnormal menstruation and practically anything untoward in female behavior. Among the indications were troublesomeness, eating like a ploughman, masturbation, attempted suicide, erotic tendencies, persecution mania, simple "cussedness," and dysmenorrhoea (painful menstruation, long held to be one consequence of masturbation). Most apparent in the enormous variety of symptoms doctors took to indicate castration was a strong current of sexual appetitiveness on the part of women. That is, castratable women evinced a quality held to be characteristic of men (Barker-Benfield 1972, p. 60).

Gynecologists argued that the surgery would make women like castrated animals—that they would become tractable, orderly, and faithful servants (Barker-Benfield 1972, pp. 60-61).

During the early 1890s, female castration was exceedingly popular. Doctors competed with each other in the number of ovaries

---

*Female circumcision was performed at least through 1937 according to Barker-Benfield (1972, p. 59). Ehrenreich and English (1973, p. 34) report that the last known clitoridectomy in the United States was performed in 1948 on a five-year-old girl to cure her masturbation.

they extirpated; some boasted they had removed from 1,500 to 2,000.[*]
Using their surgical skills, physicians shored up male authority over
women. Thus, the dictates of "science" were used to perpetuate prevailing sex roles at a time when the traditional social order was
threatened from many directions (Barker-Benfield 1972, pp. 60-61).

Controlling the Sickening Masses

The threat to the existing social order came not only from
militant feminists. During the mid-1800s, the upper classes were
concerned about the tide of new immigrants pouring into the country.
On the one hand, they sorely needed immigrants as a cheap source
of industrial labor. On the other, the Anglo-Saxon upper classes,
along with the eugenicists, argued that the newcomers were inferior,
a "degenerate breeding stock" that threatened the survival of the nation (Higham 1969, pp. 150-51). Fear of immigrants was complex,
for in certain ways, the newcomers were especially robust and sturdy.
As Ehrenreich and English (1973, p. 55) point out: "As breeders,
they seemed to outdo the delicate or 'high-strung' ladies of the better
classes."

Eugenicists' efforts to perpetuate the "great race" involved
working to restrict immigration[†] and to alter the balance of fertility
between the newcomers and the upper classes. Militant middle- and
upper-class feminists crusading for birth control shared some, but
not all, of the eugenicists' eagerness for fertility control. Margaret
Sanger (1938, pp. 374-75) pointed out that while the eugenicists emphasized more children for the rich, feminists sought first to stop
the multiplication of the unfit as a more important step toward race
betterment.

---

[*]Ironically, castration led to even more drastic gynecological
surgery, including ovarian transplants to replace the organs removed.
Of course, ovarian transplants were only possible when "normal
ovaries" were available to transplant, so ovariotomy (to obtain transplants) continued to be performed through the early 1920s (Barker-
Benfield 1972, pp. 60-61).

[†]Many physicians, active in the eugenics movement, worked
for restrictive immigration legislation or served as public health and
immigration officers, screening out new immigrants suspected of
being carriers of physical and mental diseases. For further discussion, see Higham 1969, pp. 149-57; Handlin 1957, pp. 74-110; and
Salmon 1913.

Birth control was controversial not only for political, moral, and religious reasons but because it directly involved men's control over women. Smith (1970, pp. 233-34) described masculine opposition to dissemination of birth control knowledge as "the 'last and bitterest battle waged by men to keep women in subjection.' In terror 'of what should happen to their vested interests should this last security fail,' men were fighting for their very lives." Sanger discovered the depth of masculine opposition shortly after World War I when she consulted a German gynecologist, an abortion advocate, to learn contraceptive techniques, only to have her cause roundly denounced. When Sanger asked why he opposed the safer form of limiting population through contraception, he retorted: "We will never give over the control of our numbers to the women themselves. What, let them control the future of the human race? With abortions it is in our hands; we make the decisions, and they must come to us" (Sanger 1938, p. 286).*

Physicians' social control function also involved preventing contagion and contamination by the lower classes. Ehrenreich and English (1973, p. 55) argue that lower-class women were regarded as particularly "sickening" and dangerous because they were much more likely than working-class men to come into close contact with the affluent. While the men were employed in heavy industry, the women entered domestic service, garment manufacture, and prostitution, where they could, if ill, expose their "betters" to disease. Contagious and sick many women were. Living conditions in the urban slums were squalid, and typhoid, yellow fever, tuberculosis, cholera, and diphtheria ravaged the poor, who were already weak from overwork and malnutrition.† Although a few socially minded physicians urged reform, their pleas went largely unheeded by the upper classes, until fear of cholera and other epidemic diseases motivated the well-to-do to demand public health measures (Shryock 1966, pp. 128-34).

---

*Sanger actually planned to leave considerable control in the hands of physicians. While she published pamphlets offering contraceptive advice, she strongly felt that women should be instructed personally by physicians, and she objected to plans for manufacturing or distributing contraceptives without close medical supervision (Sanger 1938, pp. 190, 414-15).

†Shryock (1966, pp. 127-29) points out that slum conditions made disease problems particularly acute, noting that the urban death rate rose ominously from 21 per 1,000 in 1810 to 37 per 1,000 in 1857—nearly an 80 percent increase within 50 years.

While epidemic diseases were fearful, prostitution was the overriding social evil of the century. In the 1860s, there were an estimated 20,000 prostitutes in the city of New York alone. Prostitution was not only a threat to the family but exposed innocent wives and fetuses in the womb to venereal disease (Ehrenreich and English 1973, p. 60; Smith 1970, p. 228).

By the late nineteenth century, the threat of disease had thoroughly stirred the upper classes into a drive for improved public health and sanitation. Women physicians were particularly active in the public health movement, promoting the improvement of the lot of the poor for the benefit of their betters. In the battle against contagion, public health officers were vested with tracking down and quarantining persons suspected of spreading disease. Public health crusaders were especially concerned with the cost of disease in terms of worker absenteeism, public relief, and public hospital costs (Ehrenreich and English 1973, pp. 62-65; see also Duffy 1968, 1974).

Ehrenreich and English (1973, pp. 72-73) emphasize that in fighting for improvements in birth control and public health, middle- and upper-class women allied themselves with a professional group that was basically oppressive to them in order to protect themselves from threats posed by the poor. The medical myths and biological fears were simply overlays giving "scientific plausibility" to underlying class concerns.

SCIENCE AND SEXISM IN CONTEMPORARY MEDICINE

Redefining "Biological Inferiority"

The social control function of the physician vis-a-vis women, which shifted in the mid-twentieth century in significant ways, remains similar in certain respects. With the advent of Freudian psychoanalysis, upper-class women no longer were confined to the cult of invalidism. Instead, women found themselves channeled into an oftentimes equally debilitating and restricting cult of analytic therapy. While in many ways this represented a genuine improvement for women, the Freudian theory of female nature was strikingly similar to the gynecological view that it replaced. Whereas women had been viewed as inherently defective because of the domineering uterus, their latest defect was the absence of a penis. Or as Ehrenreich and English (1973, p. 44) conclude: "Women were still 'sick,' and their sickness was still totally predestined by their anatomy."

This shift in attitude toward women's "biological inferiority" has had far-reaching consequences. First, women who fail to meet societal standards of behavior are likely to have psychiatrists attempt to "cure" their ills. However, feminists—including many mental health practitioners—argue that psychotherapy is simply a modern day prescription for keeping women "in their place" (see, for example, Bart 1971b; Chesler 1971, 1972; Fields n.d.; Roth 1973; Tennov 1973, 1975; Walstedt 1971; and Weisstein 1971).

Chesler (1972) argues that independent, creative, and assertive behavior in women is often viewed negatively and has been taken as evidence of "madness" by husbands, therapists, and society in general. Once again, the physician and his mental health teammates—the clinical psychologist, social worker, and psychiatric nurse—are called upon to ensure that women learn to be self-sacrificing, maternal, dependent, and passive.

Bart (1971a, 1971b, 1973) argues that females often are "cooled into" traditional roles by therapists, who view women primarily as sexual objects and mothers. Psychologist Lorna Benjamin at the Wisconsin Psychiatric Institute notes how sexism in the psychotherapeutic process pushes women into approved role behavior. For example:

> A husband is counseled not to try to understand his wife, since women are incapable of being logical.
>
> A wife is counseled to inhibit her point of view, since her husband needs to be dominant. She is told that a cuddly, soft, submissive woman is truly feminine and loveable whereas an assertive, active female is castrating and ugly.
>
> A female medical student is told not to speak up in class because "the boys don't go for that castrating crap" (Bart 1973, pp. 28, 64).

It should be emphasized that sex-role stereotypes are just as likely to be held by female clinicians as by male mental health professionals. The Broverman et al. (1970) study of 79 therapists indicated no significant differences between male and female clinicians on attitudes about normal female behavior. What was striking, however, was the double standard of health. The respondents, asked to list traits felt to be characteristic of healthy males, healthy females, and healthy adults-sex unspecified, judged what was healthy for adults-sex unspecified as similar to what was judged healthy for adult males. Healthy women, however, were seen as more submissive, less independent, less adventurous, more easily influenced, less aggressive, less competitive, more excitable in minor crises, more easily hurt, more emotional, more vain, and less objective. Traits considered pathological in one sex were "normal" for the other, to the extent that ideal concepts of health for mature adults-sex unspecified are meant primarily for men. Broverman et al. (1970, p. 7) point out how this places women in a double bind:

> For a woman to be healthy, from an adjustment view-
> point, she must adjust to and accept the behavioral norms
> for her sex, even though these behaviors are generally
> less socially desirable and considered to be less healthy
> for the generalized competent, mature adult. ... Accep-
> tance of an adjustment notion of health, then, places wom-
> en in the conflictual position of having to decide whether
> to exhibit those positive characteristics considered desir-
> able for men and adults, and thus have their "femininity"
> questioned, that is, be deviant in terms of being a woman;
> or to behave in the prescribed feminine manner, accept
> second-class adult status, and possibly live a lie to boot.

Coercion in the Name of Mental Health

Not all women have the opportunity to decide for themselves whether or not they will adjust or conform to social expectations. Roth and Lerner (1974, p. 803) point out that "therapy" can at times be cruelly and openly coercive, designed to force women into conventional sex roles. First, women are more subject than men to institutionalization on specious grounds. Because women by tradition and training are weaker, more submissive, and anxious to please, they are particularly vulnerable to such pressure from male authority figures; distinctions between voluntary and involuntary admissions may be effectively eliminated. In addition, institutional authorities tend to accept the perceptions of the husband, father, or policeman seeking a woman's commitment and to ignore or minimize the woman's version of the situation. Particular groups of women are far more vulnerable to commitment than their male counterparts: disobedient or runaway adolescent females, women involved in custody suits, single mothers receiving public assistance, and women who are in inferior economic positions when involved in family conflicts (Roth and Lerner 1974, pp. 797-801).

Institutional treatment of women often consits of conditioning and enforcing sexual stereotypes. Such an approach is lauded in psychiatric literature, for the goal of therapy is to encourage patient-inmates to adopt "appropriate" social roles. Roth and Lerner (1974, p. 802) discuss the extremes of the adjustment approach, citing a 1963 study published in the Archives of General Psychiatry:

> Dr. Herbert C. Modlin treated five "paranoid" women by
> "managing" them into submissive "feminine" roles. The

women "fancied" that men were persecuting them. Dr.
Modlin advised his colleagues to disregard their patients'
"distorted perceptions" and substitute their own "acknowledged authority." The study concludes that "the disappear-
ance of delusions coincided ... our helping her to reassert
her feminine social role."

Not all role conditioning takes such mild forms. Women patients who persist in demonstrating anger or aggressiveness are considered so deviant that isolation, confinement in straitjackets, or
even shock therapy are prescribed. In one reported incident, researchers attempted to reduce aggressive behavior in a female inmate
by shocking her repeatedly with a cattle prod whenever she made verbal threats or committed aggressive acts (Chesler 1972, p. 36).
Coercive treatment does "work" in a sense, for example:

An informant reported that his mother, who had suffered
a nervous breakdown, finally "got so bad she forgot how
to cook." After receiving a few electroshock treatments,
however, "she remembered like magic" (Lerner and Roth
1974, p. 803).
A doctor tried to rape me during a gynecological examination, but I was afraid to complain, afraid they'd say I was
lying or crazy and give me shock treatments (Chesler
1972, p. 170).

For intractables who will not or cannot adjust, drastic physical
modes of treatment are still available. Much like castration and old-
fashioned lobotomy, their modern offspring, psychosurgery, makes
women passive and docile. Dr. Peter Breggin, an authority on, and
opponent of, psychosurgery, notes that the procedure destroys the
brain's capacity to respond emotionally; impairs the function of insight, creativity, and judgment; and, occasionally, inhibits control
of bodily functions (Breggin 1972, 5567).
Approximately three times as many women as men receive
psychosurgery (Breggin 1972, 5571). And psychosurgery is on the
increase, with between 400 and 600 operations performed each year—
mostly on women, children, homosexuals, and prisoners.* Proponents

---

*According to a California neurosurgeon, 72 percent of the
psychotics and 80 percent of the neurotics operated on in 1964 were
female. At a 1970 medical conference, R. F. Heatherton of the
Kingston Psychiatric Hospital in Ontario, Canada, stated that the

of psychosurgery argue that women respond particularly well because of their passive conditioning. Furthermore, as Breggin notes, it is more socially acceptable to lobotomize women, because creativity, which the operation totally destroys, is an "expendable quality" in women (Roberts 1972, p. 14).

Psychosurgeons expect women to function only in the traditional roles of housekeeper and mother. As one psychiatrist observed, after a lobotomy: "Women do the dishes better, are better housewives and comply with the sexual demands of their husbands. ... It takes away their aggressiveness" (Roth and Lerner 1974, p. 806). Not surprisingly, evidence of successful treatment is that previously "distraught" women return to, or take up, housekeeping chores (Beam 1973, p. 9; Roberts 1972, p. 14).

Critics argue that proponents of lobotomy "twist the facts" to convince themselves and detractors of some operations' successfulness. Breggin, for example, notes that in 1970, psychosurgeons Frank Ervin and Vernon Mark from Boston City Hospital lauded a lobotomy as a great success despite the fact that the patient killed herself. The woman, who had a long psychiatric history, submitted to the operation under pressure from doctors and her mother. When the first operation failed to relieve her depression, she was given a second. Furious at the doctors, she refused a third operation; her rage was dismissed as "paranoid." Her mood seemed to improve, and when allowed out of the hospital to shop, the woman committed suicide. Breggin reports that her suicide "is seen not as the vengeful act of a mutilated soul against her mother and her physicians. Instead her suicide is interpreted as a sign that she was getting over her depression, a gratifying result of the operation" (Roberts 1972, p. 14).

Women are particularly at risk, because severe depression is regarded as an indication for lobotomy. And it is typically older women who suffer agitated depressions during midlife and menopause. Middle-aged women have always been a target for whatever "therapy" is in vogue (Roberts 1972, pp. 14-15). In the light of the growth of psychosurgery, many feminists, including physician Barbara Roberts, fear it may represent the "final solution to the women problem" (Roberts 1972; Beam 1973).

---

hospital administration refused to allow lobotomies on men because of unfavorable publicity given to lobotomy in Canada. However, the hospital did allow 17 lobotomies to be performed on women that year (Roberts 1972, pp. 14-15).

While overt forms of social control are limited, psychiatric theories have had tremendous influence in legitimating sexist ideology in other branches of the medical system. Psychological thinking, aided by the widespread use of psychoactive drugs, "helps" women bring their behavior in line with societal expectations of proper feminine behavior. Although the use of psychotropic drugs generally is associated with psychiatric practice, it is not psychiatrists, but general practitioners and internists, who prescribe the bulk of these drugs (Linn 1971, p. 133). Thus, women need not even consult mental health practitioners to be vulnerable to some form of psychiatric labeling and psychotropic therapy.

Feminists revolt against treating women with tranquilizers, because drugs "hook women" but cannot solve problems caused by women's position in society. Drugged into lethargy, women are robbed of the motivation to reexamine their lives and make needed changes. In short, psychotropic drugs remove symptoms without touching causes (Fried 1974, p. 109; "How to Get Hooked" 1972). As women depend on drugs and doubt their ability to perceive adequately, they become even more dependent on male authorities—a situation feminists decry.*

"Good Patients" and "Crazy Ladies"

Even women who never contact mental health professionals or seek help for "nervous disorders" can get caught in the web of psychological thinking unless they adhere to the "proper patient" role. Feminist medical student K. Emmott argues that "a woman who goes to a doctor must turn over her body to him and at the end of the treatment she gets it back; she is entitled to no explanations, she must not ask questions nor make suggestions" (A Woman's Place 1972, p. 46). Women who deviate from this role are regarded as neurotic.

The label "neurotic female" is difficult to avoid, for physicians expect women to be neurotic complainers. Cooperstock (1971), who studied the attitudes of internists and general practitioners, found that when asked to describe the typical complaining patient, sex unspecified, 72 percent of the physicians spontaneously described a woman, 24 percent conveyed the picture of a person sex unspecified,

---

*Seidenberg (1971, p. 28) reports that the prescription of "mind drugs" by specialists increases apprehension about one's reality-testing capacities.

and only 4 percent's description referred to a man. Freidson (1973a, p. 484) found a similar attitude among the physicians he studied in a large group practice. In sum, the doctors painted a caricature of the demanding patient as

> a female schoolteacher, well educated enough to be ca-
> pable of articulate and critical questioning and letter
> writing, of high enough social status to be sensitive to
> slight and to expect satisfaction, and experienced with
> bureaucratic procedures. In the physicians' eyes, they
> were also neurotically motivated to be "demanding."

This tendency of the medical profession to classify any questioning or complaining as evidence of mental disorder is the ultimate double bind women struggle against in the health system. Authors of the Vancouver Women's Health Booklet state that

> this "crazy lady syndrome" is perhaps our most serious
> charge against doctors. A woman runs the risk of neglect
> and poor treatment if she does not demand what she feels
> is best for her. And she is ignored as a "neurotic fe-
> male" when she does (A Woman's Place 1972, p. 47).

Psychogenic Disorders and Sexual Prejudice

Because physicians expect emotional causes, they sometimes fail to diagnose organic conditions, inaccurately misclassify whole syndromes and disorders, and improperly prescribe mood-altering drugs. Health activists frequently complain about physicians' failure to diagnose organic disorders. Typically, despite repeated complaints about physical symptoms, women are told that their problems are emotional. Some are denied treatment entirely; others are given tranquilizers, which reduce their impetus for seeking needed treatment.

In many cases, the problems are life threatening. Linda Fidell, a psychologist who researches drug usage, who receives numerous complaints from women who have experienced inappropriate treatment with psychotropic drugs, reports cases where women suffering from brain tumors and cancer were treated only with tranquilizers for "emotional problems" until it was too late to treat their organic diseases (Fried 1974, p. 109). Others complain that iatrogenic diseases are often dismissed as "nervous disorders." One woman, for example, reported being given so many antibiotics for an ear infection that she developed a serious bowel condition. Although they tested for cancer of the bowel, the doctors claimed her condition was due to "nerves." Ultimately, the problem was discovered to be a reaction to the antibiotics (A Woman's Place 1972, p. 43).

Not all physicians, of course, are so blinded by sexual stereotypes that they fail to diagnose properly. Nonetheless, in health education groups and self-help classes, women regularly recount such "horror stories." Problems reported most frequently involve symptoms arising during pregnancy or childbirth or related to contraceptive drugs and devices. (See Seaman 1969 and Seaman and Seaman 1977 for numerous examples of women whose contraceptive-induced problems went untreated.)

Postpartum symptoms are particularly likely to be disregarded as only evidence of the "baby blues." The Boston women note that following childbirth, women's legitimate complaints are often brushed aside as emotionalism—especially if a women is in any way upset. They note, for example, that one doctor refused to see a woman who complained that fecal matter was coming out of her vagina. He dismissed her complaint as fantasy, unwilling to acknowledge the possibility that his episiotomy was imperfect. Another doctor finally treated her for a ripped vagina (Boston Women's Health Course Collective 1971, p. 114).

Other gynecological problems are also likely to be ignored. The following excerpts from letters written in 1972 by patients involved in a California women's center attempt to have two university health service gynecologists investigated by the county medical society illustrate some of the difficulties women encounter when attempting to convince physicians that they need medical attention. (All names are pseudonyms.)

Case no. 1:

In March I experienced abdominal pain and low grade fever. I was admitted to the Health Service for possible appendicitis. For four days G.I. tests were administered. Dr. Harwood gave me a pelvic and said there was nothing wrong there. He suggested that my problem might be "psychosomatic" and a psychiatrist might help me. I left the Health Center as the problem had not disappeared and they were not treating me for anything. I saw two physicians at my own expense—gynecologists—and was told that I had enetremitis (sic). The IUD that I almost had to beg Dr. Harwood to remove was the originating factor for this infection. Dr. Harwood removed the IUD and then gave me a (cursory) pelvic saying he had just realized the pelvic should have been done first because of the pain from removal of the IUD. The doctors I am seeing now indicate that the inflammation should be treated with antibiotics

and that any competent gynecologist would recognize such
an inflammation. The seriousness of this infection has
reached the point of infecting my uterus, fallopian tubes
and ovaries. The gynecologist I now see says that this is
partly due to the lack of treatment in the early stages.

Case no. 2:

In mid-January I was a week late for my period so I made
an appointment at the Health Center to be tested for possible pregnancy. The day before the appointment I "spot-
ted" and so assumed that I had my period although I had
never been late before. I suspected that perhaps everything was not right. When I saw Dr. Jameson I told him
that I was interested in getting an IUD but that I was concerned about the possibility of pregnancy even though I did
have what seemed to be a period. He immediately brushed
off even the possibility of pregnancy and said that since I
had my period that day would be a good time to put the IUD
in. On the examining table I again brought up the possibility that I might be pregnant and so he mockingly said
that he would check. [Between] mid-January and late February I suffered from excruciating pain that, from my
talks with other girls, seemed completely out of proportion to the normal reaction to the IUD. I went back to Dr.
Jameson once or twice during this period and was condes-
cendingly told that some women are weaker than others
and therefore cannot stand pain and that either I could take
it or I couldn't. Unfortunately at that point I chose to take
it. At some point during late February or early March I
began to bleed very badly, though I cannot remember the
exact time sequence. I telephoned the Health Center and
was told that a very heavy period was normal with the
IUD—either by Dr. Jameson himself or by a nurse—I can't
remember. I trusted that that was true but continued to
bleed very badly—this was over a 10 or 12 day period. By
the end of that time the bleeding was severe. I was passing
cherry sized clots and saturating a pad every hour or so.
In mid-March I telephoned the Health Center frantically
one Saturday morning because I was fearful of hemor-
rhaging. Dr. Jameson mockingly said, "Oh Mrs. Lennard, don't you think you're exaggerating just a little
bit?" When I said no, and again tried to tell him exactly
what was happening he said, "well go to the drug store
and pick up some iron pills and come in Monday morning

so that we can be sure you're not losing too much blood! "
That day I stayed quiet and off of my feet all day and by
evening the bleeding became so bad (it was spurting out)
that my husband rushed me to a hospital and they removed
it. They could not believe that the doctor hadn't removed
it immediately upon being informed of the extent of my
bleeding. My physical condition remained bad and in
April my parents insisted that I come home to be checked
out by their family doctor. On examination, he deduced
that I had been pregnant at the time of the insertion of the
IUD and that my present physical condition was due to fetal
tissue that had remained in the uterus. The pathology report from the subsequent D & C in fact showed the presence
of fetal tissue.

In some instances, the alleged emotional problems are attributed to women's sexual activity—or lack of it. In health groups, wom-
en repeatedly complain that physicians show "excessive interest" in
their sexual activities. Some even report being told by young "hip"
physicians, "All you need is a good fuck." Others are less direct but
communicate the same message, for example:

Dr. M's attitude when he discovered that I was unmarried
and unattached (no boyfriends) was that I was probably a
sex-starved female with deep psychological problems that
were in turn causing my internal distress. But, just in
case, he took tests to make sure there was nothing physically wrong. Imagine his distress when he discovered that
his instant diagnosis (she's just another neurotic female)
was incorrect and that I was suffering from a lovely orien-
tal disease—flukes of the blood (A Woman's Place 1972,
p. 43).

Lesbians are particularly vulnerable to having their problems
sexualized. Members of the Radicalesbians Health Collective report
that when lesbians express emotional or physical pain not even related to sexuality, medical doctors or psychologists have told them,
"It's all because you're a lesbian" (Bart 1973, p. 70).
While physicians' beliefs about the emotional nature of wom-
en's complaints hinder their clinical competence and blind them to
organic disorders, they have also led clinicians and researchers to
misclassify certain diseases and syndromes. Lennane and Lennane
(1973) point out that certain disorders affecting only women or "caused"
by women have been regarded by the medical profession as psychogenic despite compelling evidence of an organic base. For example,

primary dysmenorrhea, nausea in pregnancy, pain in labor, and infantile colic are regarded as psychogenic despite contrary evidence. The Lennanes also argue that with these disorders, cause and effect are curiously reversed, that is, the results of pain (for example, anxiety) are viewed as the cause of pain. The Lennanes (1973, p. 292) conclude that

> although such scientific evidence as exists clearly implicates organic causes, acceptance of a psychogenic origin has led to an irrational and ineffective approach to their management. Because these conditions affect only women, the cloudy thinking that characterizes the relevant literature may be due to a form of sexual prejudice.

Mistaking cause and effect in these syndromes leads to many problems for the woman sufferer. First, the patient receives little or no symptomatic relief, which she would if the disorder was defined as organic. Tranquilizers do little to ease discomfort and tend to be addictive. Furthermore, patients are disinclined to report symptoms fully if they expect to have their problem regarded as psychogenic (Lennane and Lennane 1973, p. 292). The difficulty is compounded by the fact that the concept of psychogenesis and the nature of psychosomatic disorders is misunderstood by many patients and practitioners alike. While specialists in psychosomatic disorders understand the complex interplay between emotional and organic factors, psychosomatic is often taken to mean "imaginary."* A woman medical student reports that even medical professors misuse psychosomatic concepts.

> Once in a lecture, the lecturer said most women's menstrual cramps are psychogenic in origin. He went on in his erudite fashion, "The cramps are psychogenic or they may in fact even have pain"—proving that he doesn't understand the use of the word psychogenic (Campbell 1973, p. 73).

Because of the stigma of alleged psychogenic disorders, some women refuse to report important symptoms, which could lead to a

---

*For discussions of psychosomatic concepts, see, for example, Cushner 1965; Grinker 1974; and Jourard 1971, especially chap. 9, "Sickness as Protest."

more accurate diagnosis. Women who do report psychosomatic symptoms, however, may regret their full disclosure. As Ehrenreich and English (1973, p. 79) rhetorically ask: "How many times do we go to the doctor feeling sick and leave, after a diagnosis of 'psychosomatic,' feeling crazy?"

As long as physicians cling to the notion that certain disorders and syndromes are psychogenic in origin, research into the organic causes and effective forms of symptomatic relief is impeded or ignored (Lennane and Lennane 1973, p. 292). At best—or worst—women are given analgesics or psychoactive drugs to blunt their discomfort—a practice under fire from both feminists and certain health professionals in recent years (see, for example, Borgman 1973; Copperstock 1971; Fried 1974; Lennard et al. 1971; Linn and Davis 1971; Rogers 1971; and Seidenberg 1971).

Overall, women receive a disproportionate share of physician-prescribed psychoactive drugs (Balter and Levine 1969; Mellinger, Balter, and Manheimer 1971; Brahen 1973). There is considerable evidence that women are more likely to receive psychotropics than men even when they have the same disorder (Copperstock 1971, p. 243).

Sex-role stereotyping may be a significant factor in this prescribing pattern. In Linn's (1971) study of physicians' attitudes about the legitimacy of prescribing certain psychoactive drugs in specific situations, 87 percent of the physicians thought that it was perfectly all right for housewives to use Librium every day.* Commenting on Linn's findings, Cooperstock suggests that a reason for the disproportionate prescription of drugs to women is that many doctors see women as nonworkers. Since they stay home, it doesn't matter if they are sedated (Fried 1974, p. 92).

In her own study of prescribing patterns, Cooperstock (1971) asked physicians why they thought that they wrote more prescriptions for psychotropic drugs for women than for men. Their explanations ranged from women's biological vulnerability to differential life stress, self-indulgence, and male reluctance to seek help. The following physician quotes are illustrative:

> It's constitutional. The female's nervous system is more sensitive. They're affected by problems and emotional upsets more. That's the way the Lord made them.

---

*Physicians' attitudes toward drug usage in various situations were more strongly related to their own personal social values and moral standards than to their scientific backgrounds.

Females have more time to indulge in neurosis than men. They're bored often and frustrated. As they get older, there's the menopause, which we men do not indulge in (Cooperstock 1971, p. 243).

Recent studies show that once psychotropic drugs are introduced, it is difficult to withdraw patients from them (Arneson and Prickett 1968). And when psychotropic drugs are obtained from physicians, it leads to longer-term, more consistent usage than when the drugs are obtained from less legitimate sources (Mellinger, Balter, and Manheimer 1971). Thus, the contemporary physician, much like his turn-of-the-century opiate-prescribing colleague, may initiate a pattern of drug-taking that leads to serious dependence or addiction.

SOURCES OF SEXISM IN AMERICAN MEDICINE

Why do physicians hold such negative views of women? Certainly the stereotype of the neurotic female abounds in the society at large. But beyond this, many feminists believe that sexism is reinforced and amplified in medical education, medical literature, and in drug advertising. Medical educators and drug companies, they argue, pander to male prejudice, with no regard for the consequences.

Medical Education

Medical students quickly learn to denigrate women both formally and informally. In doing so, they follow in the footsteps of their mostly male mentors. Fidell argues that

If during medical training, many physicians get into the habit of referring to women under fifty as "douche bags," and patients over fifty as "the crock" (as it is done in one leading medical school), it is hard to see how the problems of women could be taken seriously (Fried 1974, p. 92).

Mary Howell, former associate dean of Harvard Medical School, has documented the ways that traditional medical education systematically conditions physicians—both male and female—to feel contempt for women (1973, 1974, 1975b). Howell's 1973 survey of discrimination against women in American medical schools, originally published under the pseudonym Margaret Campbell, M.D., is based on questionnaire responses from 146 women medical students in 41 U.S. medical schools and her own extensive experience and observations as a practicing physician and prominent medical educator.

Discussing the attitude of medical educators toward women patients, Howell argues that women are doubly demeaned. For patients "in general" are implicitly regarded as somewhat demanding, irrational, and less valuable as persons than physicians. When the patient is a woman, she has the added stigma of the stereotype: overly emotional, scheming, and "not worth the time" required for good patient care (Campbell 1973, pp. 72-73). Furthermore, medical education inculcates the view that women's ills are less important than those of men by virtue of their alleged psychological origins. For in the "scientific" atmosphere of contemporary medical education, psychological illnesses are slighted in the medical curriculum, to the extent that disorders assumed to be of psychological origin are of little or no concern to the physician (Campbell 1973, p. 73).

Because feminists complain so bitterly that their problems are dismissed as psychosomatic, it is important to consider how this attitude is inculcated in future physicians. The women medical students who participated in Howell's study report many incidents in which faculty members tell jokes about women based on the assumption that they are neurotic or dominated by their reproductive functions. Women are also portrayed as hysterical, as nagging mothers, and as having trivial complaints. Overall, women's illnesses are assumed to be psychosomatic until proven otherwise, whereas the psychological component of men's illnesses are largely ignored (Campbell 1973, pp. 73-74). A subtle and insidious form of prejudice is revealed in the use of pronouns. Howell observes that patients in most medical schools are referred to exclusively by the male pronoun "he," with one notable exception. In discussing hypothetical patients whose diseases are of psychogenic origin, lecturers often automatically switch to "she" (Fried 1974, p. 92).

Howell argues that there is an interrelation between discrimination against women as patients and as medical students. The culture of the medical school supports discrimination against women students in the overt forms of baiting, belittling, hostility, and backlashing (Campbell 1973, p. 22). Women students are baited in various ways. They are told that because of them, "a man probably went into chiropractic school," or that "most women don't practice." Ward residents have been known to call their male students "Dr." and their female students "Ms." Cheesecake pictures appear in lectures. Common comments have included: "Go home and bake cookies where you belong," or "A mother has no business in medical school." Single women are sometimes accused of husband hunting (Campbell 1973, pp. 23-24).

The largest number of overtly discriminatory remarks Howell's subjects reported were belittling. Medical school officials openly state that they do not think that women belong in medicine, and chiefs of staff feel free to declare that "a woman doesn't belong in the operating room except as a nurse." Female students making mistakes may be subjected to attending physicians' comments, such as, "Just goes to show, one should never take anything a woman says seriously." Many of the belittling incidents involve demeaning women as sexual objects. One woman's experience with a professor who had included a "nudie" slide in his lecture confirms what many feminists fear is an underlying male motivation in gynecology. The professor made an emotional comment that ended, "Men need to look down on women, and that's why I show the slide" (Campbell 1973, pp. 24-26).

Howell suggests that many of the hostile comments to women students reflect free-floating anger against women-as-colleagues. Because these hostile exchanges usually appear in a group setting, they are contagious and difficult to counteract (Campbell 1973, pp. 26-27). When female medical students complain or object to sexual prejudice, they, like female patients, are regarded as overly emotional or neurotic. The attitude of male students, professors, and administrators is that the women are overly sensitive and immature. One student noted that her dissatisfaction with a human sexuality course as offensive to women was discounted as evidence of her inability to deal with sex and her own sexuality (Campbell 1973, p. 27).

While feminism has encouraged the growth of female support systems within medical schools, it also may have encouraged a backlash of overt discrimination.[*] Howell suggests that male medical students and professors may react with additional hostility, because feminism has affected both their marriages and their profession. Medical men's negative attitudes toward feminism are clear in their advice to women not to "band together" and in their resentful comments that women who meet together are "conspiring" (Campbell 1973, pp. 28-29).

Women medical students are also denied from colleagueship by being treated as dependent daughters, pampered sisters, nurturant mothers, helpmates, or seductive playmates. More frequently, women students are simply forgotten or ignored, or equally disturbing, women are spotlighted—with interest or amusement, as well as with

---

[*]Shryock (1966, p. 198) argues that opposition to women in nineteenth- and early twentieth-century medicine was exacerbated by the association of feminism with women entering the field.

hostility. One notable form of stereotyping is the expectation that women are all alike—like other women—or that they are deviant and unfeminine by virtue of their professional interests. Another form is based on assumptions about appropriate, or "proper," roles in relation to men. In short, women are expected to "keep their place" or will be looked upon (progressively) as "abrasive," "bitchy," and then "castrating." Finally, traditional medical education caters to men's prurient interest in female sexuality, with the message that any man has the right to regard any woman—whether colleague or patient—as an object of sexual interest (Campbell 1973, pp. 30-43).

In the face of such discrimination and sexual stereotyping, women medical students cope in several ways. Some turn anger into a constructive support system for themselves and other women. Others recognize the problem but hold their tongues. Often, women use some form of protective denial, which serves to maintain the status quo. While some of these women simply do not "see" what is going on, others recognize discrimination and sexism but excuse it.

To the dismay of feminists, some professional women "identify with their oppressors," concurring that negative attitudes toward women are appropriate. Such professional women exempt themselves as exceptional, so that they can remain in agreement with the societally approved contentions about women as a group while tenuously avoiding "negative" views of themselves (Campbell 1973, p. 49). Such women are regarded by feminists as no different from male physicians and are sometimes called "honorary males." Feminists find these male-identified female physicians particularly difficult, for feminists are unsure whether or not to regard them as "sisters."

Medical Literature

Negative views of women appear frequently in the medical literature. As in medical education, the stereotypical imagery focuses on women's tendency toward psychosomatic illness and disturbances related to female sexuality. In line with the Lennanes's (1973) findings, standard gynecology textbooks and reference works continue to portray dysmenorrhea, nausea of pregnancy, pain in labor, and infantile colic as caused or aggravated by psychogenic factors.

Recent medical texts' portrayal of dysmenorrhea is illustrative both of physicians' attitudes toward women's reproductive disorders and textbook writers' unrealistic expectations of how clinicians practice in reality. Rather than focusing on the organic bases of dysmenorrhea, textbook authors suggest that primary management of dysmenorrhea should be "directed at the underlying psychodynamics." Since gynecologists typically spend little time with individual patients, it is difficult to imagine how physicians "manage" the "underlying psychodynamics" with anything beyond psychoactive drugs. Essentially, physicians are told to advise women to "accept their feminine role" (Shapiro 1975, pp. 10-12).* Green's (1971, p. 128) remarks are typical: "It is the attainment of both the physical and emotional maturity of a normal adult female [that enables the woman] to establish a normal relationship with a member of the opposite sex while simultaneously bidding farewell to her dysmenorrhea."

Gynecological texts, however, reveal deep ambivalence toward female sexuality. The Vancouver Women's Health Collective notes that a popular 1952 gynecology textbook suggested that women seek gynecological examinations out of curiosity or because they are nymphomaniacs (A Woman's Place 1972, p. 64). Others minimize or ignore female sexuality. Cooke (1943, p. 60), for example, assumed that women were "almost universally generally frigid."

While these older textbook writers had little but clinical experience or stereotypes on which to base their assertions, sociologists Scully and Bart (1973, p. 1047) point out that once Kinsey et al.'s Sexual Behavior in the Human Female was published in 1953, authoritative information on female sexuality was available to the medical community. Nonetheless, the Kinsey data was used selectively. In their review of 27 gynecology texts published between 1943 and 1972, Scully and Bart (1973) report that traditional views of female sexuality continued to be presented with little regard to the well-known findings of Kinsey and (later) of Masters and Johnson. During this period, at least one-half of the tests that indexed the topics stated that the male sex drive was stronger than the female's and that women were more interested in sex for procreation than for recreation. They also said most women were "frigid" and that the vaginal orgasm was the "mature" response.

Additionally, physicians are encouraged to teach their patients to adhere to traditional female sex roles to please their husbands. Scully and Bart (1973, p. 1048) note that Jeffcoate (1967, p. 726), for example, assumes that an important feature of male sex desire is the urge to dominate and subjugate women to their will; for women, acquiescence to the masterful male takes a high place. And Novak,

---

*At "The Social Responsibility of Gynecology and Obstetrics," a conference held at Johns Hopkins University in 1965, Dr. Irvin M. Cushner (1965, p. 184) made a plea for providing not only sex education but "proper sex orientation" of young women to the feminine role to avert possible psychosomatic gynecological problems.

Jones, and Jones (1970, pp. 662-63) argue that frequency of inter-course depends entirely upon the male sex drive. A woman should be advised to allow her husband's sex drive to set the pace, attempting to gear hers satisfactorily to his. If after several months or years, a woman finds that this is not possible, she should consult her physician. Scully and Bart (1973, p. 1045) conclude that gynecology texts reveal a persistent bias toward greater concern with the patient's husband than with the patient herself. Women are consistently described (from a male perspective) as anatomically destined to reproduce, nurture, and keep their husbands happy—a view that clearly maintains traditional sex-role stereotypes in the interest of men.

Prescription Drug Advertising

Another major source of traditional attitudes toward women in contemporary America is prescription drug advertising. And drug advertising is big business. The drug industry spends over three quarters of a billion dollars annually advertising directly to about 250,000 physicians. The 60 drug companies spend this enormous sum every year on direct mail, medical journal advertising, paramedical publications, closed circuit television, canned radio, exhibits at conventions, samples, premiums, and visits by detail men (drug salesmen). These methods work—physicians buy their products (Garai 1964, p. 191).

Physicians rely heavily on drug advertising for information. Seventy-three percent of the physicians Linn and Davis (1972) surveyed reported that drug ads were somewhat or very useful sources of drug information. The only source cited more frequently (84 percent) was the detail man, who personally purveys the same messages. Busy physicians, with little training or interest in pharmacology, are particularly dependent on pharmaceutical company claims, for, as Silverman and Lee (1974, p. 301) point out, drugs that most physicians were taught to prescribe early in their careers soon become obsolete and are replaced by new products. With only limited time to examine, evaluate, and keep up-to-date, physicians place increasing reliance for continuing postgraduate education on promotional materials distributed by drug manufacturers.

Drug industry critics also argue that it is in the interest of pharmaceutical manufacturers to promote use of their products for an ever-widening number of patients. One way is to extend the indications for drug therapy to encompass a variety of symptoms or syndromes the average physician or psychiatrist might not have thought of yet. Essentially, this means defining various problems of living as evidence of underlying emotional disorders, which could be alleviated with psychoactive drugs (Seidenberg 1971, p. 23). Physicians have bought this perspective—as seen in prescribing patterns during the past decade. Between 1964 and 1970, the use of minor tranquilizers alone increased by nearly 78 percent (Balter and Levine 1971).*

Persons for whom such drugs are suggested risk being labeled as sick or disturbed. The pharmaceutical industry encourages society's prejudices about women as the weaker and sicker sex in prescription drug advertising, generally portraying women negatively. The drug industry openly acknowledges the enslavement of women. Physicians are simply told to help them adjust to their lot. For example, one ad shows a woman behind bars made up of brooms and mops, captioned: "You can't set her free but you can make her feel less anxious." Another pictures a woman who is claimed to hold an M.A. degree but who must be content with the PTA and housework, which contributes to her gynecological complaints. It is suggested, of course, that both women be given tranquilizers (Seidenberg 1971, p. 26; see also A Woman's Place 1972, pp. 65-69, and Muller 1972).

Conceivably, not wanting to wash dishes, sweep, mop, or do laundry might be a sign of mental illness. Yet in many instances, reluctance to wash dishes, for example, is the anger of a wife who resents her role—surely not a form of mental illness (Seidenberg 1971, p. 30).

Just what is and is not mental illness is open to question (see, for example, Halleck 1971; Scheff 1966, 1967; and Szasz 1961, 1963, 1970). Out of their mutual self-interest, psychiatry and the drug industry have created a peculiar problem with the mood-altering drugs. Psychiatry—to strengthen its legitimacy as a medical specialty—has embraced the notion that mental problems are diseases like other diseases for which specific drugs can be prescribed. The drug industry encourages this view, advertising that all kinds of problems of living, from washing dishes to raising children, can be solved with its products (Seidenberg 1971, p. 30).

In 1972, Jane Prather and Linda Fidell, a sociologist-psychologist team, began systematically investigating the portrayal of women in prescription drug advertising, using a sample of 423 sex-identifiable ads drawn from the New England Journal of Medicine, California Medicine, JAMA, and the American Journal of Psychiatry between 1968 and 1972 (Prather and Fidell 1975, p. 23). In these advertisements,

---

*For discussion of the hazards of addiction and iatrogenic disease, see, for example, Illich 1976; Lennard et al. 1971; Mintz 1967; Seidenberg 1971; and Silverman and Lee 1974, pp. 292-95.

48 percent portrayed the patient as female; 52 percent showed the patient as male. Forty percent of the ads portrayed drugs for alleviating symptoms that were primarily psychogenic; 60 percent were aimed at relieving nonpsychogenic symptoms.

When analyzed on the basis of sex and type of disorder, women were underrepresented in the ads as suffering from organic causes and overrepresented as suffering from psychogenic disorders. Interestingly, the main source of the discrepancy was in the nonpsychoactive drug category, where there were far too few women patients portrayed. Prather and Fidell (1973, p. 6; 1975, p. 24) argue that this is strong evidence to support the claim that drug advertisers inadequately represent women as sufferers of "real" or legitimate diseases, reinforcing the physician's perspective that women's complaints are largely psychosomatic.

Sex-role stereotypes were strongly noticeable in other ways. Both men and women were portrayed in sex-stereotypical occupations. For example, although women comprise over 7 percent of all physicians in the United States, no advertisement showed a woman as a physician; nurses were always women—usually, young attractive women (Prather and Fidell 1975, p. 25).*

Men and women were portrayed as needing psychoactive drugs for different reasons. Men were shown to need them because of tensions accompanying physical disability or work, whereas women required them because of diffuse anxiety, tension, or depression (Prather and Fidell 1975, p. 24; 1973, p. 7). And such needs were presented quite differently by sex. Men's problems were presented in a very straightforward manner, sometimes portraying situations related to prestigious occupations, for example:

> A young man looking exhausted on a commuter train and the caption, "Symbols in a life of psychic tension, B.A. cum laude, V.P. at 32, ECG and complete examination normal but palpitations persist."
> A lineman in a basket near a high tension line clutching his chest, "POWER FAILURE! A lineman with angina. He has to be right there for the emergency, whenever it occurs, whatever the weather. The nature of his job and a combination of stress, extreme activity and relative inactivity makes the lineman with angina pectoris

---

*Seidenberg (1971) reports the same omission of female physicians in earlier drug advertisements.

> particularly vulnerable to an attack" (Prather and Fidell 1973, p. 11).

In contrast, women's symptoms were presented lightly, with a clever play on words or in a manner that made the woman appear silly or trivial, for example:

> A librarian reshelving books saying, "last week I felt woozy in fiction."
> A fat woman sitting on a park bench littering the area while she eats and drinks with the caption, "Is this the kind of patient you can do most for? You can't depend on her to keep America beautiful" (Prather and Fidell 1973, p. 11).

And women, rather than men, were shown in ads as suffering from socially stigmatized or embarrassing disorders, such as belching, flatulence, and diarrhea, for example: "A wedding scene with the bride at the altar in obvious anguish and the caption, "When diarrhea wrings the wedding belle" (Prather and Fidell 1973, pp. 11-12).

Many advertisements portray the role of housekeeper/housewife as frustrating. The following example also illustrates the misconception of psychosomatic disorders perpetrated by drug advertising:

> A women appearing depressed and disheveled with the caption, "The Collector: at 35 she's collected, among other things, a college degree she's never used, two children underfoot most of the day, a husband whose career takes him away most of the time, a folder of unpaid bills, and various physical symptoms—real or imagined" (Prather and Fidell 1973, p. 9).

A particularly pernicious pattern of advertising is the tendency to portray women's problems as irritating to others—husbands, families, or even physicians. (Men's problems are never portrayed as directly irritating to others.) The negative image of women in the following ads is striking:

> A picture of a grotesque looking man with the caption, "This 42 year old man actually looks like a Greek God and is good to his family and to his wife ... but this is how SHE sees him: female climacteric conjures phantoms of monsters."

A picture of a family gathering with the caption, "Treat one ... six people benefit" (Prather and Fidell 1975, p. 25).

Seidenberg (1971, p. 27) particularly decries the drug companies' explicit advice in these ads that women be tranquilized for the comfort of others, because some behavioral changes that temporarily or even permanently antagonize spouses may reflect improving mental health rather than pathology to be drugged into oblivion.

Finally, drug advertising amplifies and reinforces the messages that women's complaints are trivial and that the doctor's time is too valuable to be spent on "dubious" disorders. Fidell reports on one ad that shows a wooden chair with female hands and a female head. The ad reads, "Is she becoming a fixture in your office?" The message of the tranquilizer ad seems to be that it is legitimate to drug people who bother physicians (Fried 1974, p. 92).

MALE MOTIVATION IN OBSTETRICS AND GYNECOLOGY

A theme running through feminist analyses of sexism in medicine is that medical misogyny stems in part from men's awe, fear, and envy of female procreative powers and male anxiety over sexual identity. Some have argued that men are motivated to specialize in obstetrics and gynecology out of a dual desire to create life and to prove their masculinity among men. To fulfill these desires, medical men have devised childbirth practices, promulgated mutilating surgery, and psychologically assaulted half the population (see, for example, Barker-Benfield 1972, 1976; Barry 1972; Ehrenreich and English 1972, 1973; Groesser 1972; Rich 1975; Seaman 1972; Shinder 1972; and Stannard 1970).

Feminists argue that men's desire to procreate is evident in mythology and in the Bible.* In primitive societies, the custom of couvade allows men to play out their desire to have babies. When a

---

*For example, Hephaestus created Pandora out of earth and acted as midwife for Zeus, splitting open his head with an axe to deliver Athena. When Semele prematurely begat Dionysus, Zeus sewed the child to his thigh and carried him to term. In addition to being the sole progenitor of Adam, God delivered a female from Adam's rib cage (Stannard 1970, p. 24).

woman goes into labor, the father typically takes to bed, groans, and cries out, imitating his parturient wife. Sometimes, after delivery, the infant is placed in the man's arms, and he, not the mother, receives congratulations. The Arapesh of New Guinea use the phrase "to bear a child" for either a man or woman.* If one comments on the looks of a middle-aged man, Arapesh often remark, "You should have seen him before he bore all those children" (Stannard 1970, pp. 24-25; for other accounts of couvade, see Malinowski 1955, pp. 186-90; Matthews 1902; and Service 1963, p. 197).

Male initiation ceremonies (involving circumcision or subincision) in some primitive societies reveal men's desire to be like women. Subincision—splitting the penis the length of the urethra—makes the penis resemble a vulva. The wound is sometimes called a vagina or penis womb. After subincision (common among central tribes in Australia), boys lose control over urine flow and must squat, like women, to urinate. Arunta boys regularly reopen subincision wounds to cause bleeding—an imitation of menstruation (Stannard 1970, p. 25).

"Man-making" ceremonies themselves symbolize creation. Initiation houses are often called wombs or birth enclosures, and adult men treat initiates as newly born. Stannard (1970, p. 25) suggests that it is as if the men say that though women give birth to boys, only men can give birth to men.†

Men's imitation or appropriation of women's reproductive functions in primitive societies give credence to theories of womb envy. Fear and envy is particularly understandable, since the male's role in procreation is unknown in many primitive societies and has been fully understood in the Western world for less than a century (Stannard 1970, pp. 25-28).

When Leeuwenhoek viewed semen under his microscope in 1677, he declared that the wriggling "animalcules" were the male's

---

*The father is seen to be as necessary as the mother in creating babies; during early pregnancy, the male deposits large quantities of semen into the woman because the baby is believed to consist of male sperm and female blood. After birth, the father lies down next to the mother and child, so that the baby can receive its life-soul from either parent. During the lying-in period, the father is said to be "in bed having a baby" (Stannard 1970, pp. 24-25).

†For further discussion of male initiation ceremonies, see Bettelheim 1954; Eliade 1965; Whiting, Kluckhohn, and Anthony 1958; and Young 1965, 1962.

babies—complete little men or women to be delivered into the female
for nurturance. Thus legitimated by "science," men were viewed as
essential givers of life—women only supplied the raw material for life
nourishment. Until the mid-nineteenth century, few scientists even
entertained the idea that the sexes might contribute equally in gen-
erating a child. Even the few "ovists"—those who believed the embryo
was preformed in the ovum, not the sperm—regarded the embryo as
inert until semen transformed it into a living person. It was only in
1861 that scientists realized that the ovum was the female sex cell—not
simply nourishment for the embryo. Mendel's actual observation of
the union of female and male gametes in 1875 finally destroyed the
male illusion that he was lord of creation (Stannard 1970, p. 28).

As male illusions of procreative power were destroyed by scientific inquiry during the latter part of the nineteenth century, men's
dominant role in childbearing was re-established through obstetrics
and gynecology. While women might create life, obstetricians—armed
with anesthesia, forceps, and medical authority—could dominate and
get credit for birth, returning it to male control. Many contemporary
feminists argue that secretly and unconsciously, obstetricians and
gynecologists wish to usurp these childbearing functions that they,
and presumably all men, envy.

Seaman (1972, pp. 164-65) asserts that gynecologists' remarks
such as, "We're in labor," or, "We're four fingers dilated," reveal
physicians' wishes to be intimately involved in childbearing. John
Miller, an early proponent of prepared childbirth, himself acknowledges that obstetricians have been so clever with their tools and gad-
gets that they have rewritten the obstetrical drama to make them the
stars instead of women, even accepting the congratulations of husbands.
Miller notes the connection between these practices and women's re-
sentment of men (1962, p. 167).

Health advocates resent men's psychic and symbolic as well
as physical intrusion in childbirth, partly because it is felt to be the
proper domain of women—an inexorable part of female culture. In
addition, women fear the technical hazards associated with medicalized
birth practices, hazards some believe have evolved to boost male egos
rather than to "help" women. Barry (1972, pp. 4-5), for example,
argues that with the advent of male obstetricians, obstetrical chairs
disappeared because men were unwilling to stoop in front of a woman.
Putting women flat on their backs and strapped to a table with their
legs spread wide apart in stirrups may enhance male egos but hinders
quick and safe labor and delivery.

"Natural" or prepared childbirth professionals have done little
to return childbirth to women. Frederick Leboyer, who advocates
that obstetricians deliver babies in dimly lit hospital rooms where
they can be immersed immediately in water, argues that the psychic

revival of the birth struggle impels obstetricians to hasten the birth process. Feminists suggest that Leboyer exhibits the male need (seen in couvade) to take over the "mana" of birth and fails to recognize that the infant's passage through the birth canal can be increased and lengthened by common obstetrical practices (Rich 1975, p. 28).

Some feminists argue that male gynecologists' objections to abortion also reflect a sexual-fear-jealousy motive. Just prior to the Supreme Court abortion ruling, for example, George S. Walter, a maternal and child health consultant for the federal government, stated that

> the male physician won't let the woman decide [to have an abortion]—the pregnant woman symbolizes proof of male potency, and if the male loosens his rule over women and grants them the right to dispose of the proof when they want to, the men then feel terribly threatened lest women can, at will, rob them of their potency and masculinity" (Barry 1972, p. 10).

Shinder (1972, pp. 5-8) argues that men suffer breast envy as well. Annoyed that women's breasts develop fully and can nourish infants, men are also threatened by the power of female breasts to arouse them sexually. It was this envy and fear, Shinder argues, that led surgeons to promote cruel, mutilating "treatment" for breast cancer. Barry (1972, pp. 13-14) adds that since doctors continue to perform radical mastectomies despite compelling evidence that it is no more effective than less disfiguring procedures, it can only be concluded that "the radical is preferred and practiced for the purposeful and sadistic maiming of women."

Others emphasize men's use of medicine to secure their sexual identity and social status. Barker-Benfield (1972, 1976), for example, suggests that late nineteenth-century gynecological practices grew directly out of men's insecurity over their sexual identity.* Pressured to concentrate all energies on achievement and exhorted not to dissipate energy through unnecessary copulation or masturbation, women's sexual appetite was understandably dreaded. Women's latent boundless sexuality clearly posed a threat to male energies, and nineteenth-century gynecological surgery was an effort to control female sexuality.

---

*Although these anxieties were not unique among American men, the democratic achievement-oriented status striving in America is said to have exacerbated male anxieties.

As for doctors themselves, the operations, the lengthening records of ovaries removed, attempts to innovate and prove priority in new techniques and surgical feats (termed <u>conceptions</u>, <u>bantlings</u>, and <u>babies</u>) were all means of attaining status and manhood in the eyes of other men. A successful gynecologist might be able to hand "his" ovaries around on a plate—an affirmation of his professional identity and his manhood. The woman's body simply furnished the material for his identity (Barker-Benfield 1972, p. 65).

The underlying motivation of gynecological surgeons was not completely obscure even in the nineteenth century. In 1896, physician Robert Edes openly suggested that gynecological surgery was performed to relieve the surgeon of the anxieties women caused him rather than to relieve women's sickness. This same emotional undercurrent may underlie a contemporary physician's declaration at a medical convention that: "no ovary is good enough to leave in and no testicle is bad enough to take out" (Barry 1972, p. 13).

Psychological theories of male motivation in obstetrics and gynecology based on womb envy are held not only by feminists. Several prominent analysts, including Freud himself, raised the issue of womb envy, only to be ignored. For example, Freud's description of male pregnancy phantasies and the wish for a baby in two major papers and Bettleheim's (1954) account of rituals symbolizing male womb envy in preliterate societies have received little attention. Lederer (1968, p. 153) argues that such pertinent studies have been conspicuously neglected because the men writing psychoanalytic papers have, out of their own fear and envy of women, maintained a fraternal silence.

Friedman (1971) argues that men's envy of women's ability to create life is particularly revealed in the daily language of creativity. The terms <u>pregnant with</u>, <u>gives birth to</u> an idea, an <u>abortive thought</u>, <u>brainchild</u>, <u>this is my baby, my creation</u>, are analogous to reproductive terminology. Lomas (1964) has even suggested that the dehumanizing medical treatment of childbearing women in American society is related to male envy of female creative achievement in childbirth. And Lederer (1968, p. 153) wonders how much of the sadistic crime against women is the result of male envy, noting that in the Orthogenic School in Chicago, boys admit to envying girls their breasts, their genitalia, and their ability to bear children. Their dreams of violence include cutting off breasts and tearing out vaginas.

Gynecologists' emotional stability and maturity has also been seriously questioned. The Boston Women's Health Book authors (1973, pp. 252-53) argue that the psychological profile of most men in practice reveals a repressed, compulsive, money-oriented individual. Medical students, carefully selected by men anxious to reproduce themselves, become somewhat cynical and more emotionally detached and mechanistic during training. As a group, they are less mature emotionally and sexually than their peers, who have taken the time to live and love, which brings one to maturity.

Seaman (1972, pp. 163-64) also makes this argument, citing psychiatrist George Vaillant's study comparing physicians' social psychological adjustment with that of a control group of educated non-physician men over a 30-year period. Of the 268 subjects, 46 graduated from medical school. Overall, the physicians had more problems than the others. For example, 47 percent of the physicians, compared with 32 percent of the other men, had unsatisfactory marriages, and 17 percent of the doctors, compared with 5 percent of the controls, were hospitalized for psychiatric illness. The differences were even more striking when the physicians in primary patient care specialties—gynecology, psychiatry, internal medicine, and pediatrics—were separated out from other physicians. The primary care specialists were least like the controls, had the largest share of emotional difficulties as adults, and had experienced the most unstable childhoods. Vaillant concludes that some physicians may choose direct care specialties to give others the care that they did not receive themselves during childhood (Seaman 1972, p. 163).

Seaman (1972, p. 164) suggests that gynecologists may be unhappy men who want to mother women to prove themselves better "mothers" than their own mothers. While such a career may be an admirable altruistic resolution of a psychic conflict, the problem for women remains; women are the real mothers and entitled to some measure of self-determination.

THE DYNAMICS OF SEXISM AND CAPITALISM

Gaining self-determination in the health care system is viewed as problematic, because American medicine is not only patriarchal but capitalistic as well. Furthermore, feminists argue, patriarchy and capitalism complement each other. The dynamics of sexism and capitalism in American medicine—their interdependence and mutual support—are well illustrated by a sign hanging in a gynecologist's office in Silver Spring, Maryland. The sign reads, quite simply: "You rape 'em—We scrape 'em" (Seaman 1972, p. 155).

While this sign must have been intended to be "funny," feminists find no humor in it, for the message clearly reveals a willingness to accept rape as a "normal," functionally interdependent aspect of medical practice, an attitude feminists fear is common. The sign also supports women's complaint that men do not treat women seriously, with respect, or with compassion, especially when "problems" stem from male oppression.*

Overall, feminist health activists feel that the American health care industry is an exploitative business, where women are exploited not only as users of services but as 75 percent of all workers in the health industry. Most are clustered in low-paying, low-status positions, reflecting race and class, as well as sex segregation. As in other American industries, upper-middle-class men comprise the majority of high-status medical professionals (for example, physicians and dentists), while lower-middle- and working-class women predominate in all middle-level, clerical, and service positions, a division of labor related both to women's family roles and to their function as a reserve labor force (Navarro 1975, p. 398).[†]

Women physicians suffer from sexism and prejudice within their own profession. Channeled into traditionally female specialties of pediatrics, psychiatry, and internal medicine, women are discouraged from entering the male surgical specialties (Campbell 1973).[‡] Feminists point out, however, that women are usually nurses, not doctors. And nursing, an overwhelmingly female profession, has been molded to serve the needs of the male-dominated medical profession. In daily practice, nurses' occupational roles reflect stereotypical sex-role relationships between men and women (Clelland 1971; Fleeson 1973; Heide 1973; Kushner 1973; Levin and Berne 1972). Even when promoted to positions of great responsibility, women's autonomy and authority are severely circumstribed within male-dominated health institutions.**

---

*For feminist perspectives on the social, political, and medical aspects of rape, see Brownmiller 1975; Burgess and Holmstrom 1974; Griffin 1971; Russell 1975; and Thompson and Medea 1974.

[†]For documentation and discussion of women's position in various health occupations, see, for example, C. Brown 1975, 1976; Ehrenreich 1975; Navarro 1975; Reverby 1972a, 1972b; Wolfson 1970; Woodside 1975; and Women's Work Project of the Union for Radical Political Economics 1976.

[‡]In 1973, women comprised 7.5 percent of all practicing physicians. While only 7.5 percent of the obstetrician/gynecologists were women, 21.9 percent of all pediatricians and 13.7 percent of psychiatrists were female (Pennell and Showell 1975, p. 36).

**Clelland (1971), for example, points out that the vast majority of directors of nursing do not control their departmental budgets,

The white male physicians who dominate health institutions have rarely objected to social conditions detrimental to people's health. Until recently, health industry profiteering, poor housing, inadequate nutrition, lack of sanitation, environmental pollution, dangerous working conditions, maldistribution of services, and lack of preventive care were either tolerated or ignored. Organized medicine has imposed additional impediments to improved health by opposing free innoculations against diphtheria and polio,* free smallpox vaccination, Red Cross blood banks, federal grants for medical school construction and medical student loans, national health insurance, and Medicare (Boston Women's Health Course Collective 1971, pp. 123-217; Carter 1961). More recently, physicians in many areas have opposed the growth of nurse-midwifery, a service desperately needed by rural and inner-city women (Brown 1976, p. 12).

By fiscal year 1974, total American health expenditures reached $104.2 billion, 7.7 percent of the gross national product. The average per capita cost of $485 in 1974 was 10.6 percent higher than in 1973, and greater than in any country in the world. In 1972, the median net earnings of physicians reached $40,730. Obstetrician-gynecologists did better than the average physician; their $47,000 average income even exceeded that of general surgeons ($45,340), traditional "high income" specialists (Fatt 1975, p. 4).

According to a Department of Health, Education and Welfare survey, obstetricians' average net income (before taxes) was $64,563 in 1975; obstetricians practicing in two to five member groups averaged $75,000 per year. The survey also provided support for the theory of physician-induced demand. It confirmed that as the number of physicians per capita increased in a geographical area, physician fees tended to increase (Meyer 1977).

Increasingly, health profits are corporate profits, as medicine is converted from enterpreneurial to corporate capitalism (Boston Women's Health Course Collective 1971, p. 132; see also Navarro

---

although the nursing department typically spends 80 to 85 percent of the total personnel budget in most hospitals. Thus nurses—and nursing administrators—are often denied authority men in similar positions would demand.

*The federal program to innoculate the population against polio in 1955 was openly called "a violation of the principles of free enterprise." As a result of doctors' unwillingness to participate in the program, half the vaccine purchased by the federal government went unused the first year.

1976). Profits in health are large. For example, in its second year of operation, Healthcare Corporation, a Boston-based nursing home and medical supply company, made a net profit of $1 million (Boston Women's Health Course Collective 1971, p. 124). According to Arthur D. Little, Inc., the market for medical technology now exceeds $450 million each year. Major corporations, including Motorola, IBM, Monsanto, Litton, Lockheed, United Aircraft, Zenith, and Philip Morris, have all expanded or diversified into the health field (Boston Women's Health Course Collective 1971, p. 124; Groesser 1972, p. 13).

Obstetrics and gynecology offer a fertile field for technological tinkering for profit. If every birth in the United States were electronically monitored, 6,000 to 8,000 machines would be needed at an initial outlay of over $40 million. (Hewlett-Packard, a major manufacturer of $6,000 fetal heart monitors, is on Forbes Magazine's list of profitable firms.) With the slowdown in the space program, proposed cuts in military spending, and changes in overseas markets, some observers believe that capitalistic expansion is likely to target the domestic health area as a particularly lucrative electronics market (HealthRight 1975, p. 5).*

During the past few years, baby formula manufacturers have been selling their products to women in Third World countries, who can ill afford them and who do not have adequate means for sterilizing bottles or obtaining pure water (needed to mix the powdered formula). Encouraged to purchase these formulas to provide their babies with "the best," Third World women give up nursing their babies only to end up starving them (Margulies 1977).

Recognizing American medicine's central role in the profit system, some feminists suggest that most reforms are palliative at best, subversive at worst. At the "International Conference on Women in Health," held in Washington, D.C., in June 1975, Ehrenreich (1975, p. 21) asked:

> Can we hope to make the changes we would like to make
> in the health sector without making much more profound
> changes in our society? Can we hope for a health care
> system that is both egalitarian and effective within the
> context of a social system which is based on class, race
> and sex inequities? And if not, if more broad and

---

*For discussions of military-industrial involvement in health, see Millman 1977; Kelman 1971; and Krauss 1971.

revolutionary changes are required, then we must ask
ourselves—where do we start?

For the most part, feminist health advocates (like other social
activists in the late 1970s) either do not know where to start or do not
wish to provoke such fundamental changes in the larger society. As
in the larger feminist movement, there are some women who emphasize the need to create a socialist state. Others work for more immediate reforms—some major, others less so. And despite widespread admiration of health activists for women's roles in Chinese
medicine (believed possible only within the context of that societal
political philosophy), few see a realistic possibility of creating such
a system in this country. While some believe that a resolution such
as China's is needed, a common attitude is: "If you wait for a revolution you will never get anything accomplished. There are many organized efforts in the community to bring about change. Women health
workers can and should join in the efforts" (Brown 1976, p. 13).

Above all, then, women's self-determination is the crucial
feminist health issue. Capitalism is of concern because it severely
alters women's opportunities for obtaining quality care. The feminist
critique focuses on how and why men deny women self-determination
in health for reasons above and beyond simple capitalistic exploitation.

As shown in this chapter, much evidence supporting feminist
contentions of mistreatment and male control come from scientists
and medical professionals themselves. But prior to contemporary
feminists' interest in health, many issues were overlooked, ignored,
or disregarded as trivial, uninteresting, or unusual random problems
unrealted to women's position in society. Feminists, elaborating the
theory of sexual politics, focused attention on how sexism, like racism,
becomes institutionalized or embedded in the fabric of society, so
that individuals are not conscious of it and have no need to discrimi-
nate overtly; it becomes "natural." As both academics and activists
demonstrate, sexism is built into law, language, and scientific research—blinding even the observant from recognizing the source of
their taken-for-granted beliefs and behavior.

As feminism heightened women's (and some men's) awareness
of the sexual politics of health in a capitalist economy, the credibility
of the physician's mystique and consequent belief in the appropriateness of medical authority were seriously undermined. The only issue
remaining was—and still is—what to do to assure women's health.

5

The Structure of Obstetrical and Gynecological Health Care Worlds: Familiar Terrain and Visions Beyond

Obstetrical and gynecological health care settings both reflect and shape patients' and practitioners' conceptualizations of health and illness. That is, these organizations reflect views of health and illness and appropriate role behavior held by members of a society or subculture; participating in these institutions also creates a pattern of behavior that reinforces and leads one to take as "natural" certain basic values and beliefs about health and illness.

Institutions organized or controlled by high-status professionals incorporate, and operate on, medical-professional perspectives that are quite different from those guiding lay-controlled health organizations. High-technology university labor and delivery services, for example, are significantly different in practice and ideology from lay-organized home birth centers. A key difference between these health care worlds is the balance of responsibility and authority believed appropriate between patients and practitioners. Beliefs about the appropriate division of responsibility and authority are observable in dominant role relationships and in the social distribution of medical knowledge negotiable in each setting.

Practitioners (medical or other) want health care worlds to support their own value system, allowing them to interact in ways supporting their images of themselves. When women patients and practitioner share similar views, routine care often proceeds with little difficulty. Of course, women cannot always obtain care in settings that are congruent with their values. Sometimes, the incompatibility is due to chance. If the woman recognizes the difficulty and can find another setting, conflict may be minimized.

Often, however, women have few options: there are no other practitioners or no practitioners sharing the patient's views, or the patient has limited time or money. Even when alternatives are

available, women may be discouraged from seeking them when told
that they are unsafe or somehow "inferior." For example, women
are often pressured to believe that radical mastectomy is the only
safe or available treatment for breast cancer or that surgery must
immediately follow biopsy (see, for example, Cowan 1977; Eagan
1976; R. Kushner 1975; and Switzer 1976). Similarly, many women
are led to believe that hospitals are the safest or only reasonable
place to give birth (Arms 1975; Haire 1972; B. Rothman 1976). None
of these are unequivocally accepted truths, even within the medical
profession, although women are often encouraged to accept them as
if they were.

IDEAL TYPES OF HEALTH CARE WORLDS

The key issue feminist health activists raise is women's right
to choose and decide about their own care. Although quality of care
(including quality of medical technology) is at issue, women emphasize the need for humane practitioners working in settings that allow
women to retain their life values, especially those related to autonomy.

Practitioners' and patients' beliefs about the responsibility
and authority appropriate to each are a crucial factor limiting or encouraging women's decision-making opportunities. These beliefs
can be viewed as falling along a continuum: beliefs range from expecting physicians to assume nearly all responsibility to expecting
women themselves to assume most responsibility for routine care.

For analytic and comparative purposes, we can construct ideal
types (Weber 1947, 1958) of routine obstetrical and gynecological
health care settings, using the dimension of beliefs surrounding who
is to assume responsibility for, and authority over, certain aspects
of women's health care. In this chapter, four ideal-typical health
care worlds are described that were constructed by the author from
field observations, interviews with patients and practitioners, and
available literature. How authority and responsibility are negotiated
in these traditional-authoritarian, traditional-egalitarian, traditional-
feminist, and radical-feminist worlds can be discovered by comparing
various health care settings across salient dimensions: dominant role
relationships, the social distribution of medical knowledge, the division of labor, access to curatives, management of time and space,
and assignment of risk.

A comparative analysis of health care worlds reveals why
some settings attract certain women but not others. It also offers
insight into some of the consequences of the social organization of
routine care, revealing the structural features of medical practice
affecting style of patient-physician interaction, access to information,
and right to decision making—all of concern to feminist health activists.

Traditional-Authoritarian Worlds

At one end of the continuum are traditional-authoritarian health care worlds. (For sociological studies of these settings, see, for example, Emerson 1963, 1970a, 1970b; Ford 1975; Freidson 1961, 1973a; Rosengren and DeVault 1963; and Shaw 1972, 1974. For practitioners' perspectives, see Anonymous 1972 and Sweeney 1973. Feminist descriptions and critiques include Arms 1975; de Maehl and Thurston 1973; Gendel 1974; Haire 1972; Hirsch 1977; Proceedings of the First International Childbirth Conference 1973; Rich 1975; Seaman 1972.) Typically, public clinics and hospitals operate on a traditional-orthodox model. Many private practitioners also provide this type of care in their offices and hospitals.

Dominated by physicians who believe all authority and decision making should remain in their hands, the typical doctor-patient relationship resembles the "activity-passivity" model (Szasz and Hollender 1956), although the patient may actually be awake, conscious, and potentially quite capable of participating. Some interaction may conform to the "guidance-cooperation" model (Szasz and Hollender 1956), particularly with high-status patients. However, the patient's primary responsibility is to allow herself to be molded into raw material in a form suited to maintain the stability of conventional settings. Emerson (1970a, p. 83) argues that in these settings, women are expected to be passive and self-effacing, show a willingness to relinquish control to the doctor, refrain from speaking at length or from making inquiries requiring long explanations, and to keep their personalities from projecting profusely—in short: "The self must be eclipsed in order to sustain the definition that the doctor is working on a technical object and not a person."

Much of the female patient's incapacity to participate or function as a competent adult is physician induced—the result of overbearing attitudes inhibiting discussion, the consequences of unnecessary anesthesia in childbirth, rendering women incapable of participation, or the result of "scare" tactics designed to force women to submit to radical mastectomies despite personal doubts. That women become helpless or even hysterical in these settings is understandable; they have given up (or been deprived of) their ability to behave as competent adults.

Medical ideology stresses the benefits of passivity to the patient; supposedly being treated as an impersonal object minimizes threats to a woman's dignity and reduces possible embarrassment. What is more salient is that the staff uses this medical definition to inveigle the patient to cooperate to make the work easier for themselves (Emerson 1970a, p. 79). The system is self-perpetuating, for physicians invoke self-fulfilling prophecies that women need and want to be treated in this manner in order to continue this treatment.

Some women—particularly, women following traditional sex roles—may find these health care worlds compatible with their self-images and values, as long as the care is provided in a humane, "caring" manner by apparently sympathetic and competent physicians. However, patients' cooperation and lack of overt objection in actual patient-physician encounters cannot be taken as definitive evidence that women necessarily like or want this type of care. Arms (1975) points out that childbearing women go along with procedures simply because they have no choice. And Emerson (1970a, p. 90) argues that after gynecological examinations patients sometimes confide their great distaste for procedures to nurses, indicating that patients actually have strong negative reactions that belie their acquiescence.

Traditional-Egalitarian Worlds

In traditional-egalitarian settings, professionals assume responsibility for, and authority over, care; patients are expected to be somewhat informed and involved. Although patients are encouraged to ask questions, they are expected to follow doctors' orders. While patients make choices and decisions, physicians define the parameters within which choices can be made. In these settings, physicians vary widely in willingness to discuss reasons for following certain procedures on a level comprehensible to women; some physicians are more open than others to individual negotiation.

Role relationships largely follow the "guidance-cooperation" or "mutual-participation" model (Szasz and Hollender 1956) for routine care. (For sociological comment, see Shaw 1972, 1974. Miller 1962 and Lanson 1975 are medical proponents of this type of care; Sweeney 1973 also describes this style of practice. Feminist descriptions—both positive and negative—are included in Arms 1975; the Boston Women's Health Book Collective 1973, 1976; Hirsch 1977; Proceedings of the First International Childbirth Conference 1973; Rothman 1976; Seaman 1972; Rich 1975). Traditional-egalitarian settings can be found in clinics, hospitals, and private practices organized for prepared childbirth, as well as in some "progressive" family-planning and abortion clinics.

In the traditional-authoritarian and traditional-egalitarian settings described above, the term traditional indicates the physician's retention of the "expert" role. In the first setting, physicians adhere to conventional authoritarian professional and sex-role behavior. In the egalitarian setting, roles more congruous with contemporary views on social relationships between both men and women and professionals and clients predominate. Although the patient is more active, involved, and responsible for herself in traditional-egalitarian settings than in traditional-authoritarian settings, medical authority really is not altered; instead, it is enhanced by the active cooperation of the patient.

Most women obtain obstetrical and gynecological care in these conventional settings. Poor women usually end up in traditional-authoritarian settings (as "teaching material" or clinic patients), but so do many middle- and upper-class women. Traditional-egalitarian settings, often available to middle- or upper-class women, are rarely available to lower-class women. Poor patients are more likely than middle-class patients to be treated by residents, interns, and medical students. Physicians-in-training can be expected to take an authoritarian approach in order to minimize inroads on their shaky authority under conditions where maintaining authority is rewarded by superiors. Both Shaw (1972, 1974) and Rosengren and DeVault (1963) note how private and clinic patients receive differential treatment, even in the same hospital delivery service—prima facie evidence of the fluidity with which social worlds are constructed.

Traditional-Feminist Worlds

With the growth of women's health collectives, clinics, and self-help activities, two alternative ideal-typical settings became available: traditional-feminist and radical-feminist. In both of these settings, medical authority and responsibility are altered, but in different ways. (Social science studies of these settings include Harding, Harrington, and Manor 1973; Light and Kleiber 1975a, 1975b, 1975c, 1978; Marieskind 1976; Palmer 1974, 1976; and Peterson 1976; health movement and popular literature describing these settings include Aldrich 1974; Arms 1975; Barfoot 1973; Berkeley Women's Health Collective n.d.; Campbell, Dalsemer, and Waldman 1972; Frankfort 1972; Hirsch 1977; Rothman 1976; Stephen 1973a, 1973b; and "Women's Clinics" 1971.)

In traditional feminist clinics, female paraprofessionals provide much actual care, reducing opportunities for physician dominance. By minimizing patients' interaction with physicians, the distance resulting from the status differential between patient and practitioner is reduced. Closeness and communication between patient and practitioner is also facilitated by the important role of the all-female paraprofessional staff, creating a "fellow-woman aura," which Emerson (1970a, p. 90) and others suggest women seek in gynecology.*

---

*Rosengren and DeVault (1963, p. 292) remind us that Everett Hughes noted that both physical and symbolic "closeness" between

Palmer (1974, p. 8) argues that an all-female staff (including physicians) is critical for creating an atmosphere where questions can be asked without embarrassment. While providing exclusively female physicians is an ideal, it is often impossible. There are simply too few available who are willing to work in women's clinics—with or without pay.

In many clinics, physicians diagnose, offer advice, or perform medical procedures only <u>after</u> other workers have seen the patient and have determined that the patient needs (and is willing) to see a physician; some patients refuse physician care. Interaction between patients and paraprofessionals (often referred to as "pelvic teams") and patients and physicians typically follows the "mutual-participation" model (Szasz and Hollender 1956). Where physicians' activities are very limited, they interact in an advisory or "consultant-client" role with individual patients and/or paraprofessionals. During clinic hours, some physicians simply wait to be called by the teams to see patients, answer questions, write prescriptions, and dispense drugs. Where mutual trust is high between physician and paraprofessionals, physicians dispense many services without actually seeing the patient.

In these traditional-feminist worlds, women are expected to be interested and involved in their own health care. Whether or not they are interested on arrival, health workers attempt to involve them through group discussions and individual attention, encouraging them to assume responsibility for their health.

These settings are promoted as places where female patients can feel more in control of their own health. Often patients agree, adding that the fear and embarrassment typically felt in conventional settings (partly but not entirely related to examination by male physicians) are eliminated, leaving them freer to ask questions and take responsibility. Other patients are less eager and only reluctantly accept education to get a needed service—an attitude accepted but disliked by some clinic workers. As with the Salvation Army dinner line, one must listen to the sermon to get the soup.

Some feminists feel these settings fail to challenge many crucial aspects of traditional medical practice and professional dominance—an assessment traditional-feminist health advocates, including Beverly Palmer (1976, p. 3), a founder of the Harbor Women's Free

---

staff and patients is related to the social status of the patient. J. Roth (1972, 1973) emphasizes that despite the medical ideology of affect-neutrality, perceived social status of the client strongly affects the interaction.

Clinic, agree is accurate; that is, this type of service changes professional practices but does not seriously challenge the assumption that professionals should provide routine services.

Radical-Feminist Worlds

In radical-feminist settings, patients are encouraged to assume major responsibility for their own care (with the assistance of lay-women who organize and control self-care activities).* (For social science studies, see Jones 1973; Kleiber 1974; Kleiber and Light 1978; Edwards 1973; Marieskind 1976; Peterson 1976; Reynard 1973; Ruzek 1977a; and Smith 1973; other descriptions are available in Arms 1975; Brown 1973; Downer 1972; Farenza 1976; Fishel 1973; L. Hirsch 1972; Lang 1972; Proceedings of the First International Childbirth Conference 1973; Rothman 1972; and Yost 1974.) Radical-feminist health care settings are created in self-help gynecology and obstetrics clinics, menstrual extraction groups, and lay-operated home birth centers.

Physicians, when present in these worlds, are relegated to technician status. They are hired only to perform tasks restricted by law. Physicians are called upon to write prescriptions, insert IUDs, perform abortions, or hospitalize women for complications of labor or deliver only after lay persons have defined what needs to be done. As in traditional-feminist worlds, much routine care (often very informal) is provided by laywomen with paraprofessional training. What is distinct about these settings is that women learn to perform basic health services for themselves. Depending on the working relationship between the individual physician and laywomen controlling the setting and the task involved, "mutual-participation" (Szasz and Hollender 1956) or "consultant-client" role relationships predominate.

Overall, physicians must unlearn much of their traditional professional role and accept the status of technician or standby—waiting to act only when specific technical assistance is needed or because folkways (lay practices and/or home remedies) have failed to produce desired results. This role is difficult for them, because persons trained to use technology are eager to apply their skills.

---

*Although self-care is not new, that is poor women and women in rural areas must regularly rely on lay care, self-help is a radical feminist activity in that it "goes to the roots" of medical oppression of women. By redefining crucial life-events and activities as non-medical activities, self-help participants believe that they eliminate some central forms of oppression.

Professionals must also cooperate with, or at least tolerate, unorthodox practitioners (for example, astrologers, lay midwives, or herbalists) patients select as primary caregivers or as authorities on health matters. Even nurse-midwives—seen by many as the solution to the dilemma of physicians who have little time for, or interest in, routine birth—are shunned by some, on grounds that they act much like physicians and believe that professionals, not birthing mothers, know best and hold the power to heal (Arms 1975, pp. 155-57).

Women participating in these settings argue that they offer the only real alternative to control by the medical profession. Only in laywoman-controlled settings can women re-establish their right and responsibility to manage normal life-events, which they do not regard as medical affairs. Of course, some women are comfortable assuming maximal responsibility for their own care for certain events (routine examinations, contraception) but not for others (abortion or potentially complicated childbirth). Although, generally, the more serious the event, the more likely a woman will choose more conventional settings (where more responsibility is placed on professionals), the seriousness or potential risks involved in an event often cannot be quantified or established as absolute by "outsiders." For seriousness of risk is subjective as well as objective and involves personal values and goals.

William Silverman, former professor of pediatrics at Columbia University College of Physicians and Surgeons, point out that it is impossible for labor and delivery to be absolutely without risk. The question is how to define what the various risks are, to estimate their magnitude, and to compare these with an individual standard of benefit. The standard view is that numbers are what really count: mortality and damage statistics. The question is how to evaluate something like the effect of postpartum separation on both mother and child or to assess the impact of experiencing all of giving birth or dying—important life experiences (Arms 1975, p. 114).

Radical-feminist settings are rejected by some as antitechnological or unscientific, as well as dangerous. In fact, acceptance of technology varies tremendously in these settings, as does reliance on Western scientific medicine and less orthodox or "natural" healing principles. All, however, are highly empirical and emphasize direct observation. Efficacy is based on the subjective experience of the individual rather than being based exclusively on objective measures. This focus on personal experience stems in part from women's disenchantment with "objective" medical "facts" (discussed previously).

Both of these alternative worlds are guided by feminist principles of self-determination and the right to choice. The first setting is traditional insofar as medical authority is accepted. Women come to the clinic expecting to obtain standard medical services from sympathetic practitioners. In contrast, radical-feminist settings provide some services unavailable elsewhere—such as menstrual extraction—and also teach women to do routine procedures for themselves in innovative ways rather than relying on either lay or professional practitioners. Here, women by virtue of their female experience, are the assumed experts on many medical matters. Professional training alone is not automatically recognized as confirmation of competence.

Radical-feminist health proponents (recognizing that not all women are comfortable with self-care) often promote both types of services. For example, women involved in menstrual extraction groups (a radical-feminist activity) may also work as paraprofessionals in traditional-feminist clinics or abortion facilities staffed by licensed physicians. Lay midwives operating home birth centers (radical-feminist settings) sometimes participate in traditional-egalitarian hospital deliveries, along with licensed physicians, when a woman prefers that setting or complications indicate medical assistance is needed. (Contrary to popular belief, most lay midwives encourage rather than discourage women from seeking medical assistance when needed.)

Table 5.1 summarizes ideal-typical health care settings where routine obstetrical and gynecological services are available.

THE STRUCTURE OF HEALTH CARE WORLDS

Patients—or their agents—always make initial diagnoses, assessing when, and what type of, medical attention is needed; thus, all patients possess a modicum of medical knowledge. To assume responsibility and authority for actual care and treatment, one must possess—or be thought to possess—valid medical knowledge. Participants in all health care worlds hold views regarding the appropriate and possible social distribution of medical knowledge. Settings are also structured to perpetuate the believed-to-be-appropriate level of knowledge for all participants. Thus, to understand how participants come to assume differential degrees of responsibility and authority for health care, we must examine typical beliefs regarding the appropriate social distribution of medical knowledge; then, we can explore how the division of labor, access to curatives, and management of territories and time in each health care world sustain differential responsibility and authority.

TABLE 5.1

Health Care Settings Distinguished by the Relative Responsibility and Authority of Patient in Relation to Practitioner, for Selected Obstetrical/Gynecological Services

Service	Traditional-Authoritarian	Traditional-Egalitarian	Traditional-Feminist	Radical-Feminist
Routine examination and treatment for minor gynecological disorders	Public clinics, private offices	Progressive clinics, private offices	Feminist clinic	Self-help clinic
Contraception	Public clinics, private offices	Progressive clinics, private offices	Feminist clinic	Self-help clinic, menstrual extraction
Childbirth	Public or private hospitals	Private patient sections of public or private hospitals, "home-style" hospital birth room	Physician or nurse-midwife-attended home birth, "home-style" hospital birth room	Lay-midwife-attended home birth
Abortion	Public or private hospitals; free-standing, public, or private clinics	Progressive clinics, private offices	Feminist clinic	Refer to traditional-feminist or traditional-egalitarian setting, menstrual extraction group
Gynecological surgery	Public or private hospitals	Private patient sections of public or private hospitals	Refer to approved traditional-egalitarian setting	Refer to approved traditional-egalitarian setting

Source: Compiled by the author.

112

The Social Distribution of Medical Knowledge

Each ideal-typical health care world incorporates certain distinct assumptions about the social distribution of medical knowledge among participants. In traditional-authoritarian settings, physicians believe themselves to be the only reliable source of medical information. For them, knowledge in patients' hands is both dangerous and troublesome. Sweeney (1973, p. 155), for example, warns pregnant patients against getting any information from druggists, husbands, mothers, or mothers-in-law. He adds that once he assumes responsibility for a lady's care, she is in his ball park and has to play by his rules.

Although Sweeney does suggest women might read up on <u>normal</u> pregnancy or might even learn something from prepared childbirth classes (1973, p. 147), his basic attitude is that women are unreliable, that physicians are solely competent to understand or provide medical information and, as a consequence, solely capable of making decisions. He argues that one of the main problems of natural childbirth is that when couples go to classes, they are not told what the pain might really be like. Suddenly, labor is experienced as excruciating, and the woman shatters. The woman who goes to pieces has to be sedated, since in Sweeney's opinion, there is nothing else that can be done (1973, pp. 49-50).*

Physicians' desire to maintain a monopoly on medical knowledge goes far beyond obstetrics. Their unwillingness to provide adequate information to women about the risks and side effects of oral contraceptives (on grounds that women will be frightened or develop imaginary symptoms) is documented (Mintz 1967; Seaman 1969; Silverman and Lee 1974). Some physicians even prefer medications to remain unlabeled by pharmacists. Others refuse to reveal diagnoses, not only for fatal diseases, such as cancer, but for common disorders. One physician, defending his refusal to provide diagnostic information, told me:

> You just can't give women information without causing a
> lot of trouble. I told a patient once that she had tricho-
> moniasis [a common vaginal infection] and she went off
> to the library and read up on trichinosis by mistake.
> Then she called me back all upset saying she could feel
> all the little worms crawling around in her vagina!

---

*Shaw (1974) points out that few efforts are made to assist patients except with drugs—the easiest remedy to provide.

It never occurred to this physician that providing <u>more</u> information might prevent such problems—a view feminists hold.

Traditional-authoritarian surgeons, especially, resent medical information in women's hands and disagree that women can decide what type of surgery to undergo. For example, at a public forum in San Francisco, a prominent surgeon stated:

> The state of the art isn't such that we can do lumpectomies now despite what the <u>Ladies Home Journal</u> says (which has) caused an enormous amount of mischief. I think this is something that has gone too far ... having the women tell the doctor what he should do and not do. ... I've had several patients recently who've said, "You're not going to take my breasts off no matter what," and I said, "Well, that's fine. You can go here, there or the other place, but I'm not going to do a lumpectomy. I'm not just going to take the lump out and leave cancer behind. I think that's second best or third best." And they say, "Well do it because I want you to do it. I don't want to go to another doctor." I say, "the problem between me and you is that I can't communicate to you. You've communicated to me, but I can't convince you to accept the best treatment as I know it as a specialist. ... I have no right to do something second best and have you come in with a recurrence dying of cancer two, three, four, five years from now." Because invariably ... before they die they're looking at me with tearful eyes and saying, "Why didn't you convince me in the first place of doing the right thing?" ... I do not think it's right for a doctor—if he can't convince his patient of the right thing to do—to treat that patient with something second best.

Another group of surgeons (Farrow et al. 1971), arguing in <u>Cancer</u> for careful consideration of nonmutilating treatment, states, however, that women have no business making a decision about the extent of surgery for breast cancer on grounds that one cannot make a wise selection when disturbed by tensions and emotions.

In contrast, physicians in traditional-egalitarian health care settings believe that given adequate information, women can better manage pregnancy and delivery, report symptoms more accurately, and make truly informed decisions about their own care—even surgery. Prepared childbirth proponents encourage patient education and have faith in patients' ability to utilize knowledge. Both Grantly Dick-Read and Robert Bradley, two prominent natural childbirth proponents, argue that fear and ignorance underlies much of the pain of childbirth and that physicians should educate patients to break the fear-pain cycle.

Some traditional-egalitarian physicians argue that patients should be given adequate information to make informed choices, even on matters as serious as breast surgery (see, especially, Cope 1977, 1974, 1971; Cowan 1977, pp. 30-32; Crile 1974; and Lanson 1975). They point out that particularly in light of the controversy over the effectiveness of radical surgery as compared with other treatment modalities, patients ought to have some choice in the matter. Unfortunately, the bewildered patient is rarely informed of alternatives or has any part in deciding on a treatment. While these physicians would not perform procedures they deem harmful, they do suggest patients have the right to refuse treatment or choose less-effective treatments without risking abandonment by their physicians—as often occurs in traditional-authoritarian settings.

A major goal of the women's health movement is to change the social distribution of medical knowledge from the exclusive property of certified experts to women themselves. In the conventional settings described above, professionals are expected to learn and gain incremental knowledge through years of practice and experience. Patients are not expected to increase their stock of knowledge about their bodies or health, and patients who display acquired expertise are often regarded as troublemakers.

In contrast, all participants in traditional-feminist and radical-feminist settings are expected to increase their knowledge and expertise over time from many sources: encounters with physicians, nurses, lay health workers, and family and friends, and participation in health discussion groups and self-care clinics structured to maximize pooling of information. Furthermore, as many women (and even a few male physicians) point out, patients themselves are best able to recognize what is normal or abnormal in their own bodies. Physician Wes Skolosky of the West Marin (California) Medical Center, who attends many home births, believes that women are not nearly as ignorant of their bodies as doctors make them out to be but that they can be scared out of being able to perceive what is going on inside. He cannot recall one instance where the need to do something was not clear to the woman long before it became clear to him or his associates (Arms 1975, p. 194).

Participants in feminist settings believe that with adequate information, women themselves are most competent to choose contraceptives; decide whether or not to be sterilized; decide to have a baby at home or in a hospital attended by a physician, nurse-midwife, lay midwife, or friends; accept a hysterectomy on the basis of one physician's findings or insist on additional consultations; and choose minimal or radical surgery—or no surgery—for breast cancer. In sum, participants in feminist health care settings believe that they—and only they—have the right to decide what care is best for them, after assessing available information and obtaining different opinions and suggestions.

The feminist perspective recognizes that medical science (like other branches of science) is always in flux and that there are disagreements within the scientific community itself—a fact most physicians ignore or hide from their patients. Feminists suggest that women can be "well-informed citizens" when choosing their own health care; they can (and do) solicit information and advice from many "experts," but unlike the "man on the street" (who accepts any expert's advice), well-informed citizens weigh the advice and opinions of experts carefully before selecting a course of action.*

The Division of Labor

The division of labor in health care worlds is partly determined by beliefs about the social distribution of medical knowledge; it also perpetuates the distribution of knowledge and solidifies the ability of various participants to assume responsibility and make decisions.

Rigid distinctions between worker categories (based on formal training and certification) and patients are maintained in both traditional-authoritarian and traditional-egalitarian worlds. Although the actual division of labor is negotiated both by individuals and whole categories of workers (and differs between institutions), formal and informal norms strongly regulate the division of labor (once established).

In conventional settings, for example, receptionists answer the telephone, make out bills, greet patients, and sometimes escort patients to examining rooms. Nurses (practical, licensed vocational, or registered) occasionally perform some clerical tasks in small private offices, but more often they perform "nursing services" (dispensing medication; taking temperatures; weighing and measuring patients; and assisting in, or observing, pelvic and breast examinations for propriety's sake). Physicians reserve all medical tasks for themselves, including the right to delegate undesirable tasks to lower-status physicians (residents, interns, and medical students) or to

---

*See Schutz (1964) for elaboration of relationships between experts, well-informed citizens, and the man on the street.

nurses. Although some tasks (taking medical histories, blood pressure, and performing prenatal checkups) may be nurses' tasks in some institutions and doctors' in others, norms regulating the division of labor in any setting are constantly negotiated and enforced.

The division of labor between physicians and nurses is quite arbitrary in routine obstetrics and gynecology, preventing nurses and nurse-practitioners, in some areas, from practicing to their capacity and often trapping physicians into what they consider to be dull, tedious tasks. Rich Quint, a pediatrician who has worked under 20 obstetricians and observed 50 more, reports that most of these specialists will admit that attending normal births is a bore (Arms 1975, p. 45).

Nonetheless, obstetrician-gynecologists fight to keep delivery their exclusive domain, even if it requires transforming what might be otherwise normal births into surgical events. In the hospital—particularly in the delivery room—the obstetrician can become the star of the obstetrical drama. Deferred to and waited on by nurses and other lower-status personnel, physicians enjoy their status and omnipotence. Sweeney (1973, pp. 97-98), for example, explains:

> It's not just that we're idolized by our patients. We also
> work in offices and hospitals where we're waited on.
> Especially as surgeons, we don't get anything for our-
> selves: the nurse hands us the instruments or whatever
> we need. We drop a white coat and a nurse picks it up. ...
> We never clean anything. When we operate somebody else
> washes all the instruments. If, God forbid, a scalpel is
> dirty, we throw it at a nurse and say, "This one's dirty!
> How come this one's dirty?" ... It's an egotistical thing
> to become a doctor in the first place, to think you're com-
> petent to take other people's lives in your hands. Yet
> every single day we make decisions that affect people's
> lives. And to top it off, we enjoy it.

The division of labor in conventional settings also creates distance between clients and practitioners and restricts patients' access to medical information. For example, receptionists routinely route telephone calls to a nurse or physician only after the caller provides a reason (defined as acceptable in the setting) warranting professional attention. Because patients rarely can speak with a physician on the telephone without a "good reason" and receptionists and many nurses are not allowed to answer "medical questions" in person or over the telephone, many patient concerns fall in an area too trivial for professional attention but too technical for lower-status personnel to address. To obtain information, receive reassurance, or be referred to another specialist, it is often necessary to make an appointment to see a physician; this is expensive and time consuming, forcing women to wait—often for several weeks or months—for information.[*]

The ineffectiveness of medical communication in conventional settings is well documented. Korsch and Negrete (1972), for example, report in pediatric consultations, 20 percent of the mothers did not understand their child's illness and 43 percent did not follow physicians' advice. Social scientists and physicians alike tend to "blame the victim" for general ignorance or inattention. McKinlay (1975, p. 9) argues instead that patient ignorance is more correctly attributed to physicians and to aspects of professionalism.

Medical communication is encumbered by physicians' self-fulfilling prophecy about patients' ignorance. Pratt, Seligman, and Reader (1957) point out that when a doctor perceives a patient as poorly informed, he or she avoids elaborate discussion with the patient because of the difficulties of translating medical knowledge into understandable language and concern that the patient will be frightened. In turn, the patient reacts dully to the limited information, typically asking uninspired questions or nothing at all; this interaction then reinforces the doctor's view that the patient cannot comprehend the problem and provides a further rationale for the doctor to avoid discussion. Lacking physician encouragement to discuss the problem, the patient seems uninterested or unresponsive, leading the doctor to evaluate his or her capacities as even lower than they actually are.

Shaw (1974, pp. 110-11) describes how this pattern of imputed patient ignorance and incapacity to learn leads to gross dehumanization of postpartum obstetrical patients. Patients defined as ignorant are not even instructed in simple perineal hygiene but are cleaned in assembly-line fashion. In hospitals where patients are regarded more highly, women are taught to cleanse themselves.

Skipper, Tagliacozzo, and Mauksch (1964) argue that imputing ignorance to hospitalized patients, especially, maintains professional authority and control. Limited communication keeps interaction with patients on a strictly instrumental basis, geared toward the efficiency of the hospital. Not informing patients about their illnesses also protects personnel from unmanageable reactions from patients who "might not understand" and prove to be troublesome. Not giving out information also prevents patients from hearing "bad news" that might cause emotional reactions that could hamper their recovery. Finally,

---

[*]The average waiting time for an appointment was 10 to 11 days in the traditional clinic Marieskind (1976, p. 273) studied.

limited communication safeguards health personnel from patients discovering errors of neglect and incompetence in the medical work.*

McKinlay concludes that professionals' imputation of patient
ignorance may be a necessary structural ingredient in all professional-
client encounters. I would argue that a crucial structural factor encouraging patient ignorance is the division of labor making physicians
responsible for offering basic health information and treatment regimens on a one-to-one basis.

In traditional-feminist and radical-feminist settings, the division of labor is less hierarchical, and physicians' responsibilities
and actions are observed and evaluated by laywomen; doctors have
few opportunities to aggrandize their status. These settings, organized
around feminist principles of collectivity, minimize specialization,
certification, and hierarchical social relationships as much as possible. In many feminist groups and clinics—particularly those practicing self-help—lay members (trained by more experienced members)
rotate answering the telephone, collecting fees, keeping records,
performing pelvic examinations and laboratory tests, and teaching
newcomers. While this pattern works in small groups, clinics that
expand find it difficult to sustain job rotations and come to accept
more specialization. This is partly due to the inevitable process of
social differentiation. Over time, women become more skilled at
certain tasks than others and prefer to perform certain jobs.

When health workers are paid even minimal subsistence salaries, it is easier to insist that each person perform a share of less-
desirable tasks than when workers are volunteers. For example, in
many clinics, one must work as an unpaid member before becoming
salaried. New volunteers spend several hours each week on phone
lines making appointments and referrals and offering information.
Eventually, volunteers find these tasks boring and wish to do other
jobs. If workers are salaried, however, undesirable work can be
required as "part of the job." Some clinics actually hire out their
clerical tasks, while relying on volunteered professional services.
This reverses the pattern found in traditional health institutions,
where high-status professional work is reserved for paid employees,
while volunteers perform menial tasks.

Depending on the commitment to total sharing and collectivity
in traditional-feminist settings, physicians are or are not called upon
to share certain clinic tasks. For example, in some traditional-
feminist groups, physicians are expected to pitch in and do some

---

*See Quint 1965 and 1972 for discussion of controlling infor-
mation and interaction, especially with mastectomy patients.

"shit work"—for example, sterilizing instruments and mopping clinic floors; in others, regular attendance at collective meetings is expected. It is hard enough, however, to get physicians to volunteer medical skills without asking for this much sharing; therefore, the few physicians who do volunteer perform only specialized medical tasks: abortions, IUD insertions, prescribing, or diagnosing.

Because most interaction is between patients or clients and paraprofessionals, physicians' direct day-to-day responsibility for, and authority over, routine care is reduced. Ironically, physicians attracted to work in these settings are often committed to practicing humanistically; yet reduced to technician status or called upon only as an advisor or consultant, it is hard for them to develop rapport. After spending most of an evening clinic session sitting alone, ignored by patients and paramedics, a woman physician rather sadly commented: "The Collective members can do most of it alone and if I stay in the examining room I get bored just watching. So I come out here. They call me if they need me, but I really miss working with patients. It's hard just being called in to take a look and leave."

Overall, then, the traditional-feminist division of labor between physicians and nonphysicians is similar to that in other medical settings. Less-trained workers simply perform an array of tasks usually reserved for more formally certified personnel, relieving physicians of many tedious, simple procedures, which comprise the bulk of routine obstetrics and gynecology. Boring to physicians, these jobs are interesting to women with less training. While these settings attempt to provide more humane, responsive services, meeting women's emotional as well as technical needs, they do not seriously challenge professionals' prerogative to provide maternity care, abortion, contraception, and treatment for minor gynecological problems.

In contrast, radical-feminist settings drastically alter the division of labor, by shifting responsibility for routine care for well women from certified professional experts to women themselves. Thus, self-care clinics challenge the whole medical-professional model, in which the physician is assumed to be the only person who is competent to evaluate medical needs, propose or prescribe specific regimens or treatments, and judge the competence of other practitioners. Radical-feminist settings not only challenge these assumptions but shatter many myths about workable patient and professional roles.

It should be emphasized that radical-feminist health settings are organized to meet the medical needs of women who are "well," not "sick." Although many physicians would challenge this idea, feminists argue that women needing contraceptives, routine examinations, treatment for common vaginal infections, or even very early abortions are basically well. As well women, they believe they have the right and responsibility to manage their own bodies and learn basic health care skills.

Radical-feminist settings eliminate professionals entirely or transform their place in the division of labor to maximize women's access to each other's knowledge, assigning individuals major responsibility for their own care. Beginning with the premise that women possess considerable knowledge and expertise, routine care is structured to provide women access to each others' expertise rather than to only that of the physician. Having physicians see patients privately for hurried consultations is viewed as inefficient for routine care. Thus, rather than have physicians repeat simple instructions over and over to individual patients, women are seen in groups, where in-depth discussion and care is possible.

In radical-feminist settings, the right to perform many tasks is extended to anyone willing to learn. The need for, and reliance on, physicians is reduced. In self-help groups—the core of radical-feminist health care—with the guidance of experienced self-helpers, well women learn to perform speculum examinations on themselves and each other; recognize early signs of vaginal infections, syphilis, and pregnancy; and check on the placement of IUDs. Besides studying anatomy and physiology, women learn about nutrition and preventive care and how to treat minor disorders with home remedies. Breast self-examination is practiced, and various types of treatment for breast cancer are discussed. Contraception is considered and often debated; hazards of various methods are weighed in relation to personal concerns. Similar groups are organized for pregnant women in preparation for childbirth. In advanced self-help groups, women learn menstrual extraction to eliminate cramping and the need for contraception or abortion. Finally, by focusing on discovering what is "normal" for herself, each woman becomes better prepared to recognize problems early, when they first begin and are easiest to treat.

Distinctions between providers and receivers, experts, and lay persons are minimized although not eliminated entirely. Expertise and knowledge are highly valued, although formal certification is not. These settings foster a holistic perspective, encouraging all participants to share in observing, advising, treating, and being treated. The role or status of "patient" is replaced with the person as participant in well-woman groups.

To expand areas that are feasible for lay self-help or self-care, the FWHCs offer participatory gynecology clinics. Women in need of routine care—Pap smears, breast examination, venereal disease (VD) testing, lab tests for vaginal and urinary tract infections, sickle cell testing, and all standard contraceptives—receive services in a group setting. Four to eight women meet with several self-help

healthworkers (paramedics) and, in some clinics, a female nurse-
practitioner or nurse for two hours. The atmosphere is relaxed and
similar to that of self-help groups, where women share their medical
concerns and medical knowledge. Nurses and physicians are available for consultation. By enlisting the cooperation of certified practitioners licensed to perform restricted tasks (for example, fitting
diaphragms, inserting IUDs, or identifying or "diagnosing" routine
vaginal disorders), radical-feminist groups are able to expand their
access to curatives and medical procedures and yet operate within
the limits of the law.

In these settings, professionals serve primarily as resource
persons, answering questions, performing specific tasks, and assisting
group participants to carry out pelvic and breast examinations on
themselves and each other. Because diaphragms and IUDs are fitted
and inserted in the group, women have ample opportunity to learn
about the proper use of these devices and how to check their placement.
Procedures shared and observed by group members also make participants less dependent on professionals' individual observations or
assessments. Women receive full information rather than hurried
answers to routine questions and believe they become better-informed
consumers of health services from learning with and from each other.

In these groups, the knowledge and expertise of professionals
and self-help workers is shared rather than "dispensed" or "taught"—
a fine but crucial distinction, for sharing involves mutual exchange
of both information and ignorance ("I don't really know about that" is
as common as more definitive statements, preceded by, "In my experience"). Thus, when participants choose to take some action or
accept a procedure, it is with full knowledge of the limitations—as
well as the competence or experience—of the workers. For example,
new self-help workers tell clients that they are new or that they have
never done a procedure before except on themselves and/or on other
trainees; clients can then elect to provide the new self-helper a chance
to insert a diaphragm ring or take a Pap smear or have it done by a
more experienced worker. Such openness not only relieves the client
of wondering just how experienced or competent the worker is but
frees the worker from trying to hide her inexperience. She is relieved of the "face work" and "fronting," which distract workers from
attending fully to learning technical procedures in conventional settings. (For descriptions of the energy fledgling health professionals
expend attempting to appear experienced, see Becker et al. 1961;
Daniels 1960; Emerson 1963; Ford 1975; Mumford 1970; and Nolan
1972.)

Professionals, of course, learn to practice as advisors and
consultants and allow their work to be observed and evaluated by lay
persons—a step most professionals are loathe to take. They are also

"kept in line" by being paid "going hourly rates" or a standard fee for service by lay-controlled clinics. As hired employees rather than group members, physicians have little say in clinic policy set by lay-women free of professional domination. (How to "manage" professionals is troublesome in many clinics. The situation is particularly sensitive with female physicians—potentially "sisters" but sometimes "honorary males" that feminists find even harder to deal with than men.)

The radical-feminist model strongly suggests that routine health care for well women may be effectively transmitted by nonprofessionals or professionals in groups. This delivery mode is particularly cost-effective when lower-paid nurse-practitioners and women's health care specialists are utilized.

Patient receptivity to group care may be greater than might be assumed. In the mental health field, for example, group therapy is well accepted today, although initially, many doubted that patients would reveal emotional problems in groups, especially groups supervised by nonphysicians. Not only are psychologists, family counselors, and social workers now accepted by group therapy patients but peer psychotherapy has also become acceptable. (For an overview of the development of group therapy, see, for example, Bart 1974; Hurvitz 1974 discusses peer psychotherapy groups.)

As Emerson (1970b) notes, individuals' normative frameworks are extremely malleable. Socialized into new settings or subcultures, individuals rapidly redefine what would be termed odd behavior elsewhere as nothing unusual when the setting supports such a redefinition. Her observations (and those of others) confirm that women do, indeed take cues from self-help proponents and adapt to group examination as "nothing unusual." In the 11 groups I observed, most participants readily accepted the idea of group examination, while acknowledging how uncomfortable they were during pelvic exams in conventional settings. Occasionally, women chose not to examine themselves in the group. But rather than rejecting the concept of group examination, these women often defined themselves as being "unusual." Some claimed to be completely unable to look at their own bodies—even in private—and declared that the ability to examine oneself with other women seemed more "normal" and "healthier." The rapidity with which women accepted group examination as "normal" is striking in the reports of University of California, San Francisco, students assigned to attend a self-help clinic in 1975 for a "women and health" class. Nearly all the students mentioned being apprehensive before going. They emphasized, however, that the self-help workers created an ambience in which group examination was comfortable and natural—much to their surprise. (I had this same experience when attending my first self-help group.) Thus, gynecological group self-care can be taken seriously as a potentially acceptable health delivery mode, particularly for women seeking to assume greater responsibility for themselves.

Access to Curatives

Those with the legal or moral right to prescribe remedies or command the use of special equipment believed necessary to maintain or enhance health are in a better position to maintain authority and responsibility for care than those who do not. Thus, the balance of authority and responsibility between patient and practitioner is tipped in favor of physicians, who have legal license to prescribe drugs and perform "medical procedures." Physicians' authority is also buttressed by the belief that such drugs and procedures are effective curatives.

In traditional-authoritarian worlds, physicians maintain secrecy about their curatives, convincing patients (both directly and indirectly) that prescription drugs and devices are superior to home remedies or over-the-counter drugs. For example, oral contraceptives are often "pushed" as far superior to other methods in traditional-authoritarian settings, despite evidence that when used, the diaphragm with jelly or foam combined with condoms are equally as effective as either the pill or IUDs (Boston Women's Health Book Collective 1976, pp. 185-86; Cowan 1978; Heidelberg 1978). If women know that effectiveness is related to regularity of use rather than to simple technical superiority, they can decide for themselves how conscientious they are likely to be.

Physicians' admonishments, such as those given to pregnant women ("Don't worry, dear, we'll give you a little something to put you out") also consolidate medical authority. These reassurances prepare women to expect pain and to want physicians to prescribe hazardous drugs. Insisting on hospitalization and general anesthesia for abortion similarly increases women's dependence on physicians. Prescribing unlabeled medication for vaginitis (rarely explained as more than "an itch") leaves women ignorant—incapable of presenting future recurrences knowledgeably. Left ignorant, patients are unable to build up a stock of knowledge and are unprepared to report complications or side effects of treatment, a problem that is especially serious when women take several drugs simultaneously (often prescribed by several different doctors). Critics outside the health movement also deplore keeping patients uninformed of prescribed drugs, pointing out that lack of information can be fatal (see, for example, Graedon 1976; Lennard et al. 1971; and Illich 1976).

Physicians in traditional-egalitarian settings are less secretive about, and possessive of, their curatives. Many allow women to choose nonprescription curatives or prescription items that require little medical supervision without belittling these choices. Some physicians suggest inexpensive home remedies for symptomatic relief of minor disorders—baking soda sitz baths or vinegar douches for vaginal discomfort, alcohol for early labor.

However, others, even agreeing that home remedies may be effective, hesitate to suggest them. For example, when asked why he could not recommend unflavored health food store-type yogurt for minor yeast infestation (as do some physicians and self-help proponents), one physician said: "I couldn't do that! I'd feel silly!" In all fairness to this physician (who does suggest many simple remedies), patients themselves unwittingly encourage physicians to by-pass simple solutions by demanding "wonder drugs" and "miracle cures" (see, for example, Page 1975). Patients' inappropriate demands for penicillin, for example, are well known. On the other hand, writing a prescription is an easy way to terminate medical encounters (Stimson and Webb 1975). And some physicians prescribe drugs, particularly psychotropics, in lieu of careful listening, evaluating, and diagnosing.

Feminist settings alter the differential access of patients and practitioners to curatives in several ways. Women's reliance on restricted drugs and technology is reduced by (1) defining certain curatives as undesirable, (2) promoting unrestricted or "natural" curatives, and (3) declaring certain drugs, devices, and procedures accessible to lay persons, irrespective of the law.

Some feminist health activists argue that many common gynecological and obstetrical problems can be prevented simply by avoiding many drugs and devices (for example, oral contraceptives, IUDs, and anesthetics). Oral contraceptives and tetracycline, both associated with increased incidence of vaginitis, are examples of drugs women could avoid to remove the need for other drugs, breaking the iatrogenic chain. Women who choose to take oral contraceptives or tetracycline may be advised to correct the pH balance and bacterial content of the vagina by using mild vinegar douches or yogurt.

Reliance on conventional drugs versus herbal or other natural curatives varies, depending on the inclinations of clinic personnel in traditional-feminist settings. For example, although yogurt is commonly recommended for treating monilia, Mycostatin, gentian violet, and other more conventional Western curatives are usually available. In clinics emphasizing nondrug treatment, garlic suppositories may be recommended for bacterial infections before prescribing triple sulpha cream. Where practitioners are particularly enamored of natural cures, patients may be strongly persuaded to improve their nutrition and try simple remedies, on the grounds that such treatment minimizes exposure to substances with undesirable side effects and is cheaper. (For natural cures and home remedies commonly suggested, and often approved by licensed physicians working in the clinics, see, for example, Berkeley Women's Health Collective n.d.; Prensky 1975; Prescott 1976b; and Rennie and Rubin 1977.) Natural birth control methods are often discussed (see, for example, Hirsch 1973; "The Indians' Herbal Answer to the Pill" 1970; Jackson 1973; Lloyd 1964; Ostrander and Schroeder 1972; and "Vitamin C Abortion" 1974, 1973.

In office and clinic abortions, anesthesia is minimized; some even encourage clients to forgo anesthesia entirely if they prefer a drugless approach. For childbirth, drugs are strongly discouraged in the hospital or at home.

In traditional-feminist settings, compliance with legal restrictions on curatives varies considerably. Most provide paramedics the opportunity to "recommend" if not prescribe restricted substances; some slip beyond both the letter and spirit of the law restricting prescription to physicians. The need for prescription drugs is somewhat reduced, however, by the widespread acceptance of home remedies. Conditions requiring prescription drugs (for example, venereal diseases) are treated immediately, however. Physicians are usually available to prescribe, after consulting with the patient or pelvic team, although sometimes patients must return later to see a physician. Where trust between physicians and pelvic teams is high, presigned prescriptions for low-risk drugs may be available for very routine problems (for example, Mycostatin for monilia).

There is often ambivalence, however, over dispensing drugs, particularly those known to have potentially serious side effects. In some clinics, drugs stashed for dispensing are given without a physician's prescription only if paramedics are convinced the drug is extremely safe and the client is comfortable accepting it. In general, clinic workers agree that some drugs (for example, oral contraceptives, many antibiotics, Flagyl) ought to be restricted and available only after thorough examination and careful weighing of risks in relation to benefits. In short, paramedics and self-help workers tend to be more cautious and more conservative about dispensing drugs than many of their licensed medical counterparts. (For discussion of negotiating which drugs will be dispensed informally or quasi-legally in one clinic, see Peterson 1976).

Just what is or is not or should or should not be "medical practice" is, of course, open to debate. Sheldon Greenfield (involved in the paramedic training program at University of California, Los Angeles, for example, argues that looking at a woman's big belly and saying, "You're pregnant," is not diagnosing, nor is standing around giving support and advice during childbirth treatment in a medical sense (Arms 1975, p. 217). Participants in radical-feminist settings also disagree that certain other procedures should be restricted. Diaphragm prescribing and fitting, for example, is regarded as an appropriate task for laywomen to do for each other; in fact, the ultimate decision of which size to choose is believed most accurately determined by the woman who will use it.

A small minority of radical-feminist settings promote menstrual extraction. They believe that laywomen can perform this procedure competently and safely by taking standard hygienic precautions and keeping the cannula sterile prior to insertion. Menstrual extraction, most clearly an impingement on medical practice, challenges the right of both medical and legal professionals to restrict access to crucial services. Although not recommended as an abortion procedure (particularly since legal abortion is available to these women), should restrictive legislation be reinstated, menstrual extraction is obviously a simple "cure" for unwanted pregnancy. Currently, however, menstrual extraction is not offered as a service to the public; only members of advanced ongoing self-help groups may participate.

Territorial Prerogatives

The underlying morphology of time and space in medical settings, which serves to delineate status and define roles (Rosengren and DeVault 1963, pp. 270-71), is a crucial factor affecting participants' ability to assume responsibility and make decisions regarding care. How, then, in these four health care worlds, are space and time managed and utilized to aggrandize or limit the power of clients and practitioners?

Traditional-authoritarian and traditional-egalitarian health care worlds occupy physician-controlled territories: private offices, clinics, and hospitals. Within these territories, space is subdivided between workers, patients, and persons waiting for patients. Norms govern individuals' behavior while occupying specific spaces, and the first rule of medical (or any) territory is to occupy only that space allotted. In conventional settings, printed signs (for example, "Waiting Room," "Dr. X: Private," "Examining Room A," "Surgery") mark space categorically. Doors, walls, furniture (for example, high reception desks, chairs arranged in rows), frosted glass partitions, and accouterments help participants learn their proper place. "Good" patients quickly learn to observe special restrictions and meet practitioners' expectations. (See Goffman 1963 for discussion of norms governing behavior in public places, and Lorber 1975a for discussion of criteria in labeling patients good and bad.)

In examining rooms, patients-assigned spacial location—usually horizontal, not vertical—reinforces distinctions between patients and practitioners and underscores the modal dominance pattern. In gynecological examinations, stirrups and drapes divide space further, marking off the woman's pelvis as practitioners' territory and discouraging patients from observing and asking questions. A nurse, noting how this division alienates women from their bodies, adds that it also minimizes physicians' need to attend to other parts of the women.

> Here's this doctor hidden behind the sheet with the light shining. You can see the light and maybe you can see his head but you don't know what he's doing—he's just doing something very mysterious. It's completely alienating the woman from her own body. Basically it's as if she shouldn't see some part of herself—it's too horrible. Now while this keeps her from seeing herself, it also keeps him from seeing the expression on her face and having to deal with anything above her pubic bone while he's poking around down there.

Physicians, dashing from one cordoned off pelvis to another, become specialists, like other industrial workers: "It is as if the staff work on an assembly line for repairing bodies; similar body parts continually roll by and the staff have a particular job to do on them" (Emerson 1970a, p. 78).

During childbirth, women's space is further restricted in traditional-authoritarian settings by locking their arms and legs into stirrups and arm cuffs, thus immobilizing them entirely. Excluding nonmedical personnel (including spouses) from labor and/or delivery rooms further buttresses physicians' territorial prerogative.[*] Excluding husbands particularly reduces women's potential ability to retain responsibility, for in her vulnerable state, she has no one to trust to act in her behalf—no agent to protect her rights in foreign territory.[†]

---

[*]See Rosengren and DeVault 1963, Emerson 1970a, and Glaser and Strauss 1965, p. 162, for discussion of prohibitions against allowing nonmedical personnel, especially intimates, to be present during treatment or when the body is exposed.

[†]Roth 1973 argues that having an agent clearly improves the welfare of hospitalized patients. Freidl 1966 discusses how in Greek

In traditional-egalitarian settings, women are sometimes given more leeway within patient-assigned territory and have greater control over personal body space. For example, women may be allowed to observe pelvic examinations directly or with a mirror. Women awake and participating in prepared childbirth sometimes are allowed to place their feet loosely in stirrups and hold onto the delivery table without restraint; some may even be encouraged to remain upright or to squat, providing even more control over body space. Husbands may be allowed to remain with their wives through delivery, but only so long as they do not challenge staff actions.

Recently, some nurse-midwives and physicians have begun promoting home-style birth programs in hospitals as a compromise between home and hospital delivery. Women receive conventional prenatal care and are admitted to special "home birth" rooms located near conventional labor delivery services. They are encouraged to bring personal belongings and deliver with minimal medical intervention. Birth coaches, family members, and friends are allowed to remain for the birth, as long as all goes well. Infants remain with the family instead of being whisked off to nurseries (see, for example, McTigue 1977 and Lieberman 1977). These programs are very popular. Given a choice, 85 percent of the women delivering at Milwaukee's Family Hospital opt for these birth rooms ("Hospitals Bow to Couples Wanting Special Births" 1977).

Although home-style birth rooms in hospitals take on some properties of the individual woman's space—particularly when family and friends dilute the predominance of medical practitioners—these worlds can quickly be dismantled and transformed into conventional medical settings when complications arise. The ease with which the birth can be transformed into a medical event makes this alternative attractive to professionals and many patients. Other women, however, feel that their control over the situation is seriously diminished. One woman, for example, was removed from a home birth program against her wishes when her labor became protracted. A monitor, imposed upon her, indicated (mistakenly) fetal distress and gave the staff justification for further intervention. The birthing woman believed that the monitor was innacurate, as they often are, since a nurse was able to pick up a normal fetal heartbeat manually with a

---

village hospitals, patients' families watch doctors and nurses, not only to assure the patient's welfare but to serve as witnesses that the professionals have done their jobs properly.

stethescope. She bitterly resented being coerced into accepting medical intervention.*

Regardless of minor variations, women in traditional-egalitarian settings are subject to rules and regulations imposed by medical practitioners, who dominate these worlds. As clients seeking service on professionals' territory, patients play by the medical rules or risk ridicule, coercion, or even expulsion.

Traditional-feminist health clinics often operate out of old homes, flats, or storefronts that have hastily been converted into medical offices. While posters, plants, community announcements, old furniture, and homemade curtains create a warm, casual ambience, these clinics, like conventional ones, are the territory of practitioners and are managed for the workers' convenience. Nonetheless, these settings typically are more open to observation, and space is less categorically defined, in part because of limited facilities. Thus, reception desks are often out in the open in waiting areas, encouraging patients and workers to interact. Paramedics sometimes take lengthy medical "herstories" in open waiting areas. Laboratory equipment, supplies, money, drugs, and files are also frequently visible. Thus, patients have an opportunity to observe clinic procedures and develop some criteria against which to measure the treatment they receive.

During pelvic examinations, drapes are not used, so that patients can observe the work of pelvic team members, who offer detailed accounts of what they are doing and seeing. (Not all patients, however, choose to watch.) Comments on the color and appearance of the vaginal walls, the cervix, and any unusual conditions are directed toward the patient, as well as the team. Physicians, invited into the space to confirm or make a definite diagnosis, are not "waited on" as if the space belonged to them, as is common in conventional settings. When physicians perform clinic abortions, they must do so in the presence of women paramedics trained to comment on their performance; they often are observed by the patient's spouse or a friend as well. When attending home births, professionals clearly are on patient territory and are similarly subject to observation.

----

*The author has very little data on these settings and knows of no systematic studies underway. However, it is clear that the "home-style" features are provided only at the pleasure of the supervising staff and can be instantly cancelled at any time; for example, they have been cancelled in about 30 to 40 percent of the cases at Sacramento Medical Center (Gallyot 1978).

Radical-feminist settings aim to minimize spacial arrangements that reinforce distinctions between patients and practitioners. Although self-help groups often meet in women's health centers, where traditional-feminist activities are carried on at other times, self-help clinics are also held in women's centers, on college campuses, at public meetings of women's organizations, in churches, and in private homes. Menstrual extraction groups meet secretly in private homes on irregular schedules determined by the onset of members' menstrual periods. It is up to the woman whose menses are to be extracted to contact other members to share the event in a space agreeable to all. Self-help territory is thus wherever women meet to learn and share their medical knowledge.

Self-help prenatal care is offered in home birth centers operated in women's homes or women's clinics. Like traditional-feminist settings, these settings are informal and "homey," quite unlike conventional medical settings. Space is open—usually a single room, where women sit comfortably to talk as well as to be weighed and examined. Small curtained or screened off areas provide privacy when and if desired. Women birthing at home on their own territory have a better chance to make crucial decisions about how and where they will give birth—in bed, on the floor, lying down, or squatting (Arms 1975, p. 178).

Lay midwives and physicians (whom women are urged to consult for prenatal assessment) do tell women contemplating home birth that there are risks, but so are there risks in hospitals. All involved agree that most women choosing home birth assess their situation thoroughly and accept responsibility for the risks. Rather than seeing home-birthing mothers as irresponsible, physician Michael Whitt, who attends home births, believes these women are perhaps more responsible than those who abandon themselves to the "best" obstetricians (Arms 1975, pp. 194-95).

Some women who attempt to birth at home discover that they need the hospital for emotional security once labor actually begins. Arms (1975, p. 174) points out that it is difficult to know how a woman will react in labor or where she will feel safe. Some women simply cannot cope with hospitals; others are equally insecure at home; in either case, they may be unable to dilate and deliver because they are so frightened and upset.

If problems (emotional or physical) do develop at home, most lay midwives do not hesitate to transfer women to the hospital, but they try to stay with them. Of course, once in the hospital, it is difficult for women to maintain authority and retain the power to make decisions. As natural childbirth proponent Elisabeth Bing puts the problem:

> The mother who goes to the hospital to have her baby is
> in an impossible situation, really. If a doctor says he's
> doing something for the safety of her baby, there is nothing
> she can say. Once she is told a procedure is for her baby,
> she can offer no argument. If you were in a hospital and
> your obstetrician said, "Look, we are a little worried about
> your baby. We want to put you on a fetal heart monitor,"
> what would you say? I don't think a mother really has a
> choice (Arms 1975, p. 100).

Thus, unless a woman remains on her own territory, she will not
retain the power to control her birthing. The structure of health
care institutions insures that medical definitions of the situation prevail. Lay definitions are legitimate only in lay territory.

Structuring Time on Obstetrics and Gynecology

Critics argue that patients' time is undervalued in most health
care settings. While long patient waits are often attributed to unex-
pected medical emergencies, this is rarely the case. Samuels and
Bennett (1973, p. 304) point out that in most cases, the only excuse
the doctor has for making patients wait is that more appointments
are booked than can possibly be managed in the time allowed. If
some patients are late, the doctor is guaranteed a steady supply of
patients.

A major factor in overscheduling is the social status of patients. Clinic patients usually wait longer than private patients, in
part because clinics often schedule patients in blocks, instructing
several patients to come at the same time to be seen on a first-come,
first-served basis. While this simplifies scheduling for staff and
assures physicians a steady stream of patients, patients have long
waits—followed by short physician contacts.* One resident in a large
hospital who sees about 120 patients each day points out that the
clinic time frame makes personalized, humanistic care virtually
impossible. He has only two minutes allocated for regular prenatal
checkups and simply cannot talk with the women (Arms 1975, p. 253).

---

*See Shaw 1974, pp. 39-58, for a thorough discussion of how
clinic patients are made to wait, particularly when being seen by
medical students. For other data on client waiting time, see Marieskind 1976, pp. 271-75.

Private patients are more often scheduled sequentially, but too close together to allow for much deviation in time spent per patient. Consequently, private physicians often "run behind," leaving women waiting for hours. Knowing that there are dozens of others still waiting, women are especially hesitant to "take up too much of the busy doctor's time" with possibly simple, but personally important, questions and concerns.

Particularly considerate practitioners' staff may telephone patients or inform them on arrival that the doctor is behind, offering them the option to come another time for routine matters. Samuels and Bennett (1973, pp. 304-5) recommend that patients should not wait more than half an hour from their scheduled appointment and suggest that patients inform their physicians in writing that they will not wait longer than this.

Although feminist health advocates object to patients waiting time, few traditional-feminist clinics are able to improve the situation.* In fact, in some, waiting time is even longer than in conventional settings. In "walk-in" clinics, for example, women have sometimes waited from eight to ten hours to see a physician. Since most of these are free clinics, patients are unable to go elsewhere, because of low financial status or fear of moral or legal problems. (Women drug abusers, for example, may only be able to obtain contraceptives without risking arrest from free clinics.)

Some women's clinics attempt to make definite appointments but give up after too many "no-shows." No-shows are especially disruptive in clinics that emphasize information and educational "quality care." For in these clinics, 20 minutes to half an hour or a two-to-three-person pelvic team's time are commonly allocated to each patient; a no-show leaves many workers idle. Since patient slots in these clinics are usually very limited, some groups have entirely abandoned advance appointments in favor of various types of open scheduling.

Attempts to improve open scheduling are varied but are largely ineffective at reducing waiting time. Some schedule appointments earlier in the day—several hours in advance of clinic time—for persons with specific problems. Women who arrive in pain or have "priority slips" (documents from previous clinics stating they need to be seen again or were unseen because time ran out) are given

---

*Marieskind 1976, p. 273, notes that in some clinics that make appointments, the waiting time to get the appointment is shorter, however.

appointments and told approximately what time they are likely to be seen. Other women arriving at the clinic are then seen on a first-come, first-served basis. If they wish, patients may leave to attend to other matters.

Another approach is to publicize that only a specified number of appointments are offered and that registration begins at a certain time just prior to clinic opening. If one receives an appointment, she is assured of being seen; others must go elsewhere or try again for an appointment. Where women know the routine, they line up sometimes an hour before the clinic opens, stretching actual waiting time to several hours.

Clinic workers regret the inconvenience, but say that they have found no way to prevent it. Some add that women's willingness to wait, especially for well-woman routine care, is evidence of how superior their services are. Patients do not always agree, however, and sometimes express bitterness at being turned away or asked to wait so long. (For example, in one clinic a client raged so angrily at being refused a slot that a clinic worker was reduced to tears, bringing the entire clinic to a halt to console her. In another, a woman grumbled that three hours seemed a long time to wait just to have a diaphragm checked for fit.)

Although traditional-feminist clinics are unable to reduce waiting time, they often attempt to make it "useful." For example, some clinics have paramedics take detailed medical histories, or "her-stories," to elicit not only technical details about health and illness but to establish personal rapport. "Herstory" taking can consume half an hour in clinics promoting this technique as an essential component of quality medical care. After taking these lengthy "herstories," paramedics stay with the patient through the entire medical consultation and treatment—this is regarded as especially important in abortion care or where the woman is seen by a male physician. Paramedics in these settings, then, use waiting time to prepare themselves to act as advocates.

Other clinics use waiting time to offer "educationals." For example, during clinic waiting time, paramedics present information on specific topics, for example, birth control methods, vaginitis, sexuality, feminism. Clients are encouraged to "rap" and are given or may purchase mimeo sheets on health topics. Although initially quite popular in women's clinics, "educationals" are less frequently offered now because in the opinion of one clinic founder: "Now everything has been talked about, and we just focus on delivering good feminist health care."

Self-help group care in radical-feminist settings is the only delivery mode attributing equal value to the time of all participants. In these groups, waiting is eliminated; time spent observing procedures

performed on others is expected to make one more knowledgeable
and better able to care for one's self. Professionals' time in participatory clinics is not consumed by moving from cubicle to cubicle,
engaging in trivial conversation, or hurriedly repeating technical
information. Instead, professionals' time is used to oversee others'
work and offer in-depth, informed comment on medical matters, including their own assessment of recent research, clinical experience,
and personal hunches.

Patients can also recall symptoms and concerns throughout
the two-hour period, during which time valuable information—often
omitted in a hurried encounter—is revealed. In group prenatal care,
dietary habits and social and psychological factors presented by participants provide health professionals valuable information unavailable
in brief consultations. Although radical-feminist settings promote
this care as superior, some women do not wish to spend this much
time, preferring brief in-out encounters.

Managing time in obstetrical settings is especially problematic,
because babies notoriously appear at odd hours; their appearance is
invariably too fast or too slow to mesh properly with the rhythm,
tempo, and timing of conventional hospital labor delivery services.
(For discussion of the importance of timing in obstetrics, see, especially, Rosengren and DeVault 1963.) In traditional-authoritarian and
many traditional-egalitarian settings, workers attempt to make births
more temporally manageable. Using an amazing armament of drugs,
devices, and surgical procedures—analgesics, sedatives, artificial
hormones, anesthesia, episiotomy, forceps, and Caesarean section—
hospital personnel can stop, slow down, or speed up labor and delivery.
Of course, tinkering usually leads to the need for more intervention.
As pediatrician Rich Quint notes, "Once you step on the merry-go-
round of machines and western medicine, it's tough to step off" (Arms
1975, p. 96).

In the hospital Rosengren and DeVault studied, the staff noted
time involved in each delivery, and deviations from the model time
upset the delivery team, despite the fact that unusually long or rapid
deliveries might be well within the "normal" range from a strictly
medical perspective. Maintaining or working to achieve the "correct"
tempo became a matter of status and mark of professional adeptness.
Residents reputedly were able to deliver in about 50 minutes, whereas the private doctors were able to deliver in only 40 minutes (Rosengren and DeVault 1963, p. 282).

To maintain proper tempo, forceps and episiotomy are so routinely used that they are accepted as normal procedures. In the
United States, over 70 percent of the women delivering in hospitals
receive episiotomies, compared with 15 percent in England and only
8 percent in Holland; one-third of all American hospital births are

aided with forceps (Arms 1975, pp. 78, 82). To stabilize the tempo, anesthetists can hurry cases or delay them, depending on the kind and amount of anesthesia administered. Maintaining control over the flow of work is a source of pride to hospital personnel (Rosengren and DeVault 1963, p. 283).

While delaying birth may sometimes be justified as necessary—for example, when no delivery rooms are available or when the doctor is delivering another patient—it is often primarily for the physician's convenience and the maintenance of the normative division of labor. Babies can be and are (usually inadvertently) delivered in regular hospital beds or even elevators or wheelchairs with minimal assistance. Physicians, however, insist on "being there" to deliver their private patients—even if it means keeping the baby waiting. Arms reports numerous cases where labor was slowed down or even stopped so the physician could, for example, keep a luncheon date (1975, p. 205).

Although generally disapproved, holding a woman's legs together until the doctor arrives to "catch" the baby is common. That Sweeney (1973, p. 155) specifically instructs delivery room personnel not to hold babies back indicates how widespread this practice may be. Sweeney adds that holding back is particularly inexcusable because there is always someone who can take over—a detail sometimes concealed deviously and dangerously. He notes that when a patient is ready for delivery but her doctor is not there, she may be completely anesthetized (a risky procedure) and delivered by a different obstetrician. When her own doctor comes in with his white coat on, he may take some blood, smear it over him, and act as if he has just finished the delivery (Sweeney 1973, p. 155).

Some physicians have recommended transforming birth into a fully "planned event." Just prior to a woman's "due date," physicians can administer the synthetic hormone oxytocin to induce labor and shorten the early stages considerably. Proponents argue this offers many advantages besides a shortened labor. Parents can arrange for the care of their other children and schedule the time off from work. The mother can have a good sleep the night before, and the hospital staff and her doctor can be fully prepared and have no other commitments (Seligmann 1976, p. 59).

When birth is manipulated to create "nine-to-five" obstetrical practice, it minimizes inconvenience to everyone—except possibly the child. Roberto Caldeyro-Barcia, president of the International Federation of Gynecologists and Obstetricians, warns against short-cutting the natural labor period. Inducing labor increases the intensity of contractions, causing fetal oxygen deprivation, and results in added use of analgesics and anesthesia. Labor reduced below seven hours is also associated with increased risk of neurological damage and fetal death. Doris Haire (1972, p. 7) past president of the ICEA adds that according to the National Association for Retarded Children, there are 6 million retarded children and adults in the United States, with a predicted annual increase of over 100,000 a year. Recent research makes it evident that obstetrical medication plays a role in this staggering incidence of neurological impairment.

Women who receive prenatal care in traditional-egalitarian settings and prepare for natural childbirth find themselves sucked into hospital routines. Left unmedicated, women give birth when they are ready and require personal support and attention and perineal massage (to prevent tearing or the need for episiotomy)—tasks most physicians and already overworked staff are unwilling and unprepared to take on. Thus, physicians strongly advocating natural childbirth struggle with their patients against the demands of medical institutions. Natural childbirth patients, in fact, are so pressured to fit into hospital routines that few escape without considerable medication and intervention (Arms 1975, pp. 138-50).

Even nurse-midwives rarely have the time—or the temperament—to offer the personal care some believe desirable. For example, at Kings County Hospital in New York, the contemporary model and showcase for American nurse-midwifery, medication is not administered routinely to mothers during normal labor and delivery.[*] Yet even here, time pressures lead the staff to intervene. Margaret Strickhouser, attending nurse-midwife, believes that there is too much interference—too many vaginal exams, rupturing of membranes at five-centimeters dilation, routine use of IVs with glucose, routine Pitocin after delivery (Arms 1975, p. 252).

Some nurse-midwives feel their time is too valuable to warrant continuous supportive care, arguing that it does not make sense to assign someone who has had lengthy training and is making $12,000 to $13,000 per year to one patient for a whole day (Arms 1975, p. 252). Others disagree, but believe nurse-midwives should attend women at home rather than in the hospital or, as a compromise, in special birth centers that are separate from hospital labor delivery services. G. J. Klooseterman, chief of obstetrics at the famous Wilhelmina teaching hospital in Amsterdam, is an outspoken proponent of home delivery. He believes midwives, however, are more suitable birth

---

[*]Initially a hospital largely serving Brooklyn's immigrant population (95 percent nonwhite), Kings County now attracts a growing number of maternity patients from middle-class and wealthy areas who want an undrugged, midwife-attended birth.

attendants than physicians because home birth is so time consuming
(Arms 1975, p. 288).

Participants in radical-feminist settings feel that most nurse-
midwives are not interested in attending home deliveries because they
disapprove and/or fear losing their licenses. They also feel that lay
midwives are more suited to managing home birth, for they, unlike
professionals, operate on a different time frame. Rather than viewing midwifery as a full-time occupation, a job, or a task to be completed as quickly as possible, lay midwives look forward to births as
meaningful, spiritual life-events to experience and enjoy. The long
hours spent with laboring women are rewarding and satisfying because
of the "birth energy"; they are not draining, as are long hours worked
in a frenetic hospital delivery service.

A major difference in temporal orientation in home versus
hospital or professional compared with lay obstetrical management
derives from fiscal considerations. Nancy Mills, a well-known California lay midwife, recalls a lunch with an obstetrician who repeated at
least ten times, "Time is money." Seeing how important money was
to him, she doubts he can offer quality care, for in childbirth, attendants must patiently listen, talk, and "be there." While she believes doctors do deserve respect, admiration, and money comparable
to what they do, their contribution is blown way out of proportion
(Arms 1975, p. 170).

Lay midwives wish to be paid, but they have no desire to make
midwifery especially lucrative. Many believe that it should not just
be offered as a commercial service, for midwifery is a calling for
dedicated, spiritual women working in concert with like-minded patients. Rejecting the values of the cash-nexus society, many midwives
are counterculture people. But many others are quite conventional
middle-class suburbanites. One 40-year-old woman, a high school
teacher's wife who keeps her midwifery secret from relatives and
neighbors, has never charged money but often receives gifts. She
states that money just does not matter to her (Arms 1975, pp. 196-97).
Others refuse to accept fees to protect themselves from being charged
with practicing medicine without a license.

DEFINING AND ASSIGNING RISK

Proponents of each of the health care worlds argue that they
minimize risks. However, not everyone shares a common definition
of what is or is not a risk, including possible death. The closer one
comes to the traditional-authoritarian end of the continuum, the greater
the effort to promise risk-free care and preserve life at any cost.
That practitioners in these settings succeed is dubious. Haire (1975,

p. 33) points out that although large, university-affiliated hospital delivery services have long been touted as the safest place to give birth, a recent national survey conducted by the ACOG reveals that in general, the larger the obstetric service and the stronger the affiliation between the obstetric service and a medical school, the greater the rate of infant and maternal deaths. While some of these deaths are due to a greater incidence of high-risk mothers in larger teaching hospitals, the greater tendency to intervene in the normal process of labor and birth in these institutions in order to provide teaching opportunities may contribute to these statistics and may also result in a disproportionately high incidence of neurologically damaged children.

Similarly, radical mastectomy, which has been pressed on women to save their lives, often does not. Women whose cancer has spread to the lymph nodes have a five-year survival rate of 50 percent; the ten-year survival rate is only 25 percent. With new forms of chemotherapy, however, survival rates are expected to rise (Switzer 1976, p. 164; for detailed information on survival rates, see Levin et al. 1974). Even women who physically survive may be psychologically scarred—sometimes to the point that being alive is hardly better than death (see, for example, Shinder 1972).

That practitioners in these settings "succeed" or "fail," however, is not the issue here. What is important is that the value and belief in the possibility of preserving life underlies conventional physicians' reliance on—or more accurately their dependence on— technology that they believe will preserve life. For it is in part their belief that preserving life is possible and desirable that leads physicians to subject women indiscriminately to elaborate technology "just in case." Worshipping at the altar of science and technology, traditional physicians unquestioningly accept tenets of practice that lead them to express rather odd views. Fred Ostermann, a San Francisco obstetrician, for example, has stated: "If you tied 95 percent of women in labor to a tree in Golden Gate Park, the baby would fall out. ... But I would never do a home delivery because it wouldn't be safe" (Arms 1975, p. 174).

But "safety"—or even preventing death—is not always most valued by participants in radical-feminist settings (at the other end of the health care continuum). Rather, creating health care settings that support important life values takes precedence over other considerations. Thus, the desire to be independent, to learn to care for oneself, and to accept responsibility for mistakes encourages women to fit their own diaphragms, decide on a treatment for breast cancer, or participate in menstrual extraction groups. That one might fit the diaphragm incorrectly, choose minimal surgery and die shortly thereafter, or suffer an infection are, of course, possible. But while women are chided by traditional professionals for taking such risks, all kinds of problems and unintended consequences of treatment in traditional settings are simply accepted as "normal trouble." As anthropologist and childbirth commentator Lester Hazell points out, our society will not hold it against anyone whose baby is palsied or has intelligence stunted by too much anesthesia in the hospital, but if a child is born at home with a birthmark or club foot, the fault will be the parents' (Arms 1975, p. 208).

Accepting that there are inherent risks in any health care service, proponents of alternative settings seek to create environments that are conducive to health and well-being in holistic terms. But promoting well-being or nurturing quality of life is difficult for professionals to understand, let alone advocate, for they are enmeshed in institutions designed to ensure "safety" in technical terms. As Arms (1975, p. 105) points out, for some women, the establishment of immediate contact with their young and the opportunity to provide immediate nurture (for example, putting the baby to the breast before the umbilical cord has been severed) are more important than possible risk to the baby from a cold delivery room. They feel they are minimizing safety risks, while maximizing quality of life. However, the doctor and hospital staff—who feel they are there primarily to ensure safety—believe the mother is indulging an emotional whim that may endanger her child's health.

While participants in conventional institutions attempt to avoid any death and try to convince women that death in the hospital is only remotely possible, participants in radical-feminist settings particularly organized for childbirth accept possible death. Some in fact argue that death in birth is divinely ordained and not to prevented by artificial means. One mother pointed out after a home birth that

> we talked about risk. I knew that I or the baby could die. We decided the benefits of home birth were worth the risk. When my baby was born, she lay in a kind of primordial state before she cried. I thought she was dead and I accepted it. She cried then (Edwards 1973, pp. 1332-33).

Nonetheless, the risks of home birth—especially the risk of death—is largely exaggerated. Home birth attended by nurse-midwives or even experienced by lay midwives is far safer than most physicians admit, as long as the mother has had proper prenatal care. For example, the Frontier Nursing Service in Kentucky, which has offered nurse-midwifery to a high-risk, malnourished birthing population for many years, has an excellent record of no maternal deaths and few babies with respiratory problems (Arms 1975, pp. 184-85).

Recent studies indicate that for low-risk mothers, home birth may be as safe or even safer than hospital delivery. Hazell's (1975) study of 300 home births in the San Francisco Bay area attended by the father or lay midwives revealed no maternal deaths and generally favorable infant outcomes. Other studies have revealed similarly low rates of complications in supervised home births.[*] Physician Lewis Mehl reports that in 1,146 consecutive home births he studied, low complication rates compared favorably with 200 similar women's hospital births attended by the same practitioners (1976). Mehl and his colleagues (1975) also found no major differences in outcome when experienced lay midwives, as compared to family physicians, supervised home deliveries.

Studies of complication rates in menstrual extraction groups are currently underway by FWHCs. Preliminary statements issued at the 1974 Menstrual Extraction Conference claim that in the 30 menstrual extraction groups functioning, there have been no reports of major infections; one minor infection, possibly related to period extraction; and no perforations. Four women carried pregnancies to term after participating in menstrual extraction, suggesting that cervical incompetency (premature opening of the cervix) is not the hazard from extraction that some claim.

Nonetheless, concern remains over actual complication rates. Ephron (1975, pp. 112-13) reports that in 1971, a pregnant woman who had aborted with a menstrual extractor developed an infection and had to be hospitalized for a dilation and curettage. A feminist reporter covering the incident decided not to publicize the infection because she felt it could hurt the self-help movement.[†] Of course, minimizing publicity about possible complications is commonly accepted in traditional medical circles, particularly when problems are regarded as "rare occurrences." Clearly, what hazards are regarded as reportable incidents depend on the subjective definition of the groups and individuals involved.

Increasingly, physicians themselves acknowledge that their values may not be the same as their patients. Speaking primarily about the need for alternative birth settings, but also about health

---

[*]See Mehl 1977, pp. 35-40, for a detailed analysis of home birth research and complication rates.

[†]Frankfort referred to this incident at the "Medical Mystique" Symposium in San Francisco in March 1973. I have not been able to locate any other reports of serious complications.

care in general, Milton Silverman notes that in both birth and death, the question is how far we are willing to depart from the natural process, to use elaborate technology just to protect against potential risk. The agonizing experience of making difficult decisions is part of life; yet today, we attempt to avoid experiencing parts of life by laying down blanket rules about what is and what is not an acceptable risk (Arms 1975, pp. 113-14).

Women's health movement activists feel that the poor record of the medical profession in protecting women's health and welfare suggests that laywomen can just as competently evaluate the risks and make decisions about their own care; they can be "well-informed citizens." In traditional-authoritarian settings, this alternative is virtually impossible. There is more leeway in traditional-egalitarian settings. Some suggest that traditional-feminist settings offer the safety and surety of modern medical science combined with humanistic care; however, these services are still limited and available to relatively few women. Proponents of radical-feminist settings argue that their services can be made widely available. Furthermore, laywomen are as competent as medical professionals—or more competent—to perform basic care; medical professionals malign these efforts out of self-interest, not true concern for safety.

Health activists also recognize that not all women desire the same degree of autonomy and responsibility in their own health care. Given differences among feminists themselves, strategies for restructuring routine health care and invoking access to these health care settings are varied and aim to alter different aspects of the health care system—issues examined in the next chapter.

6

Strategies For Change

Health movement activists, concerned over the quality of care in conventional health settings, have developed a wide range of strategies for restructuring care. This chapter examines key strategies to alter the quality, quantity, content, and control of obstetrical and gynecological services on the societal level, institutional level, and in face-to-face interaction with professionals. Changes on all levels are viewed by activists as necessary and interrelated, for what a woman experiences in any encounter with the health care system is the consequence of how a complex array of interlocking values, beliefs, practices, and institutional arrangements mesh with her identity and personal position in the social structure.

Significantly, despite widespread belief among health activists that a humanistic health care system available to all women is virtually impossible to create under profit-oriented capitalism, none of the strategies directly attack the underlying economic organization of society. Instead, major efforts are directed toward removing control of obstetrics and gynecology from men and developing mechanisms for making professionals accountable to the consumer, women. Although re-establishing female authority in health may not be sufficient to provide women with the type of care they desire, it is seen as a necessary first step. Given the exigencies of combating male dominance, health activists have devised coping strategies for managing—rather than eliminating—the medical profit system. Many actions are thus designed to persuade medical practitioners, politicians, the drug industry, and regulatory agencies that it is "good business" to practice in accordance with feminist principles of self-determination and freedom of choice. Feminists argue ideologically that as they gain power, they will be able to effect more fundamental changes.

Health movement strategies for restructuring routine care can also be viewed as actions with the potential to deinstitutionalize medical authority, to transform authority relationships between patients and practitioners. Rather than relying on institutionalized professional authority, the professional would have to establish his or her authority by presenting persuasive evidence—a form resembling collegial or scientific authority.

This chapter describes strategies commonly used to improve health care and analyzes their potential to deinstitutionalize medical authority by (1) reducing the knowledge differential between patient and practitioner, (2) challenging the license and mandate of physicians to provide certain services, (3) reducing professionals' control and monopoly over related necessary goods and services, (4) altering the size of the profession relative to potential clientele, and (5) transforming the clientele from an aggregate into a collectivity.[*]

HEALTH MOVEMENT ORGANIZATIONS

Since 1969, when the first body courses were organized, feminist health organizations have proliferated.[†] By 1973, Rennie and Grimsted (1973) identified 35 health projects and 116 women's centers (many including health programs) in the United States. The Los Angeles FWHC reported that 48 feminist women's health clinics were in operation by 1976 (Farber 1976); 30 menstrual extraction groups were active (L. Brown 1975). A nationwide survey conducted by the Women's Health Forum-HealthRight in 1974 identified over 1,200 women's groups that were providing various types of health services, as well as tens of thousands of individuals who considered themselves to be active participants in the women's health movement (Marieskind 1975a, p. 218). Cowan (1977, pp. 45-52) lists 416 groups, including clinics, counseling centers, rape control organizations, rights groups, and professional associations involved in feminist health work. Women's health groups were also active throughout Europe, Canada, Australia, and New Zealand, and activities in Latin America were increasing.[‡] In June 1970, the International Women's

---

[*]As indicated in Chapter 1, these are all structural aspects of institutionalized authority.

[†]Names and addresses of major organizations are listed in Appendix C.

[‡]The effort to make the women's health movement international has come largely from self-help proponents. See "Feminist Women's Health Center Report" 1974, 1975, and Stephen 1974.

Health Conference in Rome drew participants from feminist groups in more than 20 countries ("Network Hotline" 1977, p. 6). (See Appendix C for names and addresses of such organizations.)

Most health movement organizations concentrate on the production and dissemination of information, lobbying or working through established channels to change the structure of the health care system, or offering direct services. A few organizations engage in all three types of activities. Health groups that provide direct services most frequently offer one or more of the following: (1) health education and "consciousness raising"; (2) referral; (3) patient advocacy; (4) routine gynecological care; (5) routine obstetrical care; and (6) abortion. A few groups offer extended primary care in neighborhood clinics. Although feminist psychotherapy groups are growing, typically they are separate from women's health clinics.*

Because this is a study of a specific social movement, rather than movement organizations, the focus is on strategies and tactics employed rather than on internal organizational structure. However, some organizations—particularly local clinics or self-help groups—operate collectively; others have more hierarchical structures. Even those that are collectively organized typically resort to some form of committee, task force, or rotating assignment plan to accomplish work. For example, the FWHCs are organized into colloms—a term used to describe a work group that functions as a cross between a collective and a committee.[†]

The major general feminist organizations—Women's Equity Action League (WEAL) and NOW—both engage in health-related activities but are not in the health movement's vanguard. WEAL's committee on health was established in 1976 only after women's health was a national issue attracting the attention of academics and the federal government. NOW's Task Force on Health and Reproduction was active early on abortion, and local chapters have expanded concern

---

*Feminist therapy is an important aspect of health care for women, but it is beyond the scope of this book. I have excluded it not only for practical reasons but because structurally it emerged as part of the radical or antipsychiatry movement. See, for example, Smith and David 1975; The Feminist Counseling Collective 1975; Rush 1973; and Rush and Mander 1974, for overviews of feminist psychotherapy.

[†]For health movement discussion over the need for collectivity versus hierarchy, see Downer 1974b; "FWHC Response" 1974; Hornstein 1974a, 1974b; "What is 'Feminist Health'?" 1974.

to other health issues. However, HealthRight—an influential group—
has criticized the national leadership for failing to make health issues
a priority. Specifically, HealthRight charged that NOW has refused
to emphasize health in public workshops and has failed to provide
support or recognition for local chapters' health work ("Conferences,
NOW or Later" 1975-76, p. 4).

Health movement organizations constituted primarily to produce and disseminate health information include the Boston Women's
Health Book Collective, the Women's Health Forum-HealthRight,
New Moon Communications, the National Women's Health Network,
and the San Francisco Women's Health Center. Others, including
NARAL and established abortion-related organizations, along with
newer groups—for example, the Coalition for the Medical Rights of
Women and the Women's Health Action Movement (WHAM)—concentrate
on demonstrating, lobbying, and working through established channels
to change the structure and content of the health system. The largest,
most active organizations providing both direct services and other
activities are the nationally affiliated FWHCs. The National Women's
Health Coalition (NWHC) is now inactive. The FWHC clinics emphasize self-help and women-controlled health services that minimize
professional domination. The NWHC operated within the traditional
medical-professional model, relying heavily on "experts" to set
policy and provide services. Within the women's health movement,
the FWHC is often said to be "too radical," while the NWHC was accused of not only being reformist but as being a "front" for the male
medical establishment (including USAID which supports fertility re-
duction programs to encourage modernization and industrialization,
Planned Parenthood, and other powerful population control groups).
Other direct service groups are generally independent, locally organized operations.*

STRATEGIES TO ALTER HEALTH CARE WITHIN
THE MEDICAL-PROFESSIONAL MODEL

Many health movement activities are designed to improve
quality of care and increase women's authority and responsibility
without challenging the appropriateness of professionals providing
routine services. And as already indicated, none of these strategies
directly attacks the economic organization of society—a step many

---

*Direct service organizations are listed in Appendix C.

believe to be essential. While these strategies might be termed reformist rather than radical, I believe the distinction oversimplifies the reality. For many reforms can significantly alter the structure of medical practice, with far-reaching consequences for women's health care. Furthermore, even were society socialized (as most politically oriented activists argue is necessary) or routine care placed under laywomen's control (as self-help proponents, esepcially, insist is crucial), many problems would remain: the hierarchical sex stratification of the overall medical system; sexist attitudes of physicians and researchers; patient ignorance; insulation of professionals from observability and accountability; regulation of reproductive technology; development of natalist policies; access to services; payment systems; and mechanics of adjudicating grievances.* Many reforms are intended to alleviate problems as a first, not necessarily final, step in changing the health system.

Strategies to reform existing institutions by improving or expanding the quality of health care available to women include education for patients, practitioners, and lawmakers; lobbying and legislative efforts; judicial measures; selective utilization of practitioners and institutions; and confrontation and direct pressure tactics.

Education

Women's ignorance about their own bodies and the health system are real barriers to obtaining quality care. Feminists work to eliminate this barrier by organizing health discussion groups and body courses and by producing health literature. Although the Boston Women's Health Book Collective's sourcebook, Our Bodies, Ourselves, is the best-known product of such groups, many others have produced health literature. The Vancouver, B.C., Women's Health Collective, for example, extensively surveyed local women's health needs and analyzed the Canadian health system (A Woman's Place 1972). A Colorado group published a self-health handbook (Ziegler and Campbell 1973). Members of the San Francisco Women's Health Center have produced pamphlets on breast care, vaginal infections, basic

---

*For discussion of some issues in socialized medical systems, see, for example, Macintyre 1977, Roth 1977a, and Stacey 1976 on Great Britain; Record 1974, Sidel 1975, and Sidel and Sidel 1974 on China; Field 1961, 1967 on the USSR; Weinerman 1969 on Czechoslovakia, Hungary, and Poland; and Ben-David 1958 on Israel.

gynecological examination, contraception, and diaphragm fitting and have made a film demonstrating cervical, bimanual, and breast examination. The Los Angeles FWHC has also produced a film, New Image of Myself, available in English, French, and Spanish to introduce self-help gynecology. The Berkeley Women's Health Collective (1972) booklet, Feeding Ourselves, emphasizes nutrition, food preparation, and special needs of pregnant women and infants. The Health Organizing Collective of the New York Women's Health and Abortion Project has also published a series on routine health problems, including VD and vaginitis, and "The Gynecological Check-Up," designed to educate women to evaluate routine examinations. (The checklist is reprinted in Frankfort 1972, pp. 243-50). Self-help groups distribute a wide range of literature, including organizing instructions for similar groups. The Los Angeles FWHC is currently completing an extensive self-care book.* By 1973, simple nonsexist health material was proliferating so rapidly that one activist grumbled: "I don't understand why women want to keep reinventing the wheel."

While some material is repetitive—often produced from direct self-observation and other groups' pamphlets—gathering information and writing offers a focus for women wishing to work together. Furthermore, health activists often take the view that derived knowledge, of the type available in medical texts and journals, is suspect. So body course and self-help group participants believe that their self-observations and individual investigations are needed to improve the quality of information available. The FWHC self-help book, for example, will include 32 pages of color photographs of normal cervical changes throughout the entire menstrual cycle. The authors state that this information has never appeared in a medical textbook ("The Book" 1977). And certainly, the prospect of assembling something potentially as successful as Our Bodies, Ourselves has motivated women to channel their energy into developing health material for themselves and each other.

Many health and body courses initially emphasized discussion and reading, but instruction in cervical self-examination (without other features of self-help) is now commonly offered in many basic health courses. In these courses, women learn basic female anatomy and physiology and discuss symptoms of vaginal infections, early pregnancy, VD, and contraceptive methods. Abortion, childbearing, and menopause are discussed in groups when participants choose to

---

*For lists of available self-help material see the "Feminist Women's Health Center Report" 1975.

pursue these topics. Generally, the goal is to teach women to rely more on themselves for assessing their health needs and to prepare women to utilize the health care system more effectively.

Unlike conventional "health-education" courses taught in schools by the Red Cross or childbirth educators, feminist body courses are focused consciousness-raising groups designed to shake women's acceptance of conventional medicine. Although groups vary considerably in how far they question the medical profession, all emphasize women's right and responsibility to make decisions about their own care. And they encourage women to question professionals and refuse services found unacceptable.

Like the cognitive restructuring women undergo in women's liberation consciousness-raising groups (Carden 1974; Freeman 1975; Hole and Levine 1971; Mitchell 1973, pp. 61-63), participants in body courses and self-help groups redefine personal health problems as shared problems stemming from the medical system rather than from individual weakness or culpability. Thus, contraceptive failure, botched abortions, and "unnatural childbirth" need not be viewed only as personal failures or misfortunes but as problems stemming from the oppressed condition of women in patriarchal society. Women then gradually learn that individual solutions are insufficient to improve the health care available, even to those who can afford "the best." For "the best" American medicine is often pernicious—an issue discussed along with the latest "hazards" and suggestions on how to organize for change.

Other groups organize public events directed toward the average woman, who is neither a committed feminist nor very knowledgeable about the conditions of women's health. These programs are typically panel discussions or presentations on broad health issues. The Baltimore Chapter of NOW, for example, distributes a kit on how to organize such programs. Based on its own successful health program, Baltimore NOW suggests a pediatrician present information on early adolescence, an obstetrician-gynecologist speak on "the reproductive years," and another on "the mature years." A clinical psychologist is recommended to speak on mental health. The Baltimore women invited only women clinicians to speak to honor women professionals and to provide role models to young girls contemplating career choices. The rationale for these suggestions is that having only women is a way to avoid a hostile, adversary atmosphere and make women in the audience feel more comfortable about asking questions (Baltimore Chapter NOW 1973, p. 2).

Reaching a wider public is also accomplished through feminist films. Films such as Taking Our Bodies Back, Health-Caring from Our End of the Speculum, New Image of Myself, and Self-Health are shown not only to feminist groups, community organizations, and public conferences but also in university classes.[*]

From the movement's earliest days, making information and health material available was a high priority. The Monthly Extract, founded in 1972, was expressly intended to provide a communication network and means for spreading information. By 1974, women attending the Second Women-Controlled Women's Health Center Conference in Ames, Iowa, discussed the need for a more effective informational clearinghouse and distribution system. Such a need was felt in other branches of the health movement as well, and the Our Bodies, Ourselves Fund provided a $15,000 grant to the New York Women's Health Forum to start HealthRight, a newsletter covering information of interest to the health movement's disparate segments (Hirsch 1974-75, pp. 4-5). Beginning publication in fall of 1974, HealthRight has provided ongoing coverage, but the need for systematic compliation of burgeoning information remained. With a small grant from the Ms. Foundation, the Washington-based National Women's Health Network established a national clearinghouse on women's health material. In addition, the group publishes Network News—an up-to-date newsletter on women's health issues and political action.

Educational efforts also have been directed toward medical personnel in both conventional and alternative settings. The NWHC, in cooperation with its medical advisory board (including Sadja Goldsmith, Malcolm Potts, Edward Stim, and Harvey Karman), adopted a "Patient's Bill of Rights" and a medical protocol for early termination abortion. Over 25,000 copies of the "Bill of Rights" and "Atraumatic Termination of Pregnancy" pamphlets were distributed in the United States and Canada between 1973 and 1974. Invited to participate in the 1973 annual meeting of the American Association of Planned Parenthood Physicians, the NWHC distributed professional education kits on atraumatic abortion from an official exhibition booth and spoke as panel members (National Women's Health Coalition 1974).

With foundation grants, the NWHC organized a series of one- and two-day conferences for physicians and allied professionals beginning in April 1973. The conferences, held in cooperation with university departments of obstetrics and gynecology in Los Angeles, Boston, Kansas City, and Houston, introduced physicians to atraumatic abortion techniques and raised related questions involving the psychological, legal and social problems surrounding abortion. In cooperation

---

[*]See Cowan 1977, p. 44, for titles, purchase, and rental information.

with women's groups in Vermont, New Hampshire, Massachusetts, Pennsylvania, Florida, Illinois, Colorado, Texas, and California, similar but smaller workshops were held. By early 1974, over 1,500 physicians and allied health workers had participated in these conferences (National Women's Health Coalition 1974; "Well Women Clinics Are Wave of Future" 1973).

Physician-training programs are offered by other groups, too. The FWHC's physician-training program began in 1973 in order to provide clinical training in early vacuum aspiration abortion in woman-controlled settings. The six-day course, available at FWHCs in Oakland, Los Angeles, and Santa Ana, costs $1,000 and covers orientation to woman-controlled care, clinical instruction, and supervised practice and evaluation (Feminist Women's Health Center n.d.a). Thus far, only six physicians have been trained in Los Angeles; a recent grant will expand the training program (Peskin 1976).

Other women's health group teams demonstrate self-examination in nursing and medical schools. Feminists with the Women's Community Health Center in Cambridge, Massachusetts, have taught gynecological self-help and pelvic examination, along with the regular teaching staff of a local medical school. Although a few other medical schools have trained graduate students to act as "simulated patients," this was perhaps the first group of nonprofessional women trained in self-help actually to co-teach and serve as models for both pelvic and breast examinations. Intended to replace the usual anesthetized patient or prostitute hired to give medical students experience at performing gynecological examinations, the feminist pelvic teams pointed out that having a consenting, participating well-woman pelvic model taught doctors how to deal with women as people. Their goal was to demystify the gynecological exam to student health professionals and instruct students in how to perform effective pelvic exams incurring minimum discomfort to patients. They also taught techniques to encourage dialogue between woman and doctor, emphasizing the importance of a nonhierarchical atmosphere in putting participants at ease (Norsigian 1975-76, p. 6).

The Women's Community Health Center agreement with the teaching hospitals specified that women always work in pairs, that no more than eight students be allowed per session, and that a woman could have no more than five pelvics performed on her in a session, for which she would be paid $25. Medical schools were also required to purchase and distribute to each student packets of instructional materials prepared by the health center, as well as copies of Our Bodies, Ourselves (Norsigian 1975-76, p. 6).

The dialogue and free discussion possible with an instructor-model allowed students to discuss ambivalence about performing pelvic examinations; male students reported that this made them feel more confident they would be able to talk with women patients. Proponents suggested that possibly the most important aspect was that the instructor-model taught students to expect and welcome the active participation of women patients (Norsigian 1975-76, p. 6; Women's Community Health Center 1976).

However, difficulties over distinctions between professional providers and consumers proved insurmountable. The initial program was discontinued in 1976 and revised to clarify the self-help concept. Participants are now limited to women, for self-help means reciprocal sharing, and men cannot share in a pelvic examination. The Pelvic Teaching Group now strongly discourages women's groups from participating in similar programs unless the self-help approach is maintained (Women's Community Health Center 1976).

Influencing Legislation and Public Policy

In the tradition of women's rights organizations, many groups take political action to improve or expand availability of services. Some groups, such as NARAL, continue to work through legislative channels to influence abortion-related legislation on the national level. NARAL's "Legislative Alert" provides up-to-date commentary on pending bills and urges cámpaigns to influence legislators. NARAL does more, however, than urge members to write their representatives. It tallies the volume of pro- and antiabortion mail key members of Congress receive, directing supporters to attempt to influence potential "swing votes." Letters from professionals are especially requested on the grounds that their prestige provides needed political clout (see, for example, NARAL "Legislative Alert!!!" 1976). NARAL also publicizes politicians' voting records on abortion legislation during national election campaigns.

Other health movement groups, some affiliated with larger women's rights organizations, focus on specific health reforms amenable to legislative action on the national, state, and local level. NOW's focus on abortion has already been discussed. WEAL's recent involvement in health primarily stresses need for progressive legislation in the areas of occupational health and safety and in national health insurance plans. WEAL specifically calls for insurance coverage of both reproductive and general health needs, including birth control and maternity and infant care, not only in hospitals but also in free-standing clinics and home delivery. Also supported are provision of more services for elderly women and direct reimbursement for primary health care providers other than physicians. Despite initial reluctance to take a stand on abortion, WEAL now opposes modification of the 1973 Supreme Court decision (WEAL 1976).

The Washington, D.C.-based Women's Legal Defense Fund works within the NIH to improve protection of human subjects in medical research—particularly obstetrics and gynecology. In 1974 the New York City chapter of the Committee to End Sterilization Abuse (CESA) and other women's and Third World community organizations developed guidelines to regulate elective female sterilizations in New York City public hospitals. The proposed guidelines specified a thirty day waiting period between signing a surgical consent form and performing the operation. Also required were full discussion of the operation's risks and benefits, signing the consent in the presence of a witness of the patient's choosing, and prohibition against sterilization of women under twenty-one years of age. The guidelines were accepted in November 1975 by the New York City Health and Hospitals Corporation and finally incorporated into the city Health Code, thus making private as well as public physicians and clinics adhere to the guidelines (Stamm and Williamson 1978). The Coalition Against Sterilization Abuse (CASA), formed in 1976 to ensure that liberal New York City sterilization guidelines are implemented, supports making the guidelines state law. CASA also urges congressional hearings to investigate and monitor sterilization abuse in the United States, promotes public disclosure of corporate interests behind Planned Parenthood and other population control organizations, and calls for termination of Department of Health, Education and Welfare-funded sterilization programs in Puerto Rico ("Regional Reports, New York City" 1976b).

The Women's Lobby, a national feminist organization with affiliates in 40 states, researches women's issues and testifies before congressional committees on the effects of proposed legislation. Although focusing primarily on economic issues, the Women's Lobby recently fought to defeat numerous abortion amendments in Congress, as well as bills to prohibit use of federal funds for abortion-related services. The Women's Lobby also worked on passage of the Health Manpower Assistance Act, outlawing sex discrimination in federally funded medical and dental schools ("Who Speaks for Women in Washington?" n.d.).

Major efforts are now underway to influence the design of national health insurance. In June 1974, Carol Burris, president of the Women's Lobby, testified before the U.S. House of Representatives Committee on Ways and Means. Burris outlined women's health needs typically unmet by private insurance plans and argued that most national health insurance proposals fall short of meeting these needs. While supporting many features of the Kennedy-Mills bill, Burris opposed provisions imposing deductibles, cost sharing, means tests, and continuation of the traditional role of private insurance—provisions also common to other bills under consideration. The Women's

Lobby particularly decries failure to emphasize preventive care and consumer representation. The Kennedy-Mills bill, for example, which excludes coverage to persons earning less than $400 a year, students, institutionalized persons, or persons working less than 25 hours a week, clearly discriminates against women. According to 1971 Labor Department figures, 32.3 percent of white American women and 28.9 percent of minority women work less than the 25 hours a week minimum; many of these women head families. Of all the proposals, the Griffiths-Corman bill, a health program, not just an insurance plan, was cited as the only proposal establishing health care as a right without economic deterrents to utilization of preventive and screening services—features of particular importance to women (Burris 1974).*

In response to the FDA's failure to take action on IUDs, in August 1974 several San Francisco health and consumer rights groups founded the Coalition for the Medical Rights of Women to fight for regulation on the state level. Founding groups included the American Friends Service Committee Feminist Health Project, Black Women Organized for Action, Patient Education Research Project, San Francisco Consumer Action, San Francisco Interagency Pregnancy Council, and the Western Regional NOW. The Coalition, financed by small grants from the Laras Philanthropic Foundation, the Cambium Fund, and Vanguard Foundation, has a full-time coordinator and is represented in legal action by Public Advocates and Equal Rights Advocates, two public-interest law firms. The Coalition is directed by a nine-member steering committee, with standing committees working on current issues, such as IUDs, DES, and sterilization ("Coalition for the Medical Rights of Women" 1975; Silverman 1976; Stephen 1975).

The Coalition works primarily with the state Department of Health and local health agencies but also directs attention toward the FDA and national drug companies. An issue-oriented organization, the Coalition researches and circulates information, testifies at public hearings, and petitions government bodies to improve laws and regulations governing medical services.

Health movement organizations differing greatly in structure, style, and constituency do work together on legislative efforts. For

---

*For analysis of issues involved in recent national health insurance proposals, see also Lewis 1976 and Teixera 1976. For discussion of other issues in financing reproductive health services, see especially Muller and Jaffe 1972 and Muller, Krasner, and Jaffe 1975.

example, in April 1975, women attending the Boston Women's Health Conference formed a DES Caucus to protest the widespread misuse of the morning-after pill. In three days, over 1,000 women signed a petition, organized demonstrations in Boston and Washington, D.C., and sent a delegation to Washington to visit congressional offices, the National Cancer Institute, and the FDA (Fatt 1975b).

Lobbying efforts centered around the Kennedy bill, which called for a one-year moratorium on distribution of the morning-after pill so studies of safety and efficacy could be undertaken. The Caucus also insisted on informed consent of patients before the drug was prescribed. Tentative plans were made for demanding feminist control of all research relating to drugs and devices used by woman (Fatt 1975b).

The national effort on DES was organized during the previous few years by Carol Downer and other members of the FWHCs, Belita Cowan, who testified as a DES expert before the U.S. Senate, and Kay Weiss of Advocates for Medical Information, and the Coalition for the Medical Rights of Women. Numerous local health groups participated as well. By the end of April, demonstrations and press conferences were held in seven other cities (Fatt 1975b).

Increasingly, health movement groups work jointly to influence policy and legislation on a range of issues. For example, during the Democratic National Convention in New York City on July 13, 1976, WHAM, a coalition of women's health groups, health workers, educators, and consumers, demonstrated with a march and a rally. Hoping to influence the Democratic national platform (and subsequent legislation), approximately 500 women and men attended the demonstration, which focused on abortion, day care, sterilization abuse, unnecessary surgery, unsafe drugs and devices, child and maternal health problems, and cutbacks in social services ("Regional Reports, New York City" 1976a; "WHAM Will Demonstrate on Women's Health Issues at Democratic Convention" 1976).

Nonetheless, despite effective action on specific health issues, feminist health influences on federal health legislation, policy planning, and regulatory agencies is sporadic and fragmented (Cowan 1976b, p. 4). To coordinate federal policy efforts, health activists, including Barbara Seaman, Mary Howell, Alice Wolfson, Phyllis Chesler, and Belita Cowan, founded the National Women's Health Lobby late in 1975. Conceived as a national coalition to monitor pending federal health legislation, FDA and congressional health subcommittee hearings, Department of Health, Education and Welfare regulations, and federal research on women's health problems, the founders sought a broad-based membership of 3,000 to 5,000 women and women's groups (Cowan 1976a, 1976b; Norsigian 1976).

On December 15, 1975, the newly formed National Women's Health Network held its first demonstration—a memorial funeral service in front of the FDA to commemorate the thousands of women who had died from estrogen-related complications. Speakers discussed the hazards of estrogen in various forms (oral contraceptives, the morning-after pill, DES, and estrogen replacement therapy) and condemned the FDA for negligence in failing to protect the public. The main speaker, Jim Luggen, delivered a eulogy for his wife, Dona Jean Walter, who had recently died of a pill-related pulmonary embolism. J. Richard Crout, director of the Bureau of Drugs, attended and spoke briefly, defending the FDA's actions. The demonstration drew about 100 people and was covered in the national media (Norsigian 1976).

The next day, four members of the Network testified before the House health subcommittee hearings on DES. Belita Cowan, Nancy Belden, Doris Haire, and Sherry Leibowitz presented new evidence on DES hazards, including research revealing testicular abnormalities and epidymal cysts recently discovered in DES sons. In addition to calling for restraints on use of DES, the women asked for legislation to enable low-income women to be reimbursed out of federal family-planning funds for medical screening and treatment for estrogen-induced disorders (Cowan 1976a, 1976b; Norsigian 1976).

In May 1976, the Health Network was incorporated as a nonprofit organization to monitor the activities of federal agencies, such as the FDA, HEW, and NIH, keep abreast of congressional hearings and testimony, and develop a newsletter and alert system to notify members of critical points in health legislation, policy, and regulation. Tentative plans for providing expert witnesses for government agencies were also approved ("Regional Reports, Washington, D.C." 1976).*

At the May 1976 Network meeting, more than 50 women from across the United States met in small workshops on specific health issues to identify key problems and make policy recommendations. Task force recommendations were made in the areas of (1) maternal and child health, (2) drugs and devices, (3) the federal role in health care, (4) rape and wife abuse, (5) health rights of women, (6) health rights of adolescents, (7) alcohol and drug problems, (8) special

---

*Initially, the Network was conceived of developing as a lobby to influence pending legislation. This concept gradually shifted toward the objective of monitoring public and private health regulatory agencies and the idea of developing a lobby was dropped.

problems of the elderly, ethnic minorities, rural residents, and the disabled, (9) mental health care, (10) occupational health and safety, and (11) women as health care providers. Recommendations ranged from broad policy statements to clear recommendations mandating specific action by designated public bodies (National Women's Health Network 1976, pp. 4-8); broad policy statements included, for example: "support groups for women who want to enter male-dominated health professions"; "apply for grants to do needed research on [occupational health and safety] risks"; "support of the Supreme Court decision on abortion"; and "research new and creative approaches to sex and health education in the schools."

Other statements were quite specific, suggesting possible actions. The Task Force on Maternal and Child Health, for example, offered nine specific recommendations, including:

A. HEW form a National Council on Maternal and Child Health to review and question the safety and merit of common obstetric practices and procedures. The council should be chaired by a behavioral scientist and should be comprised of consumer and consumer/advocates, obstetricians, perinatologists, neonatologists, pediatricians, midwives, zoologists, and physiologists. The number of consumer and consumer/advocates should be equal to the collective number of health professionals. ...

C. Federal funds be withheld from any hospital or health facility which does not permit patient access to medical records while in the hospital or facility, and does not make a complete copy of the medical record (including nurses' notes) available to the patient on request. ...

H. Midwives be able to function in private practice of their specialty and be reimbursed by third party payments (National Women's Health Network 1976, p. 1).

The Task Force on Drugs and Devices, for example, recommended: "Compensation for patients, injured or incapacitated by drugs and devices proved unsafe, misprescribed, poorly researched; funds from taxes levied on drug companies" (National Women's Health Network 1976, p. 2).

The newest legislative-oriented national health group, the Women and Health Roundtable, an affiliate of the Federation of Professional Women, began meeting in January 1977 to build a coalition to monitor federal health policy and its impact on women. Representatives of about 30 organizations were involved by March 1977 (Roundtable Report 1977).

Judicial Measures

Some groups seek to enforce existing laws and regulations through legal action. A particularly effective strategy, employed by the Coalition for the Medical Rights of Women, is filing administrative petitions with the California Department of Health. Under California law, such petitions may be submitted by citizens or citizens' groups to state agencies to insure implementation of existing laws—many vague or forgotten. The Coalition's first administrative petition, relating to regulation of IUDs, was filed to press state agencies to act on the 1938 California Food, Drug and Cosmetic Act authorizing the Department of Health to regulate medical devices. The department had not dealt with IUDs at all until this petition was filed (Silverman 1976, p. 14; Thomsen 1975).

Administrative petitions have also been filed to urge the Department of Health to regulate laboratory processing of Pap smears. In January 1975, the Coalition filed the Pap smear petition after investigating allegations of improper practices in the Ocean View Medical Laboratory in San Francisco, a laboratory with major contracts from the San Francisco Department of Public Health. The Coalition became involved at the request of laboratory cytotechnologists, who were concerned over inadequate record keeping, forced processing of unsatisfactory slides (including improperly prepared and stored slides), and pressure to read more slides per hour than they could handle accurately ("Testimony Heard on IUD, Pap Smears" 1976).

The Coalition was especially disturbed by reports that several women's clinics serving high-risk populations were getting statistically unlikely numbers of normal readings from Ocean View. Given the female populations served by the clinics, workers suspected false negatives. To investigate, the Coalition had a clinic send a test slide taken from a woman with known cancer of the cervix to Ocean View and to two other laboratories. Ocean View read the slide as normal, although both other labs notified the clinic of the abnormality. With legal assistance, 384 slides were recalled from Ocean View for rescreening by well-qualified experts. Of the 295 slides Ocean View released, 62 were so poorly prepared, they were unreadable, although they had been reported as normal. Six of the readable 233 slides were evaluated by experts as precancerous (Fruchter 1976).

Women with abnormal smears were contacted and rescreened. The Coalition, with the assistance of the district attorney's office, is considering a suit against Ocean View to cover the expenses involved in rescreening. As a result of the Coalition's pressure on the San Francisco Department of Public Health to review criteria for selecting, monitoring, and contracting with laboratories, Ocean View's contract was not renewed in July 1976 (Fruchter 1976).

While the state Department of Health began drafting cytology regulations in response to the Coalition's petition, the California Association of Cytotechnologists and California Society of Pathologists both suggested amplification of proposed regulations. When the Department of Health failed to respond to the professional associations' requests for stronger controls, the Coalition collaborated with the groups to resubmit stronger regulations ("Coalition for the Medical Rights of Women" 1975).

Concerned over disclosure of abusive sterilization practices throughout the country, and in California in particular, the Coalition filed an emergency petition in January 1975 demanding extensive revision to proposed federal guidelines. Provisions set forth would establish a minimal legal protection against involuntary and uninformed tubal ligation hysterectomy sterilizations—hazards of particular concern to poor and non-English-speaking women. The Coalition is also working on stricter regulation of estrogens—particularly DES as a morning-after pill—and has mounted an educational campaign to secure screening of high-risk women ("Coalition for the Medical Rights of Women" 1975).

Discouraged by the slow response from regulatory agencies, some feminist groups have taken to using the courts in innovative ways. For example, the Women's Health Care Collective of Ithaca, New York, has taken an active role in a products liability suit against A. H. Robins, the manufacturer of the Dalkon Shield. The suit, filed in Federal District Court in New York by an Ithaca woman who required emergency surgery for removal of an ovary because of an IUD-related infection, is similar to previous claims of negligence brought against A. H. Robins. The Health Care Collective, however, used the suit to gather information from women throughout the country; the intent was to build a strong case for other women to use in future legal proceedings and to pressure the FDA into regulating medical devices (Brophy 1976).

A particularly innovative use of the judicial system was initiated in October 1975 when the FWHC in Tallahassee, Florida, filed suit in U.S. Federal District Court against six local physicians and a member of the Board of Medical Examiners. The doctors were charged with conspiracy to restrain trade and create a monopoly in violation of the Sherman Anti-Trust Act.

According to Linda Curtis, director of the FWHC, the named physicians pressured a local doctor and two doctors from nearby Jacksonville to terminate their employment at the FWHC Women's Choice Clinic, which provides first-trimester abortions. Curtis (1975, 1976) believes that it is not coincidental that most of the physicians who most adamantly oppose the health center's policy of advertising services (legal in Florida) are the physicians who perform first-trimester abortions. One physician who opposes the clinic admitted that the more hazardous second-trimester abortions in Tallahassee have definitely decreased over the last year. The women attribute the decline in need for second-trimester abortions to their more available first-trimester abortions (Curtis 1975, 1976).

Since the feminist clinic opened, approximately 1,000 women from Florida, Georgia, Louisiana, and Mississippi have obtained abortions at the clinic yearly. It provides 23 percent of all Florida Panhandle abortions. The $150 fee (reduced for poor women and Medicaid patients) is substantially below the $350 charged at Tallahassee Memorial Hospital—the only facility serving the residents of three neighboring counties. Although some doctors perform early abortions in their offices, they do not offer the full range of tests and services offered at the Women's Choice Clinic or at the local hospital (Fatt 1975-76; "Tallahassee FWHC Fights Back" 1976).

Between June and September of 1975, the clinic lost three doctors in succession. The first, a young obstetrician-gynecologist new to Tallahassee, was called before a closed meeting of the Department of Obstetrics and Gynecology at Tallahassee Memorial Hospital and told his "ethics" were in question for working in a clinic that advertised. Although Florida has no law against clinic advertising as long as physicians' names are not used, the young physician felt threatened and resigned after a month (Curtis 1975; Fatt 1975-76).

Although no Tallahassee physician would work in the FWHC clinic, two residents from Jacksonville were recruited. Shortly thereafter, one resident was called by the executive director of the Florida Board of Medical Examiners, who told him he did not think residents should work at the FWHC, as they were "putting themselves in jeopardy." Several weeks later, six Tallahassee physicians (named in the suit) complained to the residents' hospital in Jacksonville that the Women's Choice Clinic did not have 24-hour abortion backup, in violation of ACOG regulations. (There were actually five doctors who provided backup to the FWHC, but they insisted on remaining anonymous for fear of collegial disapproval, denial or loss of ACOG certification, and harassment.) Since the Women's Choice Clinic could not provide written evidence of 24-hour coverage, the residents resigned (Fatt 1975-76).

Faced with the charge of violating the Sherman Anti-Trust Act, the doctors involved attempted a number of delaying tactics; none were successful. First, they filed a motion to dismiss the case from federal court on grounds that the FWHC did not engage in interstate commerce. Since the FWHC orders supplies from other states and provides health services to out-of-state residents, the motion was denied by Judge William Stafford, who was hearing the case. George Palmer, executive director of the Florida Board of Medical Examiners, named in the suit, initially refused to answer charges on the grounds that he was immune as an agent of the state. Judge Stafford refused to grant Palmer immunity ("Tallahassee FWHC Update" 1976).

In May 1976, the FWHC asked for a preliminary injunction against the Tallahassee physicians, a request denied by Stafford on the grounds that the plaintiffs could not convince him irreparable harm would accrue to them by waiting until the case came to trial. At the hearing, however, Stafford stated that the weight of the evidence thus far leaned toward the inference that the mainspring of the defendants' actions was economic. Thus, the court was of the opinion that the plaintiff had carried its burden of establishing a substantial likelihood of success on the merits of the case (Stafford 1976, p. 19).

In a surprise eleventh-hour decision, Stafford dismissed the suit against the physicians with no explanation (Richardson 1976; "A Modern Miracle of Organized Medicine—A Verdict Before the Trial" 1976). Since Stafford recently had stated that the evidence suggested that the doctors had, in fact, tried to close down the women's clinic, members of the FWHC speculated that the dismissal was a consequence of pressure from the Florida Medical Association, the AMA, and the ACOG ("A Modern Miracle of Organized Medicine—A Verdict Before the Trial" 1976; "Anti-Trust Suit: Verdict Before Trial" 1977).

The women have filed for a rehearing in federal court, but if denied, will appeal to the Fifth Circuit Court of Appeals—a procedure that could take from 18 to 24 months (Richardson 1976; "Tallahassee FWHC Fights Back" 1976). The U.S. Federal Trade Commission (FTC) and the Justice Department were urged to investigate, and representatives of the Justice Department and Planned Parenthood looked into the case (Heidelberg 1978). Numerous organizations, including the American Public Health Association, WATCH (Women Acting Together to Combat Harassment—a coalition of women's health projects), the National Abortion Council, the Abortion Rights Action League, the Southern Law and Poverty Center, and the American Civil Liberties Union, are supporting the women's case ("A Modern Miracle of Organized Medicine—A Verdict Before the Trial" 1976). The U.S. Department of Justice has been urged by several employees to join in filing an amicus brief on behalf of the women's health movement ("Anti-Trust Suit: Verdict Before Trial" 1977).

The Tallahassee case is important, for it challenges the medical establishment's right to maintain a monopoly over health services and to define "the public interest." Some observers view the suit as a landmark case, setting a precedent and guidelines for legal action against physician groups that block efforts to make abortion readily available ("Feminists' Anti-Trust Suit Rejected" 1976). The suit also indicates growing reliance on innovative legal strategies to effect change.

Selective Utilization

Selective utilization of physicians and medical facilities is a
key strategy for ensuring better care at lower cost in the short run
and encouraging physicians to improve quality of care over time, for
by channeling patients to approved physicians, feminist health groups
can "reward" approved physicians with a steady stream of patients
and cut into the supply of those judged inferior or overly expensive.

"Shopping around" for physicians does pay, as women learned
during the New York abortion law liberalization, where, as indicated
in Chapter 3, the cost of first-trimester abortions varied tremendously. After the 1973 Supreme Court decision, low-cost abortions became more available, if one knew where to go. In 1973, a San Francisco Bay area woman could pay anywhere from $135 for a first-tri-
mester abortion at the FWHC Woman's Choice Clinic in Oakland,
California (The Feminist Women's Health Center n.d.b, p. 3), to
over $850 in private hospitals (Cathedral Hill Medical Center 1974,
p. 2). While private physicians routinely recommended that women
wait six weeks from the first day of the last menstrual period for a
positive pregnancy test before being aborted, the FWHC and a few
clinics encouraged women to undergo very early pre-emptive abortions for $75.

About the same time, private physicians in the Bay area were
charging from $150 to $475 for tubal ligations. Although the "average"
ligation cost $350 to $450, women fortunate enough to be referred to
several prominent board-certified obstetrician-gynecologists paid
only $200 (Planned Parenthood Association of Marin 1973). Clearly,
neither skill nor certification determined price. Feminists seized
upon the fact of this differential quickly and sought to make the most
of it by establishing feminist referral networks.

Initially, lay referral systems were informal affairs, consisting
largely of information on cost and women's personal experiences with
individual physicians. Card files and the listing of names of doctors
to recommend to others were established by many women's centers
and health groups. Lay referral systems gradually developed into
published doctor and facility directories and personalized referral
services.

Health service directories typically provide information on
availability of services, fees, willingness to accept public or private
insurance, and some evaluation of services on the basis of other criteria. Many early health directories were printed in feminist newspapers (see, for example, Frankfort 1973b; Women's Health and
Abortion Collective 1973). Others were published in feminist community resource guides and primarily informed women where abortions, contraceptives, maternity care, and health referral were

available. Some of these directories noted specialized services, including mental health, nutritional counseling, and drug treatment (see, for example, Advocates for Women 1973; The Feminist Mental Health Project n.d.; The Inforwomen Collective 1974; Margolis 1972; Womanpower Project 1973).

Some directories identify institutions and physicians on the basis of some important criterion, such as sex, willingness to treat "counterculture" women, or acceptance of public insurance. Efforts to identify female physicians—especially those practicing obstetrics and gynecology—are widespread. For example, NOW's Butler County, Ohio, chapter prepared a directory of female medical specialists in that state. Although inclusion in the directory was based solely on compilers identifying the physician's first name as female in standard medical sources, women could use the directory to begin their search for acceptable practitioners (Butler County NOW 1973). A similar list of female obstetricians and gynecologists was published in The New York Women's Directory (Womanpower Project 1973).

Few feminists believe sex is the only important criterion in choosing a physician, pointing out that some female physicians can be worse than their male colleagues. To identify preferred physicians, feminist groups have developed standard evaluation criteria, based on direct personal experience, observation, and survey information.

To examine the doctors, some groups put their bodies on the line. Members of one New York feminist health group made appointments with board-certified obstetrician-gynecologists in Manhattan and then rated the physicians for their attitude and manner, as well as for performance of procedures outlined in the New York Women's Health Forum checklist of routine examination. More frequently, however, women simply fill out evaluation forms, describing their experience with specific physicians they have seen through traditional medical referral channels or those offered by women's groups.

Evaluation schedules vary from brief forms stating whether or not the physician's treatment was acceptable to very elaborate ones, covering everything from how appointments were made to whether or not alternative forms of treatment were suggested. The Washington, D.C., Women's Health and Abortion Collective, for example, seeks detailed information and widely circulates its physicians evaluation schedule. Completed evaluation schedules are available to women seeking referrals. (See Appendix D for sample physician evaluation schedules.)

While printed directories can reach large numbers of women, lists often fall short of what they are intended to do. In some cases, inaccuracies are a problem. Some inaccuracies result only in inconvenience—the address or telephone number is incorrect. More seriously, out-of-date lists may direct women to physicians who no longer accept public insurance, who have raised fees, or who now refuse to perform specified services, such as second-trimester abortions— services for which women have little time to "shop around." Some groups suggest that for their own protection, women using physicians for the first time should check the doctor's policies out by telephone in advance and even look the doctor up in the local Directory of Medical Specialists (available in most public libraries). The need for caution in using directories was highlighted by the discovery that Silvia Levin, a woman listed in The New York Women's Directory under "Obstetricians and Gynecologists" was not a properly certified specialist ("Medical Bulletin" 1974).

Women's health groups find published physician lists unsatisfactory for reasons other than obvious inaccuracies in information. The Vancouver Women's Health Collective, for example, removed its approved doctor list from the second edition of its health booklet because it was unable to include detailed information on doctors' manner with patients. Since the Vancouver women believe that the quality of a relationship with a doctor is based on how she/he relates to individuals, as well as her/his competence in treating a medical problem, not all women will feel comfortable with the same doctor. To facilitate consideration of interpersonal factors, women are asked to call or stop at the women's referral bureau to discuss choosing a doctor in depth with a collective member (A Woman's Place 1972, p. 121).

A woman calling the Vancouver Women's Health Collective avails herself of considerable information, for the collective regularly surveys local gynecologists, asking if they perform certain services and if they desire referrals from the Collective. Physicians desiring referrals are personally interviewed by Collective members, unless the physician has several negative patient evaluations on file. Physicians with good patient evaluations are interviewed to see if they meet Collective standards. If so, their names are put in a key referral file. Where contradictory comments are filed, the Collective makes the final decision as to whether or not to refer on the basis of the personal interview. Patients using the service are encouraged to read through the detailed comments when selecting from the approved list. (For details of the physician evaluation criterion, see Vancouver Women's Health Collective n.d.)

Other groups have similar policies and procedures encouraging women to read comments thoroughly. Comments about a doctor's performance on specific procedures are especially important to consider, for some physicians are recommended for one service but not for others. For example, in one clinic, a physician was highly recommended to perform late second-trimester abortions—especially since he was one of the few in the area who would do them at all; he

was also noted for humane treatment and sensitive attention to teen-
agers' needs. Yet the same physician was considered an abysmally
poor choice for natural childbirth; according to a midwife, he relied
too heavily on drugs and insisted on lengthier hospital stays than
seemed reasonable—even to other local obstetricians. In another
clinic, one woman physician was highly recommended by poor minority
women but not by white "hip" women, who felt they were treated in a
condescending and moralistic manner.

Clearly, to be effective, referral systems must provide considerable information, including the socioeconomic status and life-
style of patients making the evaluation, for personal characteristics
of patients elicit different responses from different doctors, despite
the ideological rhetoric of affect-neutrality in professional services.*

Direct Pressure

While education, legislation, and lay referral systems are expected to improve quality of care, health activists directly confront
and pressure the medical profession, health institutions, and individual physicians. Commonly employed direct pressure tactics include
using patient advocates, blacklisting, picketing, demonstrating, investigating and monitoring agencies, and invoking the power of the
state—sometimes in unorthodox ways.

Despite educational efforts aimed to help women assert their
needs, health activists acknowledge that stripped and draped, women
often are unable to demand their rights. To improve women's bargaining position, patient advocates accompany women to physical
examinations. In alternative traditional-feminist clinics, advocates
often take medical "herstories" and stay with the patient, asking questions, providing support, and assuring that instructions are clear.
When referred to conventional settings (for hospitalization or for
specialized services), advocates may assist patients in making arrangements and accompany them, especially if the woman is frightened or seriously ill.

Although some doctors refuse to see patients accompanied by
an advocate, women's clinics learn to refer to those who allow advocates. While some clinics provide advocates regularly, others

---

*For discussion of some effects of patient status characteris-
tics, see, for example, Rosengren and DeVault 1963; Lorber 1975a;
Roth 1972.

offer them only in extreme circumstances—and expect patients to learn how to fend for themselves by observing how the advocate inter-acts with medical personnel.

Patient advocates are often utilized in urban areas where pati-ents are non-English-speaking and/or must be referred to large pub-lic medical facilities. They are less often available in suburban areas serving middle-class women, except for abortion care. Patient advocates are especially recommended to accompany teen-agers un-dergoing abortions without their parents' knowledge or support. The Orange County and Los Angeles FWHCs, Womancare in San Diego, and WARS, for example, currently schedule women in groups for second-trimester abortions and provide advocates who remain with the women during the entire hospital stay. The advocates accompany the women into the operating room, even when general anesthesia is used, to ensure that the women are treated with respect and that all procedures are carried out as agreed upon prior to admission (Heidel-berg 1978).

Patient groups also organize to advocate within large prepaid medical plans. For example, in New York, Women for Improved Group Health Services (WIGHS) works to improve services to women within a major group health insurance plan ("Regional Reports, New York, NY" 1976, p. 7).

Feminist health activists also monitor and take action against entrepreneurial clinics. In New York, for example, the NWHC boy-cotted Hillcrest Hospital after the hospital refused to accept abortion patients regarded as "possible risks"—a practice leaving women with potential medical problems few places to obtain care. In another clinic in Queens, health activists from NWHC sat in the lobby telling patients the services were poor and handing out lists of better clinics ("Well Women Clinics Are Wave of Future" 1973).

In San Francisco, feminist health activists associated with the Inter-Agency Pregnancy Council picketed Cathedral Hill Pregnancy Control Center for laying off half of their pregnancy counselors—lay-women employed at low wages ($2.88 per hour)—after counselors de-manded changes in abortion procedures in keeping with feminist values (Brown 1974). In some areas, physician blacklists circulate among feminists either informally or publicly. One New York group so suc-cessfully blacklisted obstetrician-gynecologists that the doctors asked to be re-evaluated, claiming they had "changed their ways." Working through the women's center of a large California university, one group collected patient complaints against two student health service physicians and presented evidence to the county medical society to have the physicians investigated. Similar complaints to local medicine societies have been filed by other health groups on the basis of nega-tive physician evaluations.

Some groups attempt to enforce laws and regulations already on the books without going through traditional legal channels. For example, Robert Bregonier of Los Angeles County Harbor General Hospital allegedly permitted Harvey Karman to perform abortions there despite Karman's lack of medical credentials. For several years, the Los Angeles FWHC tried to have the county health department prohibit Karman's involvement in abortions and prescribing contraceptives at his profitable Women's Community Service Center. In October 1974, several members of the FWHC raided Karman's center, confiscating medical equipment, office supplies, and furniture. After piling the confiscated items on the sidewalk outside the state building in Los Angeles, they told Consumer Affairs official Dan Hauptman, "We have done what you should have done" (Cowan 1974e; "Feminists Raid Abortion Clinic in L.A." 1974).

Feminist groups have also inspected hospital facilities to develop quality assurance. On March 6, 1977, after viewing the film The Chicago Maternity Center Story at the first national conference of WATCH, participants conducted an unannounced inspection of the obstetrical unit at Tallahassee (Florida) Memorial Hospital. The intent was to document dangerous childbirth practices to local women and to inspire community action to bring change.

About 30 WATCH members, accompanied by a camera person from the public station, WFSU-TV, entered the hospital and visited the labor delivery area, maternity ward, and nursery. The women noted many disturbing practices: the routine use of internal fetal heart monitors, the presence of containers of Phisohex (a cleansing chemical known to cause brain damage in infants) in the obstetrical unit, and mothers who were drugged and kept in a prisonlike atmosphere; they were not allowed outside the postpartum area of the hospital. The inspection was conducted without incident in the labor and delivery area. In the postpartum area, the few women who entered the nursery were asked by the attending nurse to leave. Both groups left through the public entrance without incident ("Regional Reports" 1977, p. 7; "Feminists to Stand Trial For Reclaiming Birth" 1977).

Two days later, the Florida State attorney general ordered the film of the inspection confiscated. WATCH inspectors Carol Downer, Linda Curtis, Ginny Cassidy, and Janice Cohen were arrested on a misdemeanor trespassing charge and released from the county jail on maximum $1,000 bail. Initial community reaction to the inspection was negative, in part because of the inflammatory press coverage that followed. Community people were angry that the sterility of the nursery had been violated, and fathers were outraged that unauthorized women had entered the area from which they were completely barred. The local Childbirth Education Association, working to reform the Tallahassee Memorial Hospital birthing practices, was afraid the

WATCH inspection would set back their efforts. Public opinion began
to shift, however, when the local press began printing favorable letters to the editor and documented the fact that the Caesarean rate had
doubled in the past three years, in part because of the routine use of
fetal monitors ("Regional Reports" 1977, p. 7).

Feminist and civil libertarian groups supported the WATCH
action, and on April 24, the National NOW annual meeting passed a
resolution in support of the inspection. Other groups followed suit.
On May 21, all four women were convicted of trespassing. Downer
and Cassidy of the Los Angeles FWHC received 60-day jail sentences
and $1,000 fines. Curtis of the Tallahassee FWHC and Cohen of New
York City were sentenced to 30 days and fined $500 ("Regional Re-
ports" 1977, p. 7). The local press ("Editorials: Judge's Sentencing
Cannot Be Justified" 1977), as well as feminists throughout the country,
denounced the sentences as excessive and punitive. The women are
appealing their convictions to the Florida State Court of Appeals ("Regional Reports" 1977, p. 7; "Activists Convicted" 1977).

Health activists emphasize directly confronting male-dominated
health institutions and organizations—particularly those involved in
population control. Beginning in 1973, feminists have attempted to
participate in Planned Parenthood physicians' annual meetings. Carol
Downer of the FWHC in Los Angeles, Kay Weiss of Advocates for
Medical Information, Belità Cowan of Her-Self newspaper, and Harla
Kaplan of Houston NOW first approached Planned Parenthood in Houston at the 11th annual conference. The women were given a few minutes to speak and presented a list of demands to put women rather
than male professionals and politicians in control of fertility-related
issues. In 1974, Debra Law of the Oakland FWHC and Shelley Farber of the Los Angeles FWHC attempted to participate in the 12th
annual conference in Memphis, Tennessee. When Law attempted to
establish a booth to distribute feminist literature, she was physically
removed by guards. Law and Farber both threatened to press charges
of battery ("Feminist Women's Health Centers Meet Planned Parenthood Physicians" 1975).

By 1975, Planned Parenthood recognized the growing women's
health movement by allocating 25 minutes for a panel discussion.
Carol Downer presented a number of demands from Barbara Seaman's
keynote speech delivered at the 1975 Conference on Women and Health
in Boston—demands discussed later in this chapter. Downer also
denounced Planned Parenthood for inviting Merle Goldberg of the
NWHC to speak, because Goldberg, who had been formally denounced
at the Boston Conference for attempting to involve the media in pushing concerns not central to the group, did not, in Downer's opinion,
represent a grass-roots feminist organization. Downer also laid out
steps to insure that Planned Parenthood would once again function as

its founder, Margaret Sanger, had intended it to operate, that is, in the best interests of women ("Feminist Women's Health Centers Meet Planned Parenthood Physicians" 1975).

Seeking to influence natalist policies worldwide, Lolly Hirsch attended the World Population Conference and Population Tribune in Bucharest, Romania. Laura Brown, after initially being refused admission to the Menstrual Regulation Conference in Hawaii, finally registered and confronted participants about the relationship between imperialism and population control. She also chided the group for holding different standards for health practitioners in different countries (Hirsch 1974-75, p. 6). Representatives of the Los Angeles, Orange County, Oakland, and Tallahassee FWHCs actively demonstrated and participated in the International Women's Year Conference and Tribunal in Mexico City in 1975 (Snow 1975). Feminists' activities at these conferences—along with their reports on the activities of those active in the population control movement—have been publicized throughout the movement in order to mobilize women to secure their rights in fertility-related matters.

In sum, strategies to reform existing institutions are varied, reflecting the interests, concerns, and abilities of specific organizations and their members. As is common with reform movements, early concerns were expressed in global terms. More specific—and effective—policies and strategies evolved as the movement grew (rapidly) between 1972 and 1976. Health movement groups increasingly rely on a variety of approaches to solve what has come to be defined as the fundamental problem: putting women in control of their own health and bodies. However, it is also increasingly clear that "control of women's bodies" means something quite different in Harlem or Latin America than it does in the suburbs. The interests of white middle-class women who dominate the movement clearly can conflict with those of minority women (see Chapter 7).

ALTERNATIVE INSTITUTIONS: STOP-GAP SERVICE VERSUS COMPREHENSIVE OR COMPETITIVE CARE

Whether health activists should emphasize building alternative services or attacking and changing existing institutions has generated much debate. A major controversy revolves around how alternative services siphon off discontent, allowing conventional institutions to ignore women's needs. The problem is not new; it arose earlier in the free clinic movement—sometimes accused of letting conventional institutions "off the hook" by caring for society's outcasts. But unlike the free clinics' clientele, many users or potential users of women's clinics are middle-class paying patients, many of whom need abortions—a lucrative surgical procedure. Because these patients are neither outcasts nor unprofitable, their choice of where to seek care has an impact on traditional practitioners.*

Although most groups now agree that direct service operations and pressuring established medical institutions are both important to the development of the movement, the debate continues over how groups can best direct their efforts (HealthRight 1975, p. 4). A major factor in the continuing ambivalence may lie in women's uncertainty that they can actually work effectively on a scale larger than local projects.

Some suggest that women's clinics should expand to offer comprehensive care to compete with and eventually replace traditional institutions. Expansion into related health areas is particularly recommended to relieve the problem of fragmented care. After three years experience under New York's liberalized abortion law, for example, Merle Goldberg of the NWHC declared that single-procedure clinics are inadequate and should be replaced by comprehensive health care facilities. To meet the need, the NWHC began planning a comprehensive gynecological-obstetrical prepaid health plan in 1973. Designed to utilize fully women health professionals and paraprofessionals, the NWHC emphasized training nurses and nurse-midwives to perform routine well-women care in order to free physicians for evaluating and treating sick women (National Women's Health Coalition 1974; "Well Women Clinics Are Wave of Future" 1973).†

In California, the FWHCs now offer comprehensive obstetrical and gynecological care. A prepaid birth control plan that emphasized local contraceptive methods (diaphragm, foam, or condoms), regarded as statistically "less effective" than drugs and devices was briefly operated in 1976.‡ By offering abortion as a backup, the FWHC believed women could be encouraged to rely on less-hazardous contraceptives ("FWHC Plans Birth Control Subscriptions" 1976). The program was discontinued, however, because too few women enrolled (Heidelberg 1978). In the Seattle, Washington, area, the Fremont

---

*Freidson 1969 points out how certain specialties, including obstetrics and gynecology, are client controlled to some degree because they are dependent on lay referrals.

†The author's letters requesting further information on these services were not answered by the NWHC and it no longer has a listed telephone number.

‡Local contraceptives' failure rates are strongly related to failure to use rather than to technical inferiority. See Boston Women's Health Book Collective 1976.

Women's Clinic and Country Doctor Women's Clinic offer comprehensive primary care, including pediatrics, nutritional counseling, and geriatric screening programs, as do the Sommerville Health Project (in Massachusetts) and others.

Nonetheless, most services remain fragmented or involve the "dirty work" many physicians would prefer delegating to others. At the Second Women-Controlled Women's Health Center Conference in Ames, Iowa, Rachelle Walker and Holly Lindsay from the Elizabeth Blackwell Clinic in Minneapolis expressed concern that women's clinics may become dumping grounds for what the traditional medical system regards as "problem patients" (Hirsch 1974-75). A Sommerville Health Project member similarly has expressed the view that her group's clinic provides the primary care (routine checkups, treating minor infections, and providing contraceptives) that no one else wants to do, taking the pressure off the local medical establishment. Sommerville Project physician Judy Herman (1975) adds that the clinic's presence has had no effect on the prices at Sommerville Hospital and only a negligible effect on the way people are treated there.

While providing primary care does not threaten the medical establishment, offering surgical services does. Providing surgery puts women's clinics in direct competition with established practitioners who offer this high-priced service. Feminists believe that in many communities, the threat of competition has led to continual harassment and/or outright denial of clinic licenses. For example, the Women's Community Health Center in Cambridge, Massachusetts, ("Health Centers: Surviving Boston" 1977) and the Los Angeles FWHC ("State of California Goes Fishing Without a License" 1977) have both fought attempts to close their clinics.* The Tallahassee doctors discussed earlier may have resorted to questionably legal tactics, because there were no Florida clinic licensing regulations doctors could use to fight their feminist competitors (Fatt 1975-76, p. 7). The case against the Santa Cruz lay midwives (see Chapter 3) is also viewed by many as a response to threat of competition. In response to this type of medical harassment, a coalition of women's groups in conjunction with the FWHC founded WATCH in 1976. WATCH both demonstrates and raises funds for legal action (to prevent closure of feminist clinics by organized medicine).

_____

*On November 2, 1976, California deputy director of the Department of Consumer Affairs apologized to the FWHC for the year of investigation and harassment. The FWHC subsequently filed a $500,000 damage claim against the state.

Feminist competition threatens obstetrician-gynecologists in several ways. The effectiveness of abortion referral in reducing abortion fees in many areas suggests that organized women's groups can create market competition despite medical monopolies on this procedure. Similarly, the refusal of growing numbers of women to give birth in hospitals has stimulated financially hard-pressed maternity facilities to offer more acceptable services, including "home-style" birth programs (see Chapter 8).

By fully utilizing nurse practitioners, physicians' assistants, and nurse-midwives, feminist health centers also demonstrate the effectiveness and public acceptance (even among white middle-class women) of nonphysician providers. Public officials seeking to reduce medical costs can cite women's clinics as effective health delivery models that are capable of reducing costs while improving availability of primary care. Growing acceptance of midwife deliveries are likely to be seen as a way of containing if not lowering skyrocketing health costs (Sablosky 1976).

Doing some surgery also helps women's clinics stay financially solvent. By charging slightly less than current physician fees for abortion, competitive clinics collect enough from private insurance, Medicaid programs, and individuals to operate. Since women often work in feminist clinics for salaries considerably below those paid in conventional settings, budgetary "surpluses" from salary saving and group (rather than private) care are available to subsidize educational efforts and low-profit services. The FWHCs are particularly adept at financing their educational and political work through surgical "profits." How long women can be induced to work for substandard wages, however, is impossible to predict. Workers "burn out," and disillusionment, as well as conflict over goals, strategies, and structure, are serious problems for alternative institutions.*

STRATEGIES TO REDEFINE THE BOUNDARIES OF MALE MEDICAL AUTHORITY

Some activists believe certain functions should be removed entirely from the domain of the medical profession. They argue that medical care must be deprofessionalized and deregulated so laywomen

---

*For discussion of some of these problems, see Freudenberger 1974; "FWHC Response" 1974; Galper and Washburne 1976; and "What is 'Feminist Health'?" 1974.

have the right to perform routine gynecological and obstetrical procedures on themselves and others. Emphasizing that they are primarily concerned with meeting medical needs of well women, not wom-
en who are sick, self-help advocates believe that regardless of the
quality of care in traditional settings or the competence or humaneness
of physicians and nurses, much routine care is simply performed in
the wrong place by the wrong people—by professionals holding patriarchal values instead of by women themselves.

The core strategy to redefine the boundaries of medical authority is to promote self-help groups—advanced health groups emphasizing
gynecological self-examination, self-evaluation, and treatment of
minor disorders (as described in Chapter 5). Many self-help activities are frowned on by professionals—even by some sympathetic to
feminist health concerns. (For concern over these activities, see,
for example, Connell 1974; Frankfort 1972; and "Women's Liberation
and the Practice of Medicine" 1973.) Nonetheless, self-help proponents press their right to learn routine care, attend home births, and
perform menstrual extraction.

Downer's acquittal on charges of practicing medicine without
a license (discussed in Chapter 3) reduced concern over arrest for
these activities, yet harassment continues. The Santa Cruz midwives'
trial (challenging the appropriateness and desirability of granting
powerful professions exclusive right to provide certain services) is
an equally crucial case. But despite favorable rulings, the "right to
practice" is less likely to be conferred on laywomen than on nurse-
practitioners or other licensed and certified personnel below physicians in the health hierarchy, especially where third-party payments
are involved.

By far the most controversial self-help practice is menstrual
extraction; yet no one has been arrested for it despite ample opportunities. The procedure has been demonstrated publicly twice in San
Francisco—at the 1972 American Public Health Association meetings
and at the 1974 Menstrual Extraction Conference sponsored by the
FWHCs. However, both demonstrations were held in downtown hotels,
where the liberal local media might have portrayed arresting police
officers negatively, as media coverage has done with pornography and
prostitution arrests in the past. Organizers of the Menstrual Extraction Conference considered this possibility and believed local authorities would not arrest well-dressed women from the St. Francis Hotel
in front of television cameras, which feminists were prepared to call
in at any sign of trouble. Such arrests might have created even more
favorable publicity and support than arrests in private homes. The
medical-legal establishment ignored the challenge.

Menstrual extraction is a key issue, for it challenges both
clinical practice and the politics of professionalism; it raises serious

questions about physicians' efforts to treat menstrual difficulties and reproductive problems. The fact that laywomen—"ordinary looking housewife types," as one woman whispered in amazement at the Menstrual Extraction Conference—can successfully perform the procedure also raises embarrassing questions about high medical fees for similar services. But most important, it is a means whereby women can drive home their point that women can and must control their reproductive functions. By seizing the technology to control fertility, women can escape both medical and legal professional domination. With restrictive abortion laws imminent, this procedure may become more widespread.

While self-help proponents wish to establish their right to control certain routine services, they recognize the need for technical medical skills—skills that physicians, nurses, and other professionals possess. The problem is how to get the needed skills without the elitist, self-interested trappings of professionalism.

Mary Howell has argued that the answer might be withdrawal from established institutions to develop an all-female health school based on the principles of (1) nurturance of the patient's own healing potential; (2) concern for equity between care givers at various levels and recipients of care; and (3) concern for self-determination, which would require teaching health knowledge and skills to lay persons. Focus would be on low-technology primary care by and for women. However, starting such a school would require resolving a major dilemma: Should women continue to try to work within male-dominated institutions, and with individual men, or should women build a separate, strong, and effective women's culture parallel to that of men, as equal in access to money as possible and suited to the beliefs and values held by women for women? Howell suggests that women will ultimately make the decision to work within male-dominated institutions or to strike out on their own on the basis of men's attitudes and behavior. If men are not willing to change, not willing to be for women, women may have to be for themselves alone (Howell 1975b, pp. 52-53).

Others, too, are skeptical that reforms in the existing health system will bring needed changes and look for ways to re-establish female authority in medicine. Seaman (1975, p. 45) suggests that there is a basic violation of civil rights involved where men, who are not at risk from reproduction, control women, who are. This disparity between the controllers and the at-risk population is not paralleled in any other area of life. Seaman argues that women can legitimately demand that obstetrics and related fields be put under women's control.

Demands to do just this were issued at the Women's Health Conference in Boston in April 1975. Conferees proposed that effective immediately: (1) only women should be admitted to residencies in obstetrics and gynecology, but men currently in training or practice could remain; (2) no foundation monies should be rewarded to men to research the female reproductive system and that all new grants for reproductive research in the next five years should be designed to train women in reproductive biology; (3) all laws concerning female reproduction, abortion, and sterilization should be removed from the court and legislative systems and reviewed instead by an agency modeled after the National Labor Relations Board, the Federal Communications Commission, or the Atomic Energy Commission; and (4) the United Nations and the United States would neither sponsor nor participate in any international population conference or activity unless women were represented in proportion to their numbers in the population of participating nations (Seaman 1975, pp. 45-46). Similar policy statements to place women in control of fertility-related services have been issued by the National Women's Health Network Task Forces (National Women's Health Network 1976).

Commenting on the Boston proposals, Seaman (1975) argues that feminists, without intending to place undue hardships on men, are simply proposing to phase men out of what is rightly women's domain. Feminist attorney Kris Glen's position is that the demand for female obstetrician-gynecologists can be interpreted as legitimate because of the constitutionally guaranteed right to privacy, like separate women's bathrooms, these proposals are allowable even under the Equal Rights Amendment (ERA). Glen also suggests that sex can be a bona fide occupational qualification for the practice of obstetrics and gynecology and reproductive research on the grounds that men are socialized to regard women's bodies with contempt and that their record of past and present atrocities makes them unqualified. Demands calling for preferential awards to women researchers can be viewed as compensatory aid for scientists discriminated against in the past—allowable under the law according to a New York Bar Association interpretation (Seaman 1975, pp. 45-47).

Other feminists suggest redefining the limits of medical authority differently. Some believe that obstetrics and gynecology as a specialty should be disbanded entirely, returning women's care to nurses, midwives, and internists specializing in primary care (relying on general surgeons with gynecological experience only in extreme circumstances). For although women obstetrician-gynecologists might be more satisfactory, Marieskind (1975b, pp. 48-49) argues that it is not merely the practices and content of obstetrics and gynecology that are oppressive. By creating a reproductively oriented specialty for women, the medical system reflects the wider social ideology, which views women as sex objects and reproductive organs.

STRATEGIES' EFFECTS ON INSTITUTIONALIZED MEDICAL AUTHORITY

Types of authority relationships between patients and practitioners are important to examine, for it is on this level that women most directly experience the health care "system." These face-to-face experiences, however, must be understood in the larger context of structural features of practice, which organize and motivate individual action. Health movement strategies for change, in addition to achieving specific goals, have the potential to deinstitutionalize medical professional authority, transforming authority exercised in patient-practitioner relationships to authority similar to that found in collegial relationships—authority based on presentation of persuasive evidence.[*] Inroads on institutionalized authority in interrelated structures have a cumulative effect—jointly setting in motion a shift in laws, regulations, attitudes, values, and practices constituting the health care "system."

Knowledge Differential between Patient and Practitioner

Institutionalized professional authority is based partly on the knowledge differential between patient and practitioner. Professionals claim it is appropriate for them to make decisions on grounds that patients can never possess as much knowledge as these experts do.[†] Many health movement strategies undermine this stance, both by reducing the actual knowledge differential and by questioning the validity of certain medical knowledge.

Specifically, strategies of patient education, selective utilization of practitioners, alternative institutions, and self-help activities

---

[*]For discussion of physicians' attempts to institutionalize authority, see Freidson 1968.

[†]While overall this may be true, particularly in acute illness episodes, patients with chronic disorders often are knowledgeable about their problems and common treatment approaches. Roth (1963a) points out that patients in tuberculosis hospitals, for example, are extremely knowledgeable about various treatments. One physician the author interviewed mentioned that he made a special point of reading the daily newspaper to keep abreast of medical developments that his patients were reading about and asking him to assess for their treatment.

all increase patients' medical knowledge. Recent studies confirm that women significantly increase their knowledge of health and their own bodies in the course of using feminist health services (Reynard 1973; Marieskind 1976). Knowledge and confidence gained in feminist health activities can be—and are—used in conventional settings. (See Chapter 8 to see how widespread this is.)

Educating women about the imprecise nature of medical science also reduces women's subjective experience of ignorance vis-a-vis professionals. Feminists suggest that patients and only patients have within themselves the common sense—or wisdom—needed to evaluate benefits relative to risks before following prescribed regimens. Thus, physicians' technical stock of knowledge is downgraded from its traditional status.

License and Mandate

Claiming a mandate to protect the public's health, the medical profession demands license to restrict provision of services to its own members. By its very existence, the women's health movement challenges the medical profession's mandate in obstetrics and gynecology. Self-help practices and home birth, particularly, challenge professionals' mandate and license, showing that lay persons can quite competently perform many tasks ostensibly restricted for public protection. Alternative institutions that utilize paraprofessionals, although less dramatically, challenge professional mandate and license. Patient education and selective utilization strategies both make inroads on professionals' exclusive right to evaluate services—a key component of professional license. Legislative efforts to give nonphysicians rights to practice previously restricted tasks or to place nonphysicians on review boards challenge physicians' current monopoly over the provision and evaluation of services. Such outside observation is essential to develop any meaningful system of public accountability.[*]

Other strategies aim to enforce the conditions of license. Actions such as those taken by direct pressure groups are efforts to force professionals to fulfill their mandate to protect the public welfare (for example, DES and IUD review)—a mandate professionals

---

[*]For discussion of the social control of professions and the need for outside observation in accountability structures, see, for example, Daniels 1973; Freidson 1970, 1975; and Ruzek 1973.

invoke to justify their control over practice, but which they exercise infrequently.*

Control Over Medical Goods and Services

Physicians control patients' access to goods and services directly through the power to prescribe, admit to hospital, and certify for insurance. Indirect control is exerted in related medical industries, affecting what research will be funded, what drugs will be approved, and even how many professionals will be trained. By convincing the public that it is essential to rely on professionals, with their restricted drugs and devices to manage life-events, physicians control access to health services psychologically as well as legally.

Health movement activities reduce physicians' control over goods and services in several ways. Legislative strategies aim to give lay persons or nonphysician providers a larger voice in regulatory agencies. The work to certify out-patient clinics, community health centers, and in-home providers as legitimate recipients of public health funds is another way to dilute physicians' authority.

Physician control is simply usurped in many alternative institutions. Power to prescribe, for example, may be informally "passed down" to nurses, paraprofessionals, or laywomen themselves; "supplies" may be made accessible in violation of the law. But physicians' control is most dramatically reduced by feminists' collective definition of female life-events as "normal" rather than as "sick" states. Negating the need for and the value or efficacy of many goods and services (for example, anesthesia in childbirth, prescription contraceptives, and estrogen replacement therapy), physicians can no longer be viewed as inescapable gatekeepers to health, thereby losing much of their mystique and power.

Size of the Profession Relative to the Clientele

Restricting the profession's size relative to its clientele not only keeps professionals' services in short supply (and thereby expensive) but creates a temporal orientation, encouraging unquestioning

---

*The hesitancy of professionals—particularly physicians—to protect the public from incompetent colleagues is well documented. See, for example, Daniels 1973; Freidson 1975; and Millman 1977.

acceptance of medical authority, for the time pressure of medical practice (discussed in Chapter 5) virtually precludes presenting clients with persuasive evidence to accept a treatment regimen. Improving the practitioner-patient ratio is a necessary condition for altering authority relationships.

Pressing to increase the number and visibility of women physicians and opening practice to nurses and/or paraprofessionals increases the pool of providers, thus altering the size of the profession relative to the clientele. This change has been accomplished through legislative and judicial measures to admit more women to medical school and to expand nurse practice.* That the use of nonphysician providers will increase the time spent per patient in conventional settings, however, is by no means a certainty. Unless the nursing profession resists, practitioners may operate on a time frame identical to that of physicians, especially in large prepaid health plans, in which lowering cost per capita is a more salient priority than improving quality of care. In the private practice sector, offering more time per visit could be a means to attract a clientele, particularly for obstetrical care, for which patients often "shop around."†

Theoretically, patient-physician ratios can be altered by teaching women to care for themselves; physicians would thus have fewer "client visits." However, self-help activities may actually increase demand for services by making women more aware of their medical needs. Whether or not a long-term consequence of self-care would be to reduce visits by encouraging women to seek care early before conditions become severe has yet to be studied empirically. However, early treatment may not actually have much impact on overall usage rates.

Aggregate and Collective Clienteles

Professionals' authority is buttressed by having clienteles remain aggregates rather than collectivities. Through membership in an occupational association, the professional has prerogatives

---

*By 1976, 22 percent of all first-year students admitted to American medical schools were female ("Med Schools Prepare More Women" 1976). The increase, however, appears to be leveling off (Walsh 1977).

†This is, however, a shrinking mode of health care delivery. Between 1963 and 1973, there was a 5.4 percent decline in the number of self-employed office-based physicians and an 84 percent increase in salaried office-based physicians (McKinlay 1977, pp. 472-73).

unavailable to the unaffiliated (typical) clientele. Most important, members of an aggregate clientele are disconnected from one another, unable to "compare notes" or press complaints, except as individuals, so that problems are always subject to dismissal as isolated events or random errors.

An organized clientele, however, with a collective awareness of its constituency, is a serious threat to institutionalized authority, for professionals can now be observed and evaluated by clients sharing some common values or expectations. If dissatisfied, a collective clientele can take action against the practitioner—even pressing charges through the professional's own review boards and regulatory agencies— with greater success than a lone individual. Collectivities—especially articulate groups with access to the press—potentially wield power in democratic societies. As Krauss (1977, pp. 13-15) notes, historically, populist groups (like the Thompsonian herbalists in Jacksonian America) have sometimes reversed trends toward professional monopolies, thus allowing people to gain greater control over their lives.

The growth of the entire health movement indicates that women can transform themselves from aggregate to collective clienteles, able to influence the shape of the health care system on many levels. From lobbying and educating the public to taking legal action against professionals and demanding that certain aspects of health care be placed under women's control, feminist health activists work jointly to improve the health system rather than to "beat it" individually. In the process, health activists are beginning to renegotiate fundamental assumptions about appropriate roles for professionals in an advanced, industrial society.*

Nonetheless, barriers to change are substantial, and consumer control movements such as this one must fight constant uphill battles to make even small gains. Some resistance to needed change will probably come from consumers themselves as taxpayers and insurance premium payers. It is doubtful that consumers will be eager to absorb the cost involved in allocating more time per patient visit—a necessary condition for full patient participation. Without a fundamental shift in societal allocation of resources or a substantial shift to group care, the economics of the health industry will remain an impediment to renegotiating authority relationships.

---

*Compare Freidson 1973b and McKinlay 1977 on the role of medical professionals in society, particularly their relation to their "products."

7

Strains and Contradictions in the Multiple Realities of Reform

Both contemporary feminism and the women's health movement share attitudes, values, and beliefs, as well as strategies and tactics of protest, in common with other 1960s reform movements. The black civil rights movement, the student movement, and Vietnam War protest offered precedents for questioning established authority and institutions. Direct confrontation tactics and civil disobedience as practiced by these groups developed an air of respectability—particularly for middle-class liberals bent on furthering "good causes."*
Not surprisingly, many feminist protest activities were patterned after these earlier demonstrations.

During the late 1960s, there were many other movements that challenged various aspects of American institutions which influenced the direction of women's health protests. Some ecology and natural health movement activists predicted disaster unless worldwide fertility was reduced and the chemical environment was checked. Nader's "raiders" exposed an alarming array of hazardous consumer products and services and spearheaded the popular view that American society had been corrupted by the profit system (Nader, Petkas, and Blackwell 1972; Shostak 1974; Wellford 1972). Demands for consumer control and consumer rights, which took hold in the health care field in the late 1960s, were initially seen as an avenue for meeting the needs of the poor and ethnic minorities (Gartner and Riessman 1974, pp. 73-81). In this context, feminist health activists' concerns over

---

*For studies of these movements, see, for example, Friedman 1973; Hendel 1971; Howard 1974; Roth 1977b; and Thorne 1975.

reproductive services and technology can be viewed as extensions of growing societal concern over pronatalism, runaway technology, and the viability of the American profit system.

The influence of the youth culture and hippie movements are also evident in feminism. As in these movements, feminists proclaimed the validity of personal experience over derived knowledge and accorded individual choice supreme status. While sharing many of the flower children's disdain for "establishment" values, many feminists, however, wanted full access to the patriarchal institutions from which they had been excluded.

Desire for access to institutions and statuses perceived as corrupt and corrupting has created severe ambivalence among feminists. Within the women's health movement, the ambivalence is marked with respect to women professionals, who are seen as holding advantaged, elite positions in powerful institutions, whether or not these women are actually powerful within their professional fields.[*] Because they are perceived as already overly powerful, women physicians were not sought out or encouraged to assume leadership roles in the health movement at first.

Like participants in other contemporary movements, women's health activists grapped with difficult societal issues: race, class, capitalism, family structures, occupational hierarchies, and equal rights. But without a well-developed unifying ideology providing clear strategic approaches to social change (Freeman 1975, p. 10), feminism and specific feminist movements grew in many directions, some seemingly contradictory. Furthermore, the belief in absolute equality,[†] despite the reality of conflicting class and cultural values of women in American society, obstructed the negotiation of solutions to ongoing problems.[‡]

-----

[*]For discussion of women health professionals' actual relative powerlessness in established institutions, see especially the papers from three national conferences on women in health: "Double-Dynamics: Women's Roles in Health and Illness" 1975; "Proceedings of the Conference on Women and Health, June 27, 28, 29, 1974, Philadelphia, Pa." 1974; and "Proceedings of the Conference on Women's Leadership and Authority in the Health Professions" 1977.

[†]For an analysis of the ideology of equality, see Nelson and Olesen 1977.

[‡]See Fuller and Myers 1941, pp. 320-21, for discussion of how movements organized to solve social problems become bogged down by conflicting values.

The most fundamental value conflict within feminism at large and within the women's health movement stem from both movements' race and class composition, which conflict with their egalitarian ideology. Many of the splits between the two movements themselves are related to class and status differences between their constituencies. Although many feminists choose to believe that sisterhood will unite women of all backgrounds, the reality is that sisterhood may be powerful, but so are race, class, and status in shaping perceptions of what constitute problems as well as possible solutions.

Inability to agree on appropriate constituencies has led to bitter schisms, as well as resulting in the growth of similar organizations with different class-status memberships. For example, two organizations focus on monitoring federal agencies—the Women and Health Roundtable (an affiliate of the Federation of Professional Women) and the National Women's Health Network. The Roundtable is viewed with suspicion by some members of the Network, an organization committed to lay participation and to minimizing professional dominance, because Network members fear that the Roundtable will only concern itself with "professional" women's interests. In addition, both groups compete for scarce foundation funds for operating expenses—a situation that could create conflict and competition rather than cooperation.

THE FACES OF CONTEMPORARY FEMINISM

The general contemporary feminist movement consists of two distinct but overlapping wings—the older, or women's rights branch, and the younger, or women's liberation branch, each of which includes many segments, factions, and movement organizations that differ in emphasis, interest, and approach to change.* The women's health movement, which emerged from this more general social movement, incorporates both women's rights and women's liberation approaches in organizational form and strategies and tactics. Over time, the

---

*For discussion of the use of these terms to describe the contemporary feminist movement, see Carden 1974; Freeman 1975; Hole and Levine 1971; Jones and Brown 1970; and Firestone 1970. I would argue that there are actually several specific social movements, with their own organizations, informal networks, communication channels, and constituencies. The movement for women's rights in education and employment, for example, constitutes a separate, specific social movement.

health movement has shifted toward the direction of rights groups, although initially, it took the liberationist approach. Because many of the strains and contradictions of the women's health movement have their origins in the race, class, and status characteristics of participants, it is useful to compare health movement constituencies with those of the larger feminist movement. Briefly reviewing feminist approaches to social change will also put the women's health movement in proper context as a specific social movement with direct ties to the general feminist movement.

From their inception in 1966, women's rights groups emphasized legislative, economic, and educational reform to eradicate concrete instances of sex discrimination in social institutions by working through traditional legal and political channels. The major national organizations all have highly developed state and local affiliates: NOW, WEAL, and the National Women's Political Caucus (NWPC).* Women's rights group founders had considerable investment in established institutions and wished to improve the already privileged lot of movement members in society. The central goal of NOW, established by women active in the professions and in state commissions on the status of women, for example, was to bring women into full participation in the mainstream of American society, with all the privileges and responsibilities in equal partnership with men (Carden 1974, pp. 103-4). The moderate and conservative feminists, who dominate rights organizations, have deliberately avoided or were slow to accept extremely controversial issues, such as abortion, rape, self-defense, and lesbianism, in order to maintain their broad-based constituencies (Carden 1974, pp. 11-118; Freeman 1975, pp. 71-102; Hole and Levine 1971).

In 1973, the total membership of women's rights organizations was about 75,000 (Carden 1974, p. 3). Most members have been well-educated middle- or upper-middle-class white women. Most have pursued professional or semiprofessional careers, or have been wives of politicians or other public figures and/or have had long careers in voluntary activities. Many are married and in their twenties and early thirties, although the leadership has tended to be somewhat older (Carden 1974, pp. 19-21; Daniels 1975a; Freeman 1975, pp. 17, 84-85). Although small in number, some working-class women were

---

*Other organizations include the Women's Legal Defense Fund, the Women's Action Alliance, and The Women's Lobby. See Carden 1974 and Freeman 1975 for a thorough discussion of women's rights groups.

NOW founders and involved in early rights organizing. By the early 1970s, trade union women began organizing their own separate rights groups (Roby 1975, p. 207).

In contrast, the women's liberation branch attracted more radical women concerned with developing feminist analyses of the origins, nature, and extent of women's oppression and subservient roles in society. Many of their concerns grew directly out of their treatment in the supposedly democratic, egalitarian new left, civil rights, and antiwar movements, where they were relegated to subordinate positions and subjected to humiliating treatment. During the late 1960s, women in these movements began forming their own feminist caucuses (Burris 1973, pp. 322-57; Carden 1974, pp. 59-63; Freeman 1975, pp. 57-58; Koedt 1973b, pp. 318-21; Jones and Brown 1970; McAfee and Wood 1970, pp. 415-33).

During 1968 and 1969, the schism with the new left escalated, with many women breaking off entirely to form a separate feminist movement. They argued that a radical feminist movement must be totally separate because women's oppression both predated capitalism and is rampant in communist and socialist societies (Koedt 1973b; McAfee and Wood 1970, pp. 423-24; Jones and Brown 1970). The schism with the left was never complete, however, and many feminists have maintained the long-term goal of a socialist revolution (McAfee and Wood 1970, pp. 426-33); some have actively worked to re-establish the feminist-socialist alliance (see, for example, Mitchell 1973, p. 66). (Within the women's health movement, Marxist-socialist feminists emphasize the need for socialism to overcome the hazards that are directly related to the health profit system.)

Radical women meeting in all-female groups paid increasing attention to exploring the personal meaning of their oppression, forming personal liberation or consciousness-raising groups. Through sharing personal feelings and experiences, the women underwent dramatic cognitive restructuring, in which personal problems and concerns were redefined as the consequences of male supremacy and traditional sex roles rather than as individual failure (Carden 1974; Freeman 1975; Hole and Levine 1971; Mitchell 1973, pp. 61-63).

Consciousness-raising groups rapidly attracted women previously uninvolved in new left politics.* The women's liberation

---

*By late 1969, consciousness-raising groups could be found in most major cities. In 1970, there were at least 50 groups in New York, 30 in Chicago, and 25 in Boston (Robins 1970, p. 6). By early 1973, an estimated 15,000 women had participated in such groups, and by the mid-1970s, liberation groups were active in suburban communities, small towns, and even conservative areas of the Midwest (Carden 1974, pp. 64-65).

constituency, then, was quickly transformed from a predominantly radical socialist one into a more liberal reformist one. Participants continued to come from white middle-class backgrounds, although some ethnic minority and lower-socioeconomic group women were drawn in gradually. Most women were well educated and engaged in, or were in training for, professional careers (Carden 1974, pp. 19-21; Freeman 1975, p. 50). Although liberationists ranged in age from teen-agers to mature women in their sixties and seventies, the majority were single women in their early to midtwenties. In suburban areas, somewhat older, married women were active (Carden 1974, pp. 19-21).

The privileged middle-class image has concerned some segments of the movement, particularly those with a commitment to radical social change. Despite continuing attempts to bring disadvantaged women into the movement (McAfee and Wood 1970), working-class women tend, as already noted, to join women's rights organizations (Roby 1975, pp. 207-8).

Differences in sexual orientation created havoc and dissension. Radicals were concerned over homosexuality for political reasons, fearing it would alienate working-class women and give men a weapon to obstruct women's organizing (Jones and Brown 1970, p. 408). Lesbians resented efforts to keep their sexual orientation private so as not to mar the public image, and many chose to organize separately in gay or lesbian-feminist groups (Hole and Levine 1971, pp. 239-42; Koedt 1973a; Radicalesbians 1970; Rainone, Shelley, and Hart 1970). By 1972, lesbians were fairly well accepted within the movement, but the desirability of separatism in consciousness-raising and other activities continued to be debated (Carden 1974, pp. 68-69; Freeman 1975, pp. 99-100, 138-39; Koedt, Levine, and Rapone 1973, pp. 246-58). At the National Women's Conference in Houston in November 1977, a rapprochement on homosexuality seemed finally to have been reached.

As women's liberation groups grew, members began questioning the limits of consciousness-raising as a means of bringing about social change. While consciousness-raising was a great way to reach large numbers of women and to provide a setting where women could develop self-confidence and a realization of what they shared, some women felt that it was pointless to develop self-confidence to challenge assumptions about limitations on women's roles without then collectively doing something about these problems (Payne 1973, p. 284). Increasingly, disagreements over both ideological analysis of women's condition and how to translate ideology into specific goals plagued the movement (see, for example, Gornick and Moran 1971; Koedt, Levine, and Rapone 1973; Morgan 1970; and Tanner 1970).

Liberationists found that their idealistic organizational principles based on self-realization, equality, antielitism, sisterhood, and the authority of personal experience were difficult to implement beyond the small consciousness-raising group (Carden 1974, p. 86). Freeman (1973, p. 285-99) pointed out that structurelessness was an unrealizable goal, given the nature of social groups. To function effectively—or at beyond consciousness-raising—most liberation groups compromised and accepted a certain amount of leadership, viewing leaders as facilitators of group decisions rather than as persons to whom responsibility and authority were delegated (Carden 1974, p. 93). Nonetheless, failure to agree on organizational forms and objectives created severe internal conflicts and caused much of the fragmentation within the movement, often over the key issues of maintaining a collectivity and eliminating internal hierarchy and elitism (Carden 1974, pp. 87-99; Freeman 1975, pp. 119-29). These issues continue to concern health activists.

HEALTH: A NEEDED UNIFIER IN A DIVIDED MOVEMENT

Health and body issues have been especially important to many feminists because it is asserted that they cut across race and class lines. Women who hope to counter the image of feminism as a movement exclusively serving white middle-class women's needs were quick to so define their concerns. Ehrenreich and English (1973, pp. 85-86) popularized this view in Complaints and Disorders: The Sexual Politics of Sickness, arguing that the medical system reduces women to their biological category, stripped of occupational status, life-style differences, and individuality. Because middle-class women were becoming so acutely aware of their own medical oppression, the danger of middle-class women becoming traditional missionarylike reformers for their "inferiors" seemed unlikely; this new feminist consciousness, then, claimed Ehrenreich and English, provided women the opportunity to create a truly egalitarian mass women's health movement.

While Ehrenreich and English (1973, pp. 86-87) noted the danger that a women's health movement could become only "some women's health movement" unless the diversity of women's priorities were taken into account, this caveat (and its practical implications) went largely unheeded, although more radical health groups often discussed the importance of helping poor and Third World women. This split between the ideological concerns of leaders and active participants in the movement reflects not a rejection of broad, ideological egalitarian notions in the movement but, rather, an acting out of concerns and solutions directly rooted in participants' immediate life circumstances.

It is also difficult to mobilize groups to act selflessly on behalf of others, even when there is widespread agreement that there are others in worse straits. This is particularly so in a movement that decries paternalism and all other forms of acting in the alleged best interest of others. Middle-class women, then, are in a bind. If they act in their own class-status interest, they are accused of being selfish. If they take up the cause of the more oppressed, they may be viewed as patronizing and may also make serious errors in assessing priorities for others. To alleviate these strains, health activists have attempted to mobilize working-class and Third World women into the movement and portray the movement as responsive to all women's needs. Thus far, however, it has been difficult to attract and mobilize these constituencies.

Socioeconomic Status of Health Movement Participants

Marieskind (1975a) argues that contrary to popular belief, working-class women predominate. I believe that Marieskind overstates the case. While participants are by no means exclusively the white upper middle-class women that Carden (1974) takes them to be, neither are they primarily working class.

Clinic participants I observed ranged from middle to working class. Many women classified as "poor" are only temporarily impoverished students. In some areas, there are marked differences between clinic users and women who run health groups and participate in self-help activities. Women who operate the clinics and attend self-help activities tend to be middle class and white—even in areas serving predominantly ethnic minorities and working-class communities (Downer 1974a; Moorhead 1975).

The Somerville Women's Health Project, near Boston, Massachusetts, is often touted as a working-class clinic that offers primary care to Somerville residents (Marieskind 1975a; Reverby 1975). Project physician Judy Herman (1975) cautions, however, that efforts to reach and incorporate working-class women have not been as effective as some suggest. She points out that working-class women come as patients, participate in groups, enjoy the newsletter, parties, and benefits, but are hard to involve actively in running the project. Money is a major issue: volunteering, working for subsistence, and rotating jobs frequently are luxuries that most women cannot afford. Another serious issue is lack of skills; working-class women's ability to organize and structure work and assume major responsibility is not well developed. The women's movement cult of structurelessness has been a hindrance, doing nothing to alter the real power differential between middle- and working-class women.

Nonetheless, the Somerville project is unique in that most women-controlled health centers have not made attempting to integrate working-class women a priority (Herman 1975). In fact, some groups believe it to be unwise. One women who was interviewed worked in a West Coast clinic serving a largely middle-class student population described the problem as related to life-style differences:

> A lot of people say they want to see poor people, but I don't think we should see working-class people until our own consciousness is raised quite a bit. Working-class people just don't understand the hipness of middle-class downward mobility. They don't understand it when they come in and see people wearing clothes with patches. If they can afford to wear clothes that don't have patches, they won't. They just don't understand this whole middle-class hip thing. And this is something I've had a hard time getting across to the people in the clinic.

Even groups located in working-class areas oftentimes fail to attract the local clientele they desire. The clinic Peterson (1976) studied in Chicago, for example, saw itself as a community clinic. Yet, in a sample of 183 patients, only 28 percent were local residents. (Fifty-six percent resided elsewhere in the city, and 14 percent were from surrounding suburbs or out of state.) Furthermore, out of 129 patients for whom occupational status was known, 30 percent were students; 20 percent were professional, technical, or kindred workers; 19 percent were clericals; 3 percent were employed in sales; 2 percent were housewives; and 2 percent were unemployed. Only 16 percent were in service work, crafts, or operative occupations (Peterson 1976, pp. 91-95).

Light (1974) reports that 46 percent of the active members of the Vancouver Women's Health Collective have bachelor's degrees or higher and several hold advanced degrees; less than 12 percent have only a high school education. Nearly half have children. Of Vancouver Health Collective users, 79 percent have completed university or other professional training, whereas less than 9 percent have only a high school education or less (Steele 1974).

Reynard (1973) reports similar findings for the women she studied who attended a self-help clinic demonstration. Nearly 52 percent described themselves as professional, technical, or kindred workers; 16 percent as students; 2 percent as housewives; 10 percent as clericals; and 4 percent as managers and officials. Only 5 percent were crafts persons, operatives, or sales or service workers (Reynard

1973, p. 143). Fishel (1973) observed similar populations in other self-help clinics.

Age

Activists range in age from their teens to their upper seventies and eighties, but a disproportionate number are young—in their twenties and thirties (Fishel 1973; Moorhead 1975; Peterson 1976; Reynard 1973; Steele 1974). Nonetheless, self-help was originated by middle-aged women, and many health groups offer middle-aged and older women specialized services.* Many prominent health activists working on the national level, particularly, are older, experienced women.

Sexual Orientation

Health activists quietly ignore charges that self-help advocates are all lesbians. At early self-help demonstrations, separate clinics were offered to give lesbians a supportive setting in which to share concerns and spare them from sitting through unnecessary discussion of contraception. Nonetheless, many lesbians complain that women's clinics are riddled with "heterosex" attitudes (see, for example, Bloch 1973; Hornstein 1973). In some areas, separate health clinics have been founded by and for lesbians, who were tired of helping "straight" women or being exposed to the insensitivity of heterosexual clinic workers.

Lesbians' complaints are well founded, for heterosexual women—many married and with children—predominate and are often unwittingly insensitive. The taken-for-granted assumption that every women uses some type of contraceptive is the issue complained about most frequently by lesbians. In one clinic I observed, several active members were pregnant, and elaborate subsidies were offered to mothers to cover child care costs—a policy resented by some single, childless women. With the growth of feminist obstetrical services, the preponderance of heterosexual women has become even more apparent.

-----

*For example, the San Francisco Women's Health Center, the Berkeley Women's Health Collective, and the Aradia Clinic in Seattle all have active menopause and/or middle-age health groups. The Fremont Clinic in Seattle offers special geriatric services in its community-based clinic.

Ethnicity

The participation of minority women is a thorny issue. Marieskind (1975a) suggests that little by little, they are becoming active. Although some minority women are involved, their numbers are still small. Efforts to introduce self-help practices into women's clinics serving predominantly Asian and Latin American women in the Bay area have been largely unsuccessful; women who have tried suggest that self-care is difficult to promote because of cultural values strongly prohibiting these women from publicly exposing or touching their bodies in the presence of other women. The Orange County FWHC, however, reports that self-help clinics scheduled for groups of Spanish-speaking women, many recent immigrants from Mexico, have been effective (Heidelberg 1978).

Black women have had relatively little involvement in the health movement. The storefront settings and hand-to-mouth image many clinics present are unappealing to many black women, who are impressed by more prestigious-looking medical clinics and personnel. Furthermore, some think that black women regard many feminist gynecological issues as trivial, compared with the more serious health problems black women face (for example, sickle cell anemia, hypertension, poor nutrition, and inadequate medical care) (see Handy 1975; see also Wilson 1976-77).

The split between white middle-class goals and poor blacks' needs were apparent at the National Welfare Right's Organization (NWRO) convention in July 1973. Only 12 people attended the Philadelphia Women's Health Collective's workshop on "health issues." Three Collective members had brought stacks of pamphlets on birth control, abortion, and gynecological procedures; models of the uterine cavity; and a large chart of birth control methods and product samples, intending to perform a skit depicting a typical gynecological exam. The first speaker discussed what a competent gynecological examination should include, passed around a plastic speculum, and discussed gynecologists' authoritarian, unapproachable manner. She suggested women take a friend along for moral support and to ask questions and outlined tactics to employ to challenge the medical establishment, for example, preparing and circulating lists of good and bad doctors and refusing to pay the bill (Pollner 1973). An upstate New York welfare rights group leader interrupted, saying:

> This isn't what we're here for, at least not me. We didn't have the money to send lots of people down here. We have **financial** problems. We can't pick and choose our doctors, we don't have the option not to pay. Most private M.D.'s refuse to take us. We get whatever doctor's at the clinic,

and the clinic is crowded, and we're waiting in line a long
time, and then we're pushed through. There's no time to
ask questions. WE need money and we need services.
That's what my group expects me to tell them about (Pollner 1973).

Another added that in Mississippi, there are no doctors or clinics,
and the remainder of the workshop was spent discussing federal programs for getting conventional services (Pollner 1973). The typical
feminist health issues went largely ignored.

Nonetheless, in 1974, the San Francisco Women's Health Center conducted a four-month training program in self-health for women
on AFDC (Aid for Dependent Children). Most trainees were minority
women; several were black (HealthRight 1975b, p. 7; Wheeler 1975).
The trainees did not "take" to self-help as rapidly as the typical
middle-class women, but with some adjustments, minority women
were successfully interested in health projects (Wheeler 1975). Three
black women, Faye Roberts, Jenette Salters, and Pam Carter, previously associated with the Detroit Feminist Women's Health Center,
founded the Downtown Detroit Women's Feminist Health Center to
serve the predominantly black community (Cowan and Peck 1976,
p. 11). And at the Boston Women's Health Conference, the Third
World Caucus was active, although still convinced that the larger
movement failed to meet their needs ("Proceedings for the 1975 Conference on Women and Health" 1975, pp. 4, 21).

While working-class and minority women are increasingly involved in health movement activities, there is no evidence that their
relative proportion is increasing. For as the movement has grown
and become more "respectable," many more white middle-class professional women have also become active (see, for example, Commonwealth of Pennsylvania 1974; HealthRight 1975a, p. 3; Sandmaier
1976; Seaman 1975). Thus, while the increase of working-class and
minority women makes the movement broader based, it does not alter
the fact that the movement is largely white and middle class—especially in leadership and in focus.

Academic Appraisals of Health Work

The white middle-class interest group image is especially difficult to counteract, because women do organize into health projects
that benefit persons of roughly the same age, sex, or class despite
the ideological imperative to offer assistance to all other women.
Carden (1974, p. 76) dismisses health-related activities, including
health collectives, clinics, and self-help groups offering pregnancy

counseling, physician referral, patient advocacy, and body courses simply as self-serving measures that result in temporary self-help rather than permanent reform. Freeman (1975) also discounts the significance of most women's health activism except for abortion reform, which she readily recognizes as "political"; the only aspect of self-help gynecology discussed in detail is the debate over the safety of menstrual extraction kits (p. 158).

Carden's and Freeman's analyses of the women's health movement reflect academic feminists' propensity to focus almost exclusively on women's roles in the economic system. This concern with women's economic roles has been decried by some feminists, who fear that liberation in the marketplace alone will not solve women's problems. Mitchell (1973, p. 120), for example, argues that women's liberation can only be achieved by transforming all four structures in which they are integrated—production, reproduction, sexuality, and socialization.

Indeed, while feminism stimulated academic research in many areas, it retarded or at least reduced the tendency of scholars to explore certain issues.* Mead (1972, p. xiv) points out that many present beliefs and practices about being human—especially about the role that biological sex plays in the lives of men and women—have been unexplored. Pushing childbearing and child rearing into the background, dismissing it as a part of life that will not be onerous if husbands and the state do their part, is only part of the answer.

The "Motherhood" Issue

Academic feminists' tendency to ignore or minimize the importance of women's biological or reproductive roles is probably related to their class and status interests. As professionals, these women see restricting fertility and shifting responsibility for the care and socialization of children away from individuals as crucial to their liberation. Because they primarily seek economic, status, and power

---

*The few social and behavioral scientists, such as Bardwick (1971, 1972), and Rossi (1977) who have attempted to address or investigate biological differences between the sexes have been severely criticized (see, for example, Ehrlich and Ehrlich 1972). Recently, Mitchell (1975) has suggested that women cannot afford to ignore the work of Freud, or other scientists, simply because his work has negative implications.

rewards (rewards Blake 1971 points out upper-middle-class men typically value), these women overlook the importance of restructuring reproductive roles to make women's noneconomic roles more fulfilling (see, for example, Epstein 1971; Holmstrom 1972; Huber 1973; Theodore 1971; and Rossi and Calderwood 1973).

While a few women may be able to pursue creative, fulfilling economic roles, only 15 percent of all employed women in the United States are professionals; the majority are clustered in the low-status, low-paying "women's" professions of nursing, teaching, social work, and librarianship (U.S. Department of Labor 1975, pp. 83-96). Thus, most women work at low-level jobs that offer few monetary rewards and little challenge or chance for advancement. Not surprisingly, despite the drudgery of housework, not all women view entering the labor force as a panacea when considering their realistic opportunities. Few can afford costs of child care, even when it is available (Roby 1973; Bernard 1975; Bourne 1972; U.S. Department of Labor 1975, pp. 33-40).

These "realities of life" have generated considerable ambivalence and anxiety within the women's movement among women already enmeshed in traditional role obligations, particularly motherhood. For with the growth of feminism, many women showed indifference or even hostility toward motherhood as a career. Well-known feminists, including Simone de Beauvoir, Shulamith Firestone, and Ti-Grace Atkinson, went so far as to suggest that women would only be able to achieve parity with men when children could be produced by extra-uterine methods (Seaman 1975, p. 43). Even less radical women openly challenged the "motherhood myth" (see, for example, Rollin 1972, p. 69).

While dismal views of motherhood were taken seriously in radical-feminist circles, many women were skeptical or felt threatened or denigrated for valuing and enjoying their traditional family roles (Rivers 1975). Others decried the movement's devaluation of the skills and contributions of mothering and were saddened by some feminists' failure to recognize the joys and privileges of being with children (Heidelberg 1978). Women's liberationists were in fact so hostile to motherhood, so attached to an unspoken elitism that favored women who stayed single and childless, that many sympathetic, interested women were alienated. Many women with children wondered if liberationists were interested in including them in the women's movement at all (Abarbanel 1972, p. 362).

Nonetheless, many women with children became active, vocal feminists. While some mothers were interested in pursuing professional careers, others had neither the training nor inclination to seek fulfillment in the marketplace. Lacking options and intensely feeling the need to change the health care system because of their experiences as mothers, some of these women became the founders, active leaders, and participants in the health movement. Unlike fully-employed professional feminists, many mothers had the time needed to sustain voluntary health activities. Self-help gynecology founders Carol Downer and Lorraine Rothman, for example, were both housewives and mothers. Although Downer and Rothman were both employed at the time they became involved in the women's movement, many others were not.

The self-help clinic had great appeal, especially to women not pursuing professional careers. In fact, many nonelite women deeply resented their low status within the feminist movement and eagerly seized upon an activity where their experience in obstetrics and gynecology was regarded positively rather than as evidence of their having been duped into cultural compliance.* Their alienation from the elite feminists and attempts to transform the stigma of being "breeders" into a valued status is clear in the writing of Lolly Hirsch, a self-help movement founder with five children. Indeed, Hirsch (1972, pp. 24-25) proclaimed that the most exciting aspect of the self-help clinic was that "it came from the minds and bodies of breeders." Whereas previously, the women's movement had been carried along by academic and professional career women, who showed no concern for ordinary wives and mothers, with the advent of Carol Downer with six children and Lorraine Rothman with four, housewives, mothers, and breeders now had their own heroines. They were just like the professional and academic women who spoke at prestigious meetings and like hip young women who held speakouts. "The Self-Help Clinic was originated by, thought of, created, developed, organized, carried out to the world by bus, train, plane, letters, telephones; collated, annotated by US, US BREEDERS" (Hirsch 1972, p. 25).

Within the growing women's health movement, motherhood was reinstated as a respectable occupation. While childbearing was acknowledged as socially programmed and oftentimes restricting, it was also viewed as a potentially fulfilling experience, at least for some women. And the pregnancy and childbirth experience—with its joys and horrors—became an important feminist life-event.

---

*Members of MOTHER, a Southern California feminist group, believe that the anti-natalism of the women's movement actually plays into the hands of the multinational corporations that are pushing for population control. Thus, from this perspective, feminists exhibit their own form of cultural compliance (Heidelberg 1978).

The emphasis on childbearing is evident in the Boston Women's Health Book Collective's health course. Nearly half the 1971 edition of Our Bodies, Ourselves is devoted to pregnancy, prepared childbirth, and the postpartum period. (In the expanded 1976 edition, less than one-quarter of the book focuses on childbearing; more technical material on disease states has been added.) Similarly, the Vancouver Women's Health Collective devoted nearly one-third of its health booklet to various aspects of childbearing. In fact, a special "Childbirth Practices Study Group" carried out the extensive pregnancy needs survey and maternity services evaluation in the Vancouver area (A Woman's Place 1972).

An Uneasy Alliance

The alliance between feminists and natural childbirth proponents, however, is tenuous, for male obstetricians still dominate all but extremely radical birth groups. Furthermore, progressive reforms (for example, instructing women so as to minimize fear and pain and insisting on a calm, supportive environment) sought by prepared childbirth proponents, such as Grantly Dick-Read, leave male obstetricians in control of the situation. The most recent natural childbirth hero, Frederick Leboyer, shows great respect for the weakness and vulnerability of the newborn, but identifies with the infant to the virtual exclusion of the mother, who appears as the "monster" of uterine contractions. The psychological and psychic bond between mothers and children are all but dismissed, making Leboyer and the baby the heroes of this obstetrical drama (Rich 1975, pp. 26-28).

Tensions over these and related issues arose in 1973 at two major childbirth conferences—one on the East Coast and one on the West. The East Coast conference, the First International Childbirth Conference, held June 2 in Stamford, Connecticut, was a major event for the women's health movement, attracting around 150 participants.[*] Organized by self-help founder Lolly Hirsch and Dorothy Tennov, a psychologist at the University of Bridgeport, the conference reflected the movement's efforts to bring together feminists with common

----

[*]The entire presentations of the 29 speakers, audience additions, and news reports of the event were printed and distributed in the Proceedings of the First International Childbirth Conference 1973.

concerns despite occupational status differences.* Recognized "professional experts" and laywomen were all given equal time to present their views.

Although hospital delivery was criticized and home birth suggested as an alternative, the focus at Stamford was on limiting rather than totally eliminating drugs or hospitals. The approach was to find safe, supportive settings for childbirth, where women could be in control of their bodies at all times in order to promote an emotionally satisfying birth process. Conferees seemed to be already converted white, middle-class, "liberated" women (Miller 1973).

Despite much enthusiasm, some feminists had reservations and misgivings over the exaltation of childbirth and breast-feeding. Barbara Ehrenreich argued that the women's movement had attempted to eliminate childbearing as women's only acceptable career, fighting for safe, reliable contraception, abortions, and jobs. The central thrust of the women's movement, then, was to free women from self-definition based on reproductive functions—to make women doers, not breeders. From this perspective, Ehrenreich found something strangely nostalgic about the fascination with birth, which seemed to hark back to a time when the world was simpler and there was no women's movement to challenge women with totally new options and life-styles (Proceedings of the First International Childbirth Conference 1973, p. 23). Tennov and Gretchen Walker, another conferee, expressed similar reservations over the enthusiasm for home birth and breast-feeding as "the way" rather than as choices. The tenor of the whole conference was not as feminist as Tennov herself would have liked; she would have preferred an attitude like "get men out of female body functions" (Dejanikus 1973a, p. 7).

While the Stamford conference focused on the experience of birth and visions of how it might be, a San Francisco conference held a few weeks later focused on home versus hospital birth. Sponsored by the Continuing Education in Nursing Program at the University of California at San Francisco, feminist issues were muted. While the participants at Stamford shared common perspectives, members of the mixed group (conservatively dressed physicians and nurses, colorfully attired lay midwives, pregnant women, young children, and nursing mothers) in San Francisco were often at loggerheads.

---

*The idea for the Stamford conference originated from earlier speakouts on childbirth experiences that Tennov taped and shared with the international feminist community in London and Paris. With de Beauvoir's encouragement, Tennov returned to the United States and, with Hirsch, organized the conference.

An obstetrician who spoke against home deliveries was visibly nervous, and afterward said he was really there "to learn." A physician representing the state Department of Health was challenged on his interpretation of the legality or illegality of midwifery. Older women complained loudly that infants and small children should have been barred from the auditorium. In a lay midwifery workshop, frowning nurses questioned whether or not lay practitioners would be able to spend so much time with their patients "if they ever got popular," and regularly punctuated the midwives' presentation with disgruntled "humfs." Home birth had clearly emerged as an issue in a wider public arena, where it would confront larger professional interests. In the process, many feminist concerns fell by the wayside, along with the hope that nurses could necessarily be counted upon to support freedom of choice in childbirth.

RUDE AWAKENINGS TO MULTIPLE REALITIES

Feminists' awareness of underlying race and class conflicts came gradually and painfully. To their dismay, early reformers discovered that their demands—if met—would have cruel (even if unintended) consequences. When middle-class women complained about the hazards of the pill and demanded better testing and tighter research regulations, they learned that nonwhite women in Third World countries would just bear a greater burden as guinea pigs in medical research to evaluate side effects and complications (Brown 1973; Seaman 1975). Even the abortion issue, which unified the movement, aroused considerable criticism for its alleged racist undertones. Some segments of the black liberation movement openly charged that birth control and abortion were genocidal government programs (Hole and Levine 1971, pp. 188-89).*

The Supercoil Scandal

The complicated interplay of other race and class issues in abortion erupted in full force in Philadelphia, precipitating a major schism within the women's health movement. The difficulty began on Mother's Day, 1972, when 20 poor women—most of them black—went

---

*See Turner and Darity 1973 for a study of black Americans fear of genocide.

to Philadelphia for second-trimester abortions (because police had closed the underground women's clinic where they were initially scheduled to be aborted). In the ensuing days, conflict over who should control abortion and who should determine whether or not women can give truly "informed consent" to participate in medical experiments revealed sharp differences within the movement over the definition of these situations. It also laid bare illusions that sisterhood could easily conquer race and class differences and forced participants to examine the implications of their goals, strategies, and tactics.*

When the Chicago abortionists were arrested on May 3, 1972, 250 women were left waiting for abortions—over 50 of them in their second trimester. Merle Goldberg, executive director of the NWHC, unsuccessfully attempted to arrange hospital abortions. She finally arranged for Baron Gosnell, a physician, to perform the abortions at his Philadelphia clinic, with the assistance of Harvey Karman (a non-physician abortionist-inventor) and Benjamin Graber (another physician), who flew in from Los Angeles (BenDor 1974, p. 8).

Within the feminist community, Karman was viewed as a savior by some and a charlatan by others. He had invented the widely acclaimed thin, flexible cannula used in early vacuum aspiration abortions (BenDor 1973a; Dejanikus 1973b; Goldsmith 1972; Karman and Potts 1972) and in 1970 was honored by NOW for his work in securing abortions for women (Hart 1970, p. 49). An established underground abortionist, Karman had assisted women's groups (including Jane in Chicago) to establish their own clinics. Goldberg was a long-time Karman friend and supporter (BenDor 1973a, p. 1).

Others found fault with Karman on various counts. Some Jane members disliked his style (BenDor 1973a, p. 1), and self-help founder Carol Downer (who had learned abortion techniques by observing procedures in his Los Angeles clinic in 1970) felt his abortions were unsafe (BenDor 1973b). Animosity between Downer and Karman escalated in 1972 when menstrual extraction became a public controversy.

Karman has been accused of taking credit for inventing menstrual extraction (BenDor 1973a, p. 1) and creating intentional confusion between self-help gynecology, "do-it-yourself" abortions, and his own activities (Feminist Women's Health Center 1973, p. 3-6).

---

*There are many versions of the story (see, for example, Ben-Dor 1973a, 1973b, 1974; Borman 1974; Chapman 1973b; Copsey 1973; Dejanikus 1973b; Philadelphia Women's Health Collective 1973b; and Women's Health Consumers Union 1973).

FWHC detractors argue that Karman is basically an agent of the antifeminist population controllers who sides with professionals, the USAID, and Planned Parenthood (The Feminist Women's Health Center 1973, pp. 3-6).

Karman was known for engaging in abortion activity to generate publicity, and many observers felt that his willingness to perform the Philadelphia abortions grew out of a desire to provoke interest in his latest abortion technique.* Instead of using saline infusion—the typical procedure in second-trimester abortions—the Philadelphia abortionists used Karman supercoils. (Plastic strips are inserted much as an IUD, which gradually coil and unwind inside the uterus. The coils are removed within 24 hours, and the woman typically aborts spontaneously; remaining fetal material is removed with a Karman cannula.) Goldberg justified using Karman's experimental procedure on the grounds that saline abortions were unavailable and the situation was an emergency; supercoils had been used in another emergency—the Bangladesh rape crisis.† Goldberg contacted the Philadelphia Women's Health Collective to arrange for housing for the Chicago women (Dejanikus 1973b, pp. 2-3).

Half an hour before the Chicago women arrived, Phyllis Ryan of Choice, a clergy abortion referral service that did not typically refer to Gosnell's clinic, learned that second-trimester abortions were to be performed there. Ryan was particularly disturbed that neither physician involved was experienced with supercoils and that Gosnell did not even have a hospital affiliation (Dejanikus 1973b).

Goldberg and Karman claim that on arrival, the Philadelphia district attorney's office called and threatened a bust. (The district attorney's office denies having made any such call.) While the abortions were performed, Philadelphia Health Collective members met outside with Goldberg to discuss the technique. While the Philadelphia women claim they were concerned over the experimental nature of

---

*In 1969, he attracted nationwide attention by going on television to publicize his new flexible cannula and announcing his willingness to provide free abortions. He was subsequently arrested on 13 counts of felony abortion, freed on bail, and rearrested for performing another abortion in 1971 (BenDor 1973a, p. 1).

†Karman actually claims to have designed the device about 20 years ago, has used it in thousands of abortions, and believes that supercoils are safer than saline. He regrets that the negative publicity has made it impossible to compare supercoils to saline abortions (Copsey 1973, p. 37).

the procedure, Karman suggested that the women really objected because they felt he was "invading their turf" (Dejanikus 1973b, p. 2).
The crucial issue, however, became whether or not the women who
had been aborted had been informed of the experimental nature of the
procedure and had had the opportunity to make an informed choice.
The most serious charge was that the Chicago women were ignorant,
uninformed guinea pigs (BenDor 1974, p. 8).

Ruth Sergal, a Chicago abortion counselor accompanying the
women, argued that the women knew that the supercoil was experimental but did not care. Because the Chicago underground abortionists had been arrested, they felt that the Philadelphia clinic was their
only hope (BenDor 1974, p. 8). Sergal added that Goldberg led her
to believe that good hospital arrangements were available for emergencies. Afterwards, Sergal described the disastrous incident.

> We got there in the middle of an abortion war between
> Gosnell's clinic and Choice. Everything was chaotic—
> these Choice people came to break down the Clinic door.
> Harvey had brought Drs. Phyllis and Eberhard Kronhaus-
> en, the Swedish sexologists, to watch us and they kept
> saying what a perfect FATHER Harvey was to talk to
> adolescent girls. ... and then there was Merle, who was
> getting crazy because of all the tension, trying to talk to
> the people outside. It was like a Dali painting, all absurd.
>
> Then the deliveries took longer than they were sup-
> posed to—it was awful. We had to lock everybody in
> against the threat of arrest; there were constant phone
> calls.
>
> It's a freaky thing to watch a late abortion. Some
> of the Health Collective women got pretty upset as this was
> their first time watching an abortion. They got scared
> and sided with Choice and Phyllis Ryan. They all wanted
> the patients to go to a hospital for exams before returning
> to Chicago, so they took the air out of all the tires on our
> bus, and another had to be found.
>
> The Chicago patients were super, though. They
> were really together and supported each other and never
> complained. One of them now works with us as an abor-
> tion counselor, and several later referred relatives to us
> for abortions (BenDor 1974, p. 8).

Of the women undergoing the supercoil procedures, one required immediate hospitalization, at which the hospital director notified the Department of Public Health, which called in federal officials
from the Center for Disease Control (CDC) in Atlanta. The CDC

investigation revealed that 9, or 60 percent of the 15 women, had complications—3 of them major. The woman hospitalized immediately underwent a hysterectomy; another was hospitalized twice for serious infections, and a third required treatment for severe anemia (Dejanikus 1973b).[*]

The NWHC argued that the alleged complications did not result specifically from the supercoils. In one case, the woman already had chronic pelvic inflammatory disease; the abortion activated the condition, as it is known to do. The anemic woman was a teen-age runaway already suffering from malnutrition. The woman required a hysterectomy, it was argued, as a result of a laceration received while undergoing a dilation and curettage in the hospital (BenDor 1974, p. 8). Goldberg argued further that the supercoil method was viewed as "promising" by some abortion experts, and although the complication rate was high, the sample was too small to make statistical comparisons meaningful (Dejanikus 1973b).[†]

Incensed over the incident, the Philadelphia Women's Health Collective issued a position paper, "The Philadelphia Story: Another Experiment on Women" (1973b). Ryan, along with Hayes Wimberly, a district attorney's office detective, charged Karman on 11 counts of performing illegal abortions and 11 counts of practicing medicine and surgery without a license (Copsey 1973, p. 35). Karman was convicted on two counts and fined $500 ("Karman Found Guilty" 1974).

Although concerned over the supercoil technique, many women were outraged that the district attorney had been contacted and felt that there was no excuse for cooperating with the police to bring Karman to trial. From their perspective, trials are male institutions—inappropriate places in which to argue women's causes. A woman's tribunal was suggested as a more appropriate alternative for making Karman accountable for his activities. By letting women's cause be argued by the male state's agents, the women left themselves wide open to Ti-Grace Atkinson's accusations at a NWHC press conference; Atkinson charged that "only a pig calls the pigs" and accused the

----

[*]In contrast, the complication rate for saline abortion is only 27.9 percent, based on a sample of 6,000 cases (Dejanikus 1973b). See also Tietze and Lewit 1973.

[†]Others disagree. Sidney Wolfe of the Nader-affiliated Health Research Group in Washington, D.C., called the incident "human experimentation at its worst" in his testimony before the Kennedy "Hearings on Human Experimentation" in March 1973 (Dejanikus 1973b; Wolfe 1973).

Philadelphia women of "dragging their sisters' vaginas into court" (Chapman 1973b, p. 6).

Invoking the power of the state to "enforce the rules" engendered bitter debate. The situation was exacerbated by the fact that the Philadelphia Health Collective's key supporters were the FWHCs—the strongest opponents of state interference in women's medical affairs. In promoting both cervical self-examination and menstrual extraction, these women had argued that such procedures should not fall under the jurisdiction of male authorities; ironically, Carol Downer recently had been acquitted in Los Angeles on charges of practicing medicine without a license—the same charge for which their arch-enemy Karman was indicted.[*] As long as the male-dominated legal machinery exists, there is the temptation to use it for various purposes, including persecuting sectarian enemies, a strategy that weakens rather than strengthens a movement.

The women who had had the abortions were angry over the Philadelphia feminists' interference and insulted by the position paper's racist assumptions, which made them out to be ignorant victims. At Karman's trial, two aborted women testified for the defense (Chapman 1973b, p. 2). Eight of the Chicago women, along with four counselors and the NWHC, prepared depositions, ostensibly to be used in a libel and slander suit against the FWHC and the Philadelphia Women's Health Collective (Women's Health Consumers Union 1973). According to various reports, Choice and Sister, a Los Angeles paper that reprinted "The Philadelphia Story," were also to be named in the suit (BenDor 1974, p. 8; "Supercoil Suit" 1973). Despite widespread publicity about the impending lawsuit, however, investigative reporters were unable to verify where the suit had been or was to be filed ("Letters—Controversy Over Controversy, OOB Replies" 1973, pp. 14-15).[†]

---

[*]Heberle (1951, pp. 11-14) points out that social movements are always integrated by a set of constitutive ideas or an ideology that may be logically inconsistent but which is almost always functionally consistent with the political and economic needs of a given group. These seeming inconsistencies are in fact pragmatic responses to ongoing situations. For example, members of many movements perceive the court as an instrument of repression, yet seek protection and/or redress through the judicial system.

[†]Inquiries which the author sent to the Women's Health Consumers Union at 2405 Roscomare Road, Suite 20, Los Angeles, California (which publicized the suits), were returned by the post office marked "addressee unknown."

In an abbreviated version of the deposition, dated July 7, 1973, circulated by the Women's Health Consumers Union in Los Angeles (reprinted in Majority Report 1974, p. 6), the Chicago women who were aborted related that they had wanted to go out and tell off the feminists but the counselors thought it was better to ignore them. When they read in the Chicago papers that the abortions had led to the arrest of Karman, that they had been unaware of the TV cameras, and that they had been "used" because they were black and poor, they were angry. They were particularly incensed that Karman, who had helped them, was now being punished by women who did not help them ("Statement of Chicago Women" 1974).

Some felt that the serious complications were directly caused by Ryan's and other health groups' interference (Women's Health Consumers Union 1973). The Center for Disease Control (CDC) investigators agreed, noting that the tense circumstances, anxiety, and fatigue may have contributed to the high morbidity (Copsey 1973, p. 35).[*] The CDC subsequently notified the FDA of supercoil hazards. When the FDA contacted the manufacturer, Milton Roberts, president of Medical Concepts, the coils were no longer being promoted or distributed (Copsey 1973, p. 35).

Amidst the charges and countercharges, some issues were clear. The conditions for performing the abortions were poor. Whether or not the poor conditions were due to the actions of the feminist groups or the facilities or personnel involved was only one level of the controversy. Analyzing the situation, Chapman (1973b, p. 6) argued that the reasons for the poor conditions went deeper than short medical supplies or the alleged culpability of Goldberg, Karman, and others. The core problems were the state's power to control women's bodies with restrictive abortion laws and the medical profit system. Broadening the issues, Chapman (1973b) argued that what feminists should be concerned with was not whether the abortions were experiments but that the potential for experimentation exists in a racist and class-ridden health care system. The issue was not just that Karman earned royalties from the supercoil but that large profits can be made from drugs and devices in the abortion industry.

---

[*]The CDC report added that the small number of cases and unusual circumstances made it impossible to make a definitive judgment of risks, but the method clearly carried risk.

The Social Control of Medical Practice

While feminists could take ideological comfort in Chapman's broad view of the roots of women's medical oppression, they were obviously deeply divided over how to overcome it. A key issue revolved around the appropriate role of the state in any activity involving fertility control. Many feminist health collectives and clinics insist that abortions can and should be evaluated and regulated on the basis of "safety." Who should enforce standards, and how the standards should be enforced, is less easily agreed upon. The Philadelphia women argued after the incident that it was essential to investigate and share information concerning abortion and birth control techniques and to continue developing a network to share this information in order to gain control over local medical practices (Dejanikus 1973b, p. 11).

It is crucial to gain control over medical practices, evaluation, and enforcement of standards. However, the issues of "whose standards" and who should be responsible to enforce such standards are knotty problems. Some women are enthusiastic over having the FDA assume responsibility for drug and device safety. Others feel that the FDA has let women down so many times that women must take quality control into their own hands (Dejanikus 1974, p. 11).

When Ryan and the Philadelphia Health Collective members determined that the supercoil abortions fell short of their standards, they learned some painful truths. Not all women—even feminists—agree on what constitutes good quality care or informed consent. Nor do all share the same definition of what is acceptable under less than ideal circumstances. The attempt to stop the abortions is reminiscent of early twentieth-century women physicians' support of the outlawing of midwifery. When the power of the state is invoked to "keep up standards," poor women may have nowhere left to turn for medical care. The incident also underscores the fact that women with limited options are sometimes grateful for whatever help they can get. Under such circumstances, "informed consent" has a hollow ring.

The supercoil incident also rekindled questions about what constitutes "experimentation" and how it is best controlled. The issue had arisen earlier over menstrual extraction, with detractors arguing that it was perhaps another case of women being used as guinea pigs in medical experiments (Frankfort 1972, pp. xiv-vi). Menstrual extraction proponents disagreed, arguing that women have the right to participate in experiments as long as they are fully informed of the risks and have assurance that the research is controlled by women (Downer 1972; Brown 1973). In the light of the supercoil incident and concern over menstrual extraction, the Philadelphia Health Collective proposed guidelines to evaluate any potential experimentation on women. These guidelines (particularly applicable to endometrial aspiration research) suggest that (1) researchers be in regular contact with feminists with health skills to review their progress and control decisions about their experimentation; (2) women pay close attention to financial arrangements to see if large sums accrue to researchers, backers, or marketers or if funds are channeled back into the women's health movement for further research, clinics, and education; (3) women determine if subjects are given complete information about the experimental nature of the method, including all possible risks and alternative procedures available (Dejanikus 1973b, p. 11).

When guidelines such as these or regulations to govern research, clinical practice, or licensing of practitioners are proposed, however, the consequences are far more complex than meet the eye. The underlying issue of who will decide on risks versus benefits and who will have the structural opportunities to make choices or define the situation often creates bitter conflict. Ultimately, regulations, guidelines, and licensing laws all serve to unequally distribute access to, and control over, services. It is not possible to impose such controls without these consequences. The question, then, is not whether or not specific laws or regulations are in "women's best interest" but, rather, in which women's interest and under what specific circumstances?

As was obvious in the supercoil incident, how one defines the situation depends on one's position in the social structure. Similarly, recent debate over whether sterilization regulations that require a waiting period between signing consent and having the surgery provides a safeguard against coercive sterilization or infringes on women's rights to medical services on demand depends on one's social position. Third World women, most often the victims of unnecessarily complicated or unwanted sterilization, are frustrated over some white middle-class feminists' opposition to a mandatory waiting period. While waiting may be inconvenient or ideologically repugnant to women with options and choices, poor, non-English-speaking women feel that their more advantaged sisters should give more consideration to their plight.

These differences in priorities have been clouded over by persistent adherence to the feminist ideology of "sisterhood of absolute equality." As Nelson and Olesen (1977, p. 13) point out, the principle and possibility of perfect equality is an unexamined, taken-for-granted assumption in both Western liberal thought and feminism. While there are conflicting notions of how equality will be achieved, the assumption is that it is possible. As a consequence, feminists have failed to confront the reality of inequality in social life, inequality that is embedded in the fundamental processes of social differentiation.

While feminist health activists can ignore social differentiation, including divergent perspectives grounded in race, class, and status differences, or decry existing differences, the reality is that both worldwide and in American society, women have highly unequal health needs and access to health resources.

Productive conflict over how best to allocate health services can emerge only with full recognition of the scarceness of resources and the diversity of need—neither of which are likely to change significantly with the existing international political economy. Gaining some measure of control over health services for women will of necessity require compromises, coalitions, and acknowledgment, if not acceptance, of the reality of inequities.

SOME PARADOXES OF SOCIAL ORGANIZATION

Paradoxically, although most health activists believe some form of socialized medical system is needed, the much criticized, fragmented American health care system provides structural opportunities to create alternative health care systems in competition with the dominant mode of health production. Thus, while socialized systems are idealized, such systems are less open to change than the pluralistic American system, which does allow for innovation and challenges to the status quo. While rarely discussed in the movement, some activists acknowledge that feminist health work is facilitated by capitalism because health profits can be used for political work, which is obviously impossible where the state controls most services. Furthermore, women in socialized systems are often even more at the mercy of what the male-dominated bureaucracy offers than are women using the free enterprise health system (see, for example, Macintyre 1977 and Roth 1977b). The flexibility of the Chinese medical system vis-a-vis women or other groups that do not share overall societal goals has yet to be documented. According to Susan Rennie, the Chinese push birth control pills with little concern for side effects and do not strongly promote vasectomy (Cowan 1978). Similarly, in Cuba, the socialized system seems to be moving in the direction of high technology Western medicine, replacing midwives with obstetricians (Kaiser 1978).

Another paradoxical issue relates to scarcity versus surplus of personnel. On the one hand, feminists want to reduce the scarcity of professionals to lower costs. On the other hand, a surplus of health workers can depress wages and make women health workers even more subject to institutional manipulation and less able to press demands for change when faced with hordes of unemployed workers willing to accept subservience or docility simply to have jobs. In addition, a surplus of physicians with "idle time on their hands" could result in unnecessary surgery or other procedures, unless strong controls were imposed to monitor practice.

A third issue is that to effectively change institutions from within, the movement needs inside sympathizers in powerful positions in established institutions. Such persons are especially effective at turning an organized client group into a resource for established groups, including regulatory agencies. Thus, sympathetic insiders may discreetly or openly invite outside pressure groups to present testimony, rouse crowds, and stimulate letter-writing campaigns, to which established groups must respond. This worked well in the larger feminist movement on women's rights issues (Freeman 1975, p. 237). However, "insiders" with power often function in a style repugnant to more egalitarian-oriented grass-roots feminists. How to make use of women in powerful positions without appearing corrupted remains troublesome and crucial as increasing emphasis is placed on monitoring federal agencies. In these arenas, women must come to terms with the political processes of bargaining and trading off, although both may be seen as corrupt and corrupting.

Finally, feminist demands for female healers fit uncomfortably well with certain stabilizing trends in the larger health and stratification systems.

> As medical technology develops and changes, particular tasks are constantly downgraded; that is, particular tasks are delegated by the physician to the nurse. The nurse in turn passes them on to the maid. But occupations and people are being upgraded (Hughes 1958, p. 73).

In short, the process of upgrading and downgrading is a means for renegotiating the division of labor and status rewards without actually altering the stratification or differential reward system.

To the extent that self-help and feminist clinics succeed in returning routine care to women's control, obstetrician-gynecologists will be relieved of boring "dirty work" and will be able to focus on seriously ill patients, where their authority is less easily challenged. Upwardly mobile nurse-practitioners who desire more independent practice may be channeled into highly specialized obstetrical and gynecological practice to work out accommodative relationships with female gynecologists and lower-level female paraprofessionals. Such positions would offer women career lines apart from the mainstream of medical power and prestige and reduce status contradictions by keeping the new practitioners separate—away from troublesome situations (Hughes 1958, p. 149). Whether the benefits of isolating female healers is worth the price of stabilizing the system has yet to be seriously debated.

8

Social Movements and Social Change

Egalitarian social movements are generated, at least in part, as reactions against dominant social trends toward imperialism, industrialization, and bureaucratization. These movements strive to modify such trends to create more humane forms of social relations and social institutions. But this effort requires coming to terms with the trends themselves. In the face of imperialism, social movement leadership must learn to think in national, not regional or local, terms. Eventually, movements must attempt to become international in scale, because many problems are rooted in worldwide structures and conditions. Egalitarian social movements must also learn how to control and use the technology of advanced industrial societies. No movement can ignore either the revolutionary potential or counter-revolutionary possibilities of mass communication, nor can it wish away technology deemed harmful. Finally, movement leadership must develop effective planning—by no means the exclusive prerogative of bureaucratic institutions. In short, to be successful, social movements must enlarge their scale, use technology appropriately and effectively, and institute some form of rational planning (Roberts and Kloss 1974, pp. 166-68).

STAGES OF DEVELOPMENT

Social movements to not arise full-blown but exhibit temporal courses of development with identifiable stages. Thus, social problems and social movements can be viewed as in the process of "becoming," passing through the stages of awareness, policy determination, and reform (Fuller and Myers 1941, p. 321). The women's health movement follows a natural history (or has had developmental phases) similar to other movements that attempt to solve social problems. In this process, the movement has undergone several transformations in relation to expansion of scale, use of technology, and reliance on various forms of planning.

Constructing Awareness of Women's Health Issues

In the initial stages of a social movement, considerable attention goes to amassing tales of the inhumanity of a group's adversaries (Blumer 1951, p. 210). In the women's health movement, this account involved documenting medical misogyny and sexism in science. Laywomen, health professionals, and academics wrote critiques for a wide range of audiences. To raise discontent, stir people to action, and create a potential membership base, a shared perspective must be generated. To do this, an effective communication network is essential (Dahrendorf 1959, pp. 182-89; Friedman 1973; Wilson 1973, pp. 138-39). Access to the press is clearly the first step. By 1975, there were over 1,950 feminist newspapers and journals (Freeman 1975, pp. 110-11).

Several major feminist newspapers have provided outstanding coverage of women's health issues. Off Our Backs, the first national feminist paper, has provided timely health care information and investigative reporting with the guidance of veteran health editor Tacie Dejanikus. Under the editorship of Belita Cowan, Her-Self, an Ann Arbor monthly, was a prime source of reliable health information until it ceased publication in 1977. Feminist monthlies and quarterlies, including Ms., Marjoity Report, The Second Wave, Journal of Female Liberation, and Up From Under, all feature health issues.

In 1975, Her-Self received a grant from the New Women's Survival Catalog Fund to subscribe to five major medical journals. Several Her-Self members had professional health science training, so the newspaper could offer informed comment on technical medical matters. Because Her-Self allowed other feminist papers to reprint articles, its health coverage reached an audience far beyond the newspaper's regular readership (Her-Self 1975, p. 9).

Reviewing scientific journals in order to bring news to an interested public is a technique of information dissemination that social movements must develop when attempting to change social institutions dominated by scientists and professionals.* It has been expanded by

---

*For example, the ecology movement, the antipsychiatry movement, the national health and hygiene movement, and groups

the Community Women's Health Center in Cambridge. This group
Xeroxes copies of scientific reports, newspaper clippings, and con-
ference presentations for subscribers to their "Health Packets."
HealthRight also disseminates recent research findings.

The existence of several feminist publishing and distributing
houses also facilitates dissemination of health-related information to
a wide audience. KNOW (founded in 1969 by Pittsburgh NOW members
to reprint feminist tracts and articles at cost) distributed many early
health movement materials. The Feminist Press published and distributed Ehrenreich and English's Witches, Midwives, and Nurses:
A History of Women Healers (1972) (initially printed by Glass Mountain
Pamphlets), and Complaints and Disorders: The Sexual Politics of
Sickness (1973). The Feminist Press also assured distribution of Dr.
Mary Howell's Why Would a 'Girl' Go Into Medicine? A Guide for
Women under the pseudonym Margaret Campbell, M.D.

Thus, by the early 1970s, there were many outlets for feminist
health information.* As noted in Chapter 3, articles on health hazards
appeared in the feminist periodicals much earlier than in conventional
ones. For example, Xeroxed copies of Kay Weiss's reviews of the
scientific literature on DES appeared first through feminist literature
outlets (n.d., 1972, 1974) and were then published in feminist periodicals (1973, 1974). In 1975, Weiss's article on DES appeared in
the Journal of the American Medical Women's Association. The

---

working to restrict nuclear power plants, halt IQ testing, and bring
"basics" back to public education similarly search for scientific
studies to inform their constituencies of new developments and build
arguments for change.

*The situation had been different just a few years earlier when
two women physicians—Frances Kelsey of the FDA and Helen Taussig
of Johns Hopkins Hospital—tried to alert both the medical profession
and the public to thalidomide-induced birth defects. Taussig's letter
to the JAMA warning physicians about thalidomide was not published
nor did the American press publicize the hazard, although it was well
covered in Europe and Canada (Mintz 1967, pp. 62-63; Silverman
and Lee 1974, pp. 94-98). On July 15, 1962 the Washington Post finally broke the story of how Kelsey had kept thalidomide off the
American market. Media representatives justified the delay on grounds
of confusion over brand names and news judgment. Mintz (1967, p. 64)
observed, however, "One is struck by the frequency with which news
that might adversely affect powerful business interests encounters
indifference and lethargy."

indifference of the conventional media and professional journals to potential news items from scientific sources creates a vacuum, which social movements fill through movement communication networks. While many issues (for example, DES, contraceptive hazards, and dangerous obstetrical practices) would eventually work their way into the general media, the feminist press engineered their being defined as "newsworthy." As demand for health news increased, the mass media accepted women's health issues as newsworthy.

Although some health problems had been reported in the medical literature for decades, women did not define them as problems until contemporary feminism stirred them to see the social world in new ways.* The women's health movement was able to coalesce quickly into a separate, discernible movement because the existing feminist communication network widely publicized health issues. At the same time, this network created awareness of the growth of new health movement activities and organizations. Thus, it gave direction to any new or potential members wishing to express a sense of discontent over the status quo in women's health care.

As awareness of issues become widespread, an initial movement constituency begins to form. At first, there is little differentiation between practitioners, leaders, and the lay membership that dominates the movement's direction (Roth 1977b, p. 114). Emphasis on lay control was particularly pronounced in the self-help wing, where professionals were inherently suspect. In some circles, complete exclusion of professionals was considered on grounds that they were potentially dangerous to the movement. At the First National Conference of the Gynecological Self-Help Clinics of America in Iowa City, Iowa, in 1972, participants debated this issue, emphasizing that professional and career women have vested interests that necessarily limit their freedom of expression, their activities, and their public positions, because they always face the danger of professional ostracism (Hirsch and Alleyn 1972, p. 2). The ultimate decision to

---

*Feminist reconstruction of social reality is not unique to health issues; it has occurred in nearly every life arena (see, for example, Daniels 1975b). Commenting on the newly discovered problematic aspects of marriage for wives, for example, Jessie Bernard (1973b, pp. 329-30) commented that most of the facts had been known for a long time. She had reported many of them herself a generation ago. This time around, however, they looked different because the message of the radical young women had reached her and permitted a different analysis of the same data.

attempt cooperative relations with these women rested on the argument that "professional women and laywomen alike will ultimately be a lone naked patient of the medical profession" (Hirsch and Alleyn 1972, p. 2).

While professionals were cautiously accepted, their derived medical knowledge remained suspect and received little status in many health groups. Individual laywomen's presentations of their experiences with health problems were accorded the same respectful attention as "experts," presentations in conventional settings. In both small groups and large public arenas, official medical science and expertise was challenged and often denounced. Personal experience, not professional pronouncements, carried legitimacy. This initial rejection of orthodox medical science led outside observers to label the movement as "quackery" or as "a new form of anti-intellectualism."

Health activists rapidly became embroiled over ends and means involved in alternative solutions to problems as they proposed and acted on various strategies for change. Between 1971 and 1975, bitter factional disputes over strategies and tactics, as well as organizational form, consumed tremendous energy. Because feminist ideology so strongly discouraged hierarchical organization and insisted upon collective decision making, the growth of rational planning was severely hampered. Expanding health collectives, for example, became bogged down trying to decide how much, if any, authority could be delegated to individuals, committees, or subcommittees. Some clinics adopted more conventional organizational forms, while others attempted to become more collective. Those that abandoned strict adherence to collective decision making—the most notable examples were the nationally affiliated FWHCs—benefited from coordinated rational planning and expanded most rapidly.

Determining Policy

The middle or policy-determining stages of social movements are characterized by efforts to grow in size and to moderate or compromise some of the original doctrine (Roth 1977b, p. 114), as well as to negotiate overall direction. Despite some groups' insistence on collective functioning, the need for overall planning and coordination is increasingly recognized. The growing emphasis on legislative and judicial strategies for change suggests acceptance of more independent action by committees, task forces, and other conventional organizational forms. The action of such groups as the NWHC, HealthRight, the FWHCs, and the Coalition for the Medical Rights of Women indicate that more deliberate planning of strategies and tactics is in the offing.

By the time a major health movement conference was held at Harvard Medical School in April 1975, the movement had become broad based, with increased participation of professional and academic women. The conference itself was intended to open and extend communication between women involved in self-help activities and alternative clinics, women in the health professions, women hospital workers, students, and community women. Sponsors included diverse groups, such as the New England Chapter of the American Medical Women's Association, the Boston Women's Health Book Collective, Planned Parenthood, the Somerville Women's Health Project, and women medical students' organizations from eastern medical institutions. Nearly 3,000 women attended dozens of workshops on various aspects of gynecological care, sexuality, childbirth, the history of women and medicine, the politics of health care, and the health needs of lesbians, Third World women, and women at various stages of the life cycle ("Health Conference" 1975; Hirsch 1975, pp. 16-17; "Proceedings for the 1975 Conference on Women and Health" 1975).

In the middle stage, social movements become more formal and more concerned with credentials and legitimacy vis-a-vis established adversaries. Movement groups spawn their own experts and lobbyists and move into more traditional lobbying territory. Insurance schemes, prepayment plans, and government policy over licensure and certification become more central concerns of challenging health groups (Roth 1977b, pp. 116-18). Many clinics have moved to gain state licensing and certification for their paraprofessionals and seek public family-planning funds. Groups such as the National Women's Health Network, the FWHCs, the Women and Health Roundtable, and the Coalition for the Medical Rights of Women increasingly attempt to provide expert witnesses and testimony to government agencies on these technical matters.

By 1976, interest in women's health was sufficient to publish a new journal, Women & Health, at the State University of New York's College at Old Westbury. Intended as a forum for exploring multi-disciplinary interests in women's health, the journal reflects the linking of academic research with social action. The editorial board, itself, reveals this comingling. The founder and editor, Helen Marieskind, holds a doctorate in public health. Nine of the 25 members of the initial editorial board hold academic appointments in the fields of public health, sociology, biology, law, and social welfare. Five are clinicians in medicine and nursing; three direct health programs; and another four are health planners or consultants. Three feminist health writers, Barbara Seaman, Norma Swenson, and Judy Norsigian, as well as self-help founder Carol Downer, also sit on the board (Women & Health 1976, p. 2).

Although local and regional groups are essential to the women's health movement, increasing emphasis is placed on national organizations and international issues. At the International Women's Health Conference in Rome in June 1977, women from over 20 countries met to exchange materials and establish networks ("Network Hotline" 1977, p. 6). Health activists recognize that fertility and population control, drug development and testing, childbirth procedures, and licensing of health personnel are all national and international issues that are connected to the material interests of established elites. Recent health packets distributed by the Community Women's Health Center in Cambridge, Massachusetts, have included news clippings on abortion, sterilization, childbirth practices, and breast versus bottle feeding in Latin America, Africa, and Europe. HealthRight and Network News also cover international women's health issues.

However, directing attention to international issues creates conflict within the largely white, middle-class movement. The women who have worked exceedingly hard in this group are distressed by criticism that the changes they seek (subjectively experienced as crucial to their well being) are considered to be trivial or unimportant. When confronted with the needs of poor women, however, American middle-class women's concerns are simply not those of most women of the world. After attending the International Women's Year Conference in Mexico City, health activist JoAnne Fisher (1975), for example, reflected that as a North American woman, she is part of only 2 percent of the world's female population. She wondered if feminist concerns about better and more nutritious food, contraceptive options, cold speculums, orgasmic difficulties, drugs in childbirth, and the general quality of medical care are really significant when compared with those of women who have no food, face cultural as well as technological barriers to contraception, and have virtually no medical care. She concluded that "one woman's pain, regardless of its intensity, does not invalidate another woman's pain. ... Understanding our own oppression is important in helping us to identify with the oppression of our sisters" (Fisher 1975, p. 6). Nonetheless, Fisher urged that women become cognizant of the effects of change on the lives of other women and develop a clearer international consciousness, particularly around issues involving pharmaceutical testing, breast versus bottle feeding, contraceptive technology, natalist policies, health research, and representation of women in health and population agencies.

That women will be able to transcend racial, religious, and class interests in health is yet to be seen. Goodwill alone will never eradicate these differences, in part because goodwill often fails to take into account the subjective perspective of those to whom it is extended. Furthermore, until women dominate or more strongly influence the health arenas they seek to control, it will be difficult to assess the ability of white middle-class women to work cooperatively to assist Third World and working-class women to achieve their health goals. As it is now, white middle-class women can sidestep these issues with the argument that they are powerless; had they the power, they could be called to account.

The upcoming battles over halting the sale of infant formula to women in Third World nations, securing public funds for abortions for poor women, and adopting, implementing, and monitoring government regulations to prevent forced sterilization are critical tests—for they stand as indicators of efforts at cooperation across class and race lines. Unless the larger women's health movement is able to mobilize resources to press these issues, ideological commitment to poor and Third World women will remain just that, and activists will have to re-evaluate their goals and priorities in relation to various constituencies. To mobilize support for securing abortion rights and protection from coercive sterilization, the movement will have to develop close working relations with other health reform groups not noted for their sympathy with traditional feminist issues—welfare rights groups and ethnic minority organizations. This effort will show what kinds of long-term workable alliances are possible.

While the concerns of Third World women are often linked to lack of services or medical technology, there is growing concern that Western technology may be spreading too rapidly and accepted without question. In Brazil, for example, six out of ten private deliveries are by Caesarean section ("Health News Briefs" 1977, p. 11). Although some health groups reject modern medical technology for childbirth and routine care, it is rejected on the grounds that it is harmful or unnecessary in these situations; technology per se is not rejected. Thus, the movement strives to establish a more effective and judicious use of technology—a goal the medical profession itself now acknowledges is necessary to curtail the spiral of iatrogenic disease.*

---

*For discussion of some technical, ethical, and professional issues in medical technology, see, for example, Illich 1976; Leach 1972; Mendelsohn, Swazey, and Taviss 1971; and Sartwell 1974. McKinlay 1977, pp. 475-76, points out that while it has been claimed that in 1910, a random patient contacting a physician had better than a 50-50 chance of benefiting from the visit, we are reaching the point where a random healthy person contacting any random health worker has better than a 50-50 chance of contracting a disease or suffering unnecessarily as a result of the encounter.

Health activists skirt the technology issue to a degree by focusing on low-technology primary care. Women can legitimately claim some expertise and realistically develop proficiency in low-technology areas, if not in the more complex specialties. The continued dominance of male physicians in high-technology specialties is almost taken for granted—or perhaps ignored—because it is clearly beyond the ability of a movement such as this to do anything about it.

Charges that some segments of the movement represent a flight toward mystical healing schemes (for example, Marieskind and Ehrenreich 1975) are interesting because the medical profession itself is increasingly interested in such practices. Termed a "holistic health revolution" by some observers, nutrition, herbal remedies, self-reliance, homeopathy, chiropractic, acupuncture, and other traditional Eastern healing practices are gaining proponents among orthodox medical practitioners (see Gustitas 1975; Leonard 1976; Pixa 1975; and Samuels and Bennett 1973). Women's health groups promoting these practices may be more forward looking than detractors realize.

Institutionalization of Reform

Social movements do not continue indefinitely with the vigor and mass participation that characterize their early stages. Health movements are no exception; some health movements peter out and die, as did the naturopathic movement in the United States. Others become amalgamated by more conventional institutions, as did osteopathy and homeopathy, or assume specialty roles within established health systems, as chiropractic is doing now. Still others that retain their autonomy as separate healing systems become controlled by their own professional experts and can become "establishment"; today's scientific medicine was once only one of many competing forms of healing (Roth 1977b, pp. 118-21).

Successful movements utlimately become institutionalized in some manner and enter a reform or, in Fuller and Myers's (1941) scheme, final stage of development. As groups rely more on conventional forms of political action, such as lobbying and building enduring organizations and associations, social movements gradually become established interest groups and promote their now more socially acceptable causes. Labor unions, civil rights groups such as the NAACP, and moral reform groups such as the Women's Christian Temperance Union are all institutionalized social movement organizations. Contemporary scientific health care is an excellent example of an institutionalized stage of a health movement (Roth 1977b, p. 120). Segments of the women's health movement are entering this phase, as evidenced by those movement groups and organizations now willing to analyze programs and policies and participate in long-range policy planning with established health institutions and government agencies.

MOVEMENT IMPACT

The success and impact of the women's health movement is still difficult to assess. As with any social movement that incorporates and amplifies larger societal drifts and whose constituencies are involved in overlapping reform movements, attributing specific changes to movement activities is not possible. Some changes, such as broad attitudinal shifts, are particularly difficult to measure, partly because outside of carefully controlled laboratory situations, individuals often have different notions about how and why their attitudes have changed. Nonetheless, the evidence suggests that the women's health movement has been influential in gaining for women more control over both their own individual health care and over the direction obstetrical and gynecological care is taking in the society at large.

Attitudinal Changes of Patients and Practitioners

The movement has clearly influenced the attitudes of many women toward themselves and has altered women's expectations and definitions of what constitutes "quality care." This attitiduinal shift is noticeable even among women uninvolved in movement activities and unaware of the origins of their changing values.

By the early 1970s, conventional women's magazines, including McCalls, Vogue, Mademoiselle, Redbook, Woman's Day, and Family Circle, were all publishing health material that challenged orthodox medical approaches. In the June 1973 issue of McCalls, Judy Klemesrud wrote that "the love affair between women and their gynecologists ... is on the rocks and it may be awhile before it is patched up." Women's magazines' advice to women to remember that they, not doctors, "own" their bodies, to "shop around" for a doctor, to be assertive about their rights, is counter to their previous stance that medical authority is sacred. Of course, unlike feminist periodicals, most popular magazines did not theorize on the roots of medical misogyny or challenge the competence or general good will of most practitioners (see, for example, Edmiston 1973; Gendel 1974; Klemesrud 1973; North 1972; Ramsey 1973; and Switzer 1976).

Interest in health issues has also spread to major universities, where special courses on women and health are offered in women's studies and health science departments. These academic courses usually include feminist perspectives on women's health issues, as well as standard medical and social science material.*

The medical profession itself acknowledges the changing attitudes of women patients—often with confusion and bewilderment (see, for example, Kaiser and Kaiser 1974; Luy 1974; "Physicians and Feminist Patients: Conflict Grows" 1973; Pollner 1975; Rau 1974; Stephen 1973b; "Support, Information Ob. Gyn. 'Best Response' to Women's Lib" 1975; and "Women's Liberation and the Practice of Medicine" 1973). Michael Daly, professor and head of the Department of Obstetrics and Gynecology at Temple University Medical Center, notes that obstetricians and gynecologists, who see themselves as devoted to helping women, find it ironic and perplexing that feminists are critical of the medical profession at large, especially of obstetrics and gynecology, "once termed the happy specialty." Furthermore, with modern contraceptives, gynecologists have provided women with their new sexual freedom. Why, then, these doctors ask, are so many women—even the more docile, soft-spoken ones—suddenly questioning every procedure, every prescription? The majority of his colleagues, says Daly, are very concerned about these changing attitudes and really try to understand the criticisms so forcefully verbalized (Rau 1974).

Some physicians attribute changes in patient attitudes and behavior directly to feminism and the women's health movement. For example, John Kerner, chief of Obstetrics and Gynecology at Mt. Zion Hospital in San Francisco, claims that "there's a very verbal and impressive group of women involved in the women's health care movement in San Francisco who have had an impact. ... Patients are asking more questions" (Stephen 1973b). Another Bay area physician, John Schaupp, believes that "women are asking questions and relating in a much more intelligent manner than they used to. They seem to know more about their bodies and have read enough to be able to propose questions which have merit" (Stephen 1973b).

Three physicians and a family planning specialist discussing patient demands arising out of the women's health movement at a symposium reported in Contemporary OB/GYN generally agreed that

---

*Pat Hanson of Russell Sage College, Albany, New York, is researching the curriculum used in such courses. See Olesen 1977a for a roster of academics involved in teaching and research on women's health. A survey of women's courses is being conducted by Sociologists for Women in Society (SWS Newsletter 1977, p. 11).

women from all classes and socioeconomic levels are asking more questions and expecting more explanations, although they do not necessarily identify with the movement itself (Chez 1974).

Some physicians find adjusting to these "new patients" difficult. To ease the transition, one southern California state university health service sponsored a symposium for health professionals on how to relate to women patients involved in women's health clinics (Bullough 1975). And at the District 8 meeting of ACOG in Los Angeles in early 1975, Robert Kinch advised his colleagues that obstetrician-gynecologists' best response to the women's movement was to be more supportive, more informative, and more accepting of patients' decisions about elective and therapeutic procedures. He also warned against using cold speculums, handling patients roughly, or engaging in such mannerisms as humming, which may annoy women ("Support, Information, Ob. Gyn. 'Best Response' to Women's Lib" 1975).

Although agreeing certain changes in practice are needed or are already being implemented, other doctors have denied any relationship between feminism or the women's health movement and their changing ways. San Francisco gynecologist Robert Smith, for example, believes that women want to know more about their bodies than they once did, but thinks that "it may be the result of the mass media as much as the women's movement" (Stephen 1973b).

Other physicians argue that they, not women, initiated recent changes. For example, Benny Waxman, associate professor of obstetrics and gynecology at George Washington University in Washington, D.C., told Medical World News that

> "gynecologists don't do it [pelvic exam] that way anymore. At least here we don't. We teach our students to empathize, explain, communicate. What Women's Lib is saying confirms our attitudes and teachings, but we like to think we are acting independently" ("Women's Liberation and the Practice of Medicine" 1973, p. 33).

Physicians' claims of independent action for change suggests just how strongly physicians desire to claim full authority for, and control over, their professional turf; even the idea that change might be stimulated from outside threatens boundary maintenance. By incorporating feminist demands and then taking credit for originating change, traditional experts can relegitimate control over their social world and simultaneously reduce discontent. Indeed, the main consequence of professional responsiveness to feminist demands will be the increasing proportion of physicians practicing in the traditional-egalitarian mode. Such an outcome tends to maintain, rather than undermine, professional control.

The benefits of having active, involved patients are gradually recognized by obstetrician-gynecologists. For example, ACOG's "great debate" over whether the feminist movement has had a positive or negative effect on obstetrical and gynecological care largely turned into a consensus on benefits. Virginia E. Johnson, co-director of the Reproductive Biology Research Foundation, St. Louis, argued on the "pro" side that feminism has helped women develop self-confidence, self-definition, and commitment to themselves as individuals. This development enables women to clearly express their needs as patients and contributes greatly to both diagnosis and prognosis. Women with these qualities are also less likely than traditional women to see their physicians as surrogate husbands or mothers and are far less vulnerable to physician countertransference, a situation in which the physician imposes an emotional relationship on a woman for his or her own fulfillment (Pollner 1975).

James A. Merrill, professor of gynecology and obstetrics at the University of Oklahoma College of Medicine, added that other assets of the feminist movement included focusing attention on the demeaning nature of gynecological care as a special example of the social and political position of women. It has forced gynecologists to re-examine their general attitudes, inadequate communication, and any other inappropriate behavior; Merrill also credited vocal feminists with success in altering hospital policies concerning sterilization and maternity care, demonstrating that minor surgical procedures can be performed on an outpatient basis, and showing that nonphysician female health personnel are not simply acceptable but actually improve the quality of gynecological care (Pollner 1975).

Neither Evalyn S. Gendel, assistant director of the Bureau of Maternal and Child Health, Kansas State Department of Health and Environment in Topeka, nor Kermit E. Krantz, head of the department of gynecology and obstetrics at the University of Kansas Medical Center College of Health Sciences and Hospital in Kansas City, assigned to argue the detriments of feminism, actually did so.

Gendel, playing the "devil's advocate," did not agree with the statements she was making, and sarcastically reported negative arguments many of her colleagues had expressed. These included physician concern that feminist women would no longer accept without question what they were told and might even seek second opinions, which would both delay treatment and constitute a breach of trust. Others expressed concern that patients would ask them to quote recovery rates, which would mean they would have to look them up and then perhaps face patient questioning of the recommended therapy. Some feared that women would insist on being examined by nurse-practitioners, who can do good physicals but whose practice might destroy the traditional doctor-patient relationship. Still others were concerned that women might start learning about their bodies, might use speculums themselves, and might even ask to watch cervical examinations, when, in the opinion of these physicians, women do not need to know what their cervixes look like. Women upset hospital routines when they insist on rooming-in, local anesthesia, full information on medication, and access to medical records. "Finally, if we can't call them 'sweetie' and 'honey,' we may actually have to remember their names," noted Gendel. Krantz made little attempt to outline serious objections (Pollner 1975).

Johnson criticized the "con" debaters for failing to present some realistic and valid points and for treating the subject so lightly. Merrill added that too many gynecologists still resent expectations that they explain why treatments are suggested or what the prognosis is. In addition, some gynecologists still regard women somewhat as the property of their husbands and so tell women very little and then call husbands to provide a full report "just as a veterinarian would do after he treats a prize bull" (Pollner 1975).

At the conclusion of the debate, the moderator, Audrey J. McMaster of the Oklahoma Health Science Center College of Medicine, Oklahoma City, noted that this was the first time that two participants in an ACOG "great debate" had been women and that all audience questions had been directed to the two male panelists (Pollner 1975).

Changes in Health Care Delivery

In addition to providing new health care delivery units, women's alternative services have stimulated changes in traditional delivery modes. As Merrill noted at the ACOG "great debate," feminists have been successful in forcing changes in sterilization procedures, maternity care, the availability of outpatient surgical services, and the utilization of paramedical personnel. And as indicated in Chapters 2 and 6, feminist abortion clinics have lowered prices in some areas.

The greatest changes have been made in obstetrical services. In 1971, only 10 percent of the 7,000 hospitals in the United States offered childbirth education classes; today, it is rare to find a large hospital without them. Most classes use the Lamaze technique—breathing exercises designed to help women relax and to minimize need for medication, or the Bradley method, popular in California, which teaches women to concentrate on the pleasurable and sexual sensations of childbirth rather than on breathing exercises (Seligmann 1976, p. 60).

Even these "concessions" have been inadequate in the eyes of many feminist health activists and natural childbirth proponents, who would prefer to rely more on midwives than obstetricians. Many urge a return to birthing at home ("Editorial: The Home Birth Movement" 1977; McTigue 1977; Mehl 1977; Pearse 1977; Peterson and Mehl 1977; "NAPSAC Meeting Held, Home Birth Advocated, Decried" 1977). In an effort to counter what professionals fear is an alarming increase in home births, five major medical organizations embraced a plan for sweeping changes in hospital maternity care at an ACOG meeting in Chicago in May 1977 (Lieberman 1977; Parachini 1977).

Richard H. Aubry, head of the Interprofessional Task Force on the Health Care of Women and Children, contended that the public is telling professionals that they want birth more under their control and that health professionals must listen. In response to public demand, the ACOG, the American Academy of Pediatrics, the American College of Nurse-Midwives, the American Nurses' Association, and the ACOG's own nursing association approved position papers calling for new delivery procedures that would lead to a "revolution over the next five years" in the way babies are born in hospitals. The newly approved policy statements included the provisions that all hospitals offer birth preparation classes; that fathers be permitted to remain with women through the entire birth process, including delivery; that hospitals offer optional homelike "birth rooms"; that restrictions on children visiting mothers and newborns be lifted; and that hospitals accelerate the release of mothers and infants after birth so that they can quickly return to the more psychologically secure home. The ACOG again reiterated its opposition to home birth on the grounds that it is overly hazardous (Parachini 1977). (See Pearse 1977 for ACOG opposition to home birth.)

In some areas "home-style" birth programs are entirely instigated and staffed by professionals. Others, however, have developed as cooperative efforts between conventional institutions and feminist groups. Members of the San Francisco Women's Health Center now operate self-health clinics at the county General Hospital and were instrumental in instituting a birth program there that offers care by nurse-midwives. Because the Interprofessional Task Force supports these programs, newly instituted ones will be fully controlled by professionals. The relative proportion of services in which lay feminist groups are active will rapidly decrease.

Feminists are being incorporated into conventional settings in other ways. One Bay Area physician, impressed by health group participants' ability to communicate with women, now hires feminist health group veterans as office assistants. In addition to performing usual office tasks, feminist assistants teach patients to examine themselves; these assistants also offer support during procedures.

The eagerness of professionals to endorse these new procedures and practices is a good indicator of consumers' real power in determining how, if not what, services should be available. To a great

extent, obstetrician-gynecologists are economically motivated to provide what consumers demand. Hospitals, suffering even more than
individual physicians from the declining birth rate and increase in
home birthing, particularly in large metropolitan areas, often compete with each other to attract clients to fill their maternity wards.
Providing "consumer-oriented services" is one way to attract cus-
tomers.* In rural areas, where there are limited facilities, physicians and nurses seem genuinely concerned that women will birth at
home unless hospitals are more acceptable. Rural women are often
a great distance from medical assistance; thus, both patients and
practitioners are highly motivated to work out new accommodative
relationships.

Eliminating Sexism in Medicine

The medical profession has shown some responsiveness to
feminist charges of sexism in literature and in education. For example, the advertising, promotion, and printing of Williams and Wilkins'
1971 textbook, The Anatomical Basis of Medical Practice, were discontinued after Estelle Ramey, a prominent feminist endocrinologist
and professor of physiology and biophysics at Georgetown University
School of Medicine, charged that the book violated both medical ethics
and standards of professional behavior. In addition to complaining
to the publishers, Ramey sent her comments regarding the inappropriate use of provocative showgirl models and jocose references to
sexually attractive patients to numerous medical and scientific organizations ("Women's Liberation and the Practice of Medicine" 1973,
pp. 37-38).

Another textbook author told his colleagues at a public meeting
of obstetricians and gynecologists that after considering the Scully
and Bart (1973) study, he was rewriting his chapter on female sexuality for his next edition; Bart was personally invited to the session
at which he made the announcement. In San Francisco, Ernest Page,
head of the Department of Obstetrics and Gynecology at the University

---

*For example, in 1973, Milwaukee's Family Hospital was only
delivering 12 to 15 babies per month. The ob-gyn department was in
danger of folding unless it responded to consumer demands for home-
style birth. After converting to a "family-centered" program, deliveries increased to 70 to 80 per month and the active staff doubled
("Hospitals Bow to Couples Wanting Special Births" 1977).

of California Medical Center, told staff physicians at grand rounds
that "My book 'Human Reproduction,' a basic text, hasn't been burned
yet. [But] there are certain areas dealing with feminine psychology
and sexual attitudes that would have to be revised" (Stephen 1973b).

In response to criticism from feminists of their portrayal of
women in drug advertising, Smith, Kline, and French agreed to use
equal numbers of men and women in future advertisements (Fidell
1974). Nonetheless, women continue to appear in stereotypical roles.
A recent article in Medical Economics (Morgan 1976), entitled "Must
You Coax Her into Lithotomy Position?" replete with cartoon carica-
tures of women patients, indicates that sexism has in no way been
eliminated, even in official journals.

L. Thompson Bowles, who heads the Association of American
Medical Colleges (AAMC) Medical Curriculum Committee, predicts
that the Boston Women Health Book Collective's Our Bodies, Ourselves
will become required reading in American medical schools. Medical
school professors now find it more difficult to display the more overt
forms of sexism in the classroom, although subtler forms are still
common.* Nonetheless, medical educators are increasingly sensitive
to these issues and no longer so openly condone sexist treatment of
women students. Some are even making public apologies for their
faculty members' inappropriate behavior. For example, Vernon
Wilson of Vanderbilt University School of Medicine sent an official
letter of apology to a woman interested in applying to medical school
who had received a letter from a faculty member suggesting she pursue some field more appropriate for a woman, such as nursing.
Wilson apologized for the thoughtlessness of his colleague's statements
(which he claimed did not reflect his institution's view) and emphasized that the physician who wrote the letter had neither a direct role
in admission policies nor was in a position to speak for Vanderbilt.
Both the offending letter and Wilson's apology were published in
HealthRight 1977b, p. 27 .

Women physicians are taking an active role in improving conditions of medical education (Jacobs 1978). Support groups for wom-
en students have developed in many schools, including the University

---

*See Shapiro 1977 on counseling women on how to manage non-
actionable sex discrimination in medical schools. The newsletter of
the Women in Medicine Committee, American Medical Student Association, also offers suggestions for women to combat sexism. See,
for example, Jacobs 1978, pp. 3-4.

of California at San Francisco and Irvine and at Stanford University.*
Medical women's conferences have recently addressed feminist issues of humanizing care, reducing elitism, and developing more
egalitarian relations with lower-level health workers (Howell 1975b,
1976). And at Harvard University, the Reduced-Schedule Residency
Program collects information on, publicizes, and promotes less than
full-time residency programs to encourage women to complete specialty training (Shapiro and Driscoll 1977a, 1977b). According to
Bowles, these flexible schedules are increasingly available (Marieskind 1976, p. 204).

Controlling Hazardous Drugs and Devices

The success of the women's health movement in getting professionals and regulatory agencies, as well as women themselves, to
reassess the use of hazardous contraceptive drugs and devices is one
of the most significant outcomes of the movement. Beginning with a
feminist demonstration and disruption of Senator Gaylord Nelson's
hearing on oral contraceptives on January 23, 1970 (Seaman and Seaman 1977, p. 270), feminist health activists have waged major battles
against powerful drug interests and professional pride to combat the
wave of iatrogenic disease that "experts" ignored or denied. It was
in large part because of Seaman's efforts that women began questioning their doctors' assurances that the pill was "safe." She was also
instrumental in getting the FDA to require written warnings to be inserted in oral contraceptive packages. After testifying and badgering
the FDA for over five years, Doris Haire finally convinced the FDA
to withdraw approval for DES used as a lactation suppressant and to
withdraw approval for the use of Pitocin for elective induction of labor (Cowan 1978). Current efforts to restrict the use of DES and to
properly check on women exposed to DES in utero are now urged by
feminist health activists, with the cooperation of a growing number
of physicians concerned over the carcinogenic effects of synthetic
estrogens. (Efforts to curb the use of sex hormones are discussed
in recent works by Cowan 1977 and Seaman and Seaman 1977.)

---

*For discussion of how these operate, see, for example, Hil-
berman et al. 1975 and Walsh 1977.

Government Recognition of Women's Health Issues

The view that women's roles as providers and consumers of health care is a significant social issue has gradually been adopted by government agencies. The merging of academic, professional, and lay social action interests is a noteworthy feature of government-sponsored health activities on both the state and national levels.

In June 1974, the Pennsylvania Commission on the Status of Women, the Governor's Office, and the Southeast Region of the Pennsylvania Health Department cosponsored a major women's conference to raise public awareness of health issues, identify needs of women consumers and providers, and formulate actions and strategies to deal with problems. Well-known feminist health activists, as well as professionals, were featured speakers and drew an audience of 1,200 from widely divergent groups ("Proceedings of the Conference on Women and Health, June 27, 28, 29, 1974, Philadelphia, Pa." 1974). Conferences on women's health issues are now proliferating throughout the United States. Brief descriptions of these conferences are included in every issue of Women and Health, HealthRight, and Network News.*

The federal government has directly funded women and health conferences, indicating growing interest in Washington over issues initially raised by the militant segments of the women's health movement. The Health Resources Administration (HRA) funded five conferences between 1975 and 1977, focusing on an array of issues. The International Conference on Women in Health, held in Washington, D.C., in June 1975, had as its goals increasing information on the status of women in health careers in the United States and other countries, identifying data sources, and stimulating comparative research (Pennell and Showell 1975). At "Women and Their Health: Research Implications for a New Era," a conference held in San Francisco in August 1975, conferees (mostly academics and professionals) discussed substantive and methodological issues in research on women's health (Olesen 1977b). A third conference, "Double Dynamics: Women's Roles in Health and Illness," held in Philadelphia in December 1975, was designed as a first step to assist federal agencies develop long-range plans to improve conditions for women in the health

---

*It would be interesting to tabulate the number of conferences held and the array of topics covered since 1972, when this movement gained momentum.

system through the Office of Health Resources Opportunity (OHRO) within the larger HRA. Recommendations were made on issues involving women as paid providers, consumers, extramarket providers, and decision makers ("Double Dynamics: Women's Roles in Health and Illness" 1975). "Women's Health: Research, Policy and Communication," a conference held at the University of California, San Francisco, in May 1977, was an effort to encourage dialogue between academic researchers, health professionals, educators, students, and consumers. Each of the symposium panels included a mix of participants, and community health groups were invited to lead workshop sessions ("Proceedings of the Conference on Women's Health: Research, Policy and Communication" 1977). Another conference held at the University of California, Santa Cruz, focusing on "Women's Leadership and Authority in the Health Professions," sought to evaluate the state of research, programs, and policy on women in health work and to identify strategies for change ("Proceedings of the Conference on Women's Leadership and Authority in the Health Professions" 1977).

While these conferences may not have initiated specific action on the part of the federal government to improve conditions in the health system, they did serve several useful functions. They all legitimated women's concerns over health issues, generated the production and dissemination of much scholarly work on specific issues, and facilitated the development of informal networks around health.[*] They also provided professional women, who less often actively participate in lay movement groups, opportunities to discuss strategies and tactics for pressuring public and private groups to respond to women's concerns.[†]

Significantly, the groundwork for OHRO funding of the Program for Women in Health Sciences (PWHS) at the University of California, San Francisco, was laid at the 1975 OHRO-funded conference in Philadelphia.[‡] The PWHS, a demonstration project designing model

---

[*]See Daniels 1977 for discussion of the importance of a national informal feminist health network and Freeman 1975, p. 228, on how informal women's networks develop within federal agencies. The author participated in all except the Washington conference; other conferees also have been involved in several of these programs.

[†]See Ruzek 1977b for a description of practical strategies and tactics discussed by participants at the Santa Cruz conference.

[‡]Lucy Ann Geiselman, dean of Continuing Education, University of California at San Francisco, and Martha White, associate

programs to facilitate women's career development and consumer participation in health, sponsored both the May and June 1977 conferences in San Francisco and Santa Cruz.

Women and Health Policy Making

As Freeman (1975, p. x) points out, public policy is the means whereby government stimulates, responds to, and/or curtails social change. Yet feminists, alienated from traditional political activity, often could not relate to anything so mundane as petitioning the federal government or writing letters to legislators. The government was seen as too remote, its response too distant, to make this avenue of protest attractive. Eventually, liberal feminists succeeded in mobilizing these conventional forms of political action to combat sex discrimination in higher education (Freeman 1975, pp. 191-202).

Initially, health activists found approaching the government on issues aside from abortion equally unappealing. Efforts to influence policy within the federal government were particularly discouraging to activists in the Coalition for the Medical Rights of Women, who abandoned working in Washington, D.C., in favor of directing efforts at California state and local government agencies. As noted in Chapter 6, they have had considerable success in working with state Department of Health representatives, and in 1976, the Coalition's first coordinator, Jenny Jennison, joined the staff of Jerome Lackner, state Director of Health.

Of course, government consists of hundreds of subgovernments, including standing and ad hoc task forces, advisory committees, and consultants, as well as elected officials and bureaucrats (Freeman 1975, pp. 226-28). In recent years, feminist health activists have played an increasing role in government, although this aspect of the movement has not been widely discussed nor have systematic studies been undertaken. *

---

research psychologist, School of Nursing, University of California, San Francisco, cofounded the program. Geiselman is the project director.

*The data I have on these developments are limited largely to efforts in which I myself have been involved or have learned about informally. I have made no effort to study them systematically, although a traceable pattern exists. Task forces and local and state commissions have been formed, and testimony has been collected. Further research is needed in states other than California, as well as in Washington, D. C.

At the state level in California, feminists have become active in state advisory committees as regular members, consultants, and public pressure groups. For example, the governor's Drug Abuse Prevention Advisory Council (DAPAC) and the Technical Advisory Council (TAC) appointed a subcommittee on women and drugs in 1974, later named the California State Committee on Women and Drugs (CSCWD). One CSCWD member was appointed an official consultant to the DAPAC/TAC and provided information on women's issues to the state Office of Narcotics and Drug Abuse. CSCWD members also cooperated in getting formal recognition and funding for a Northern and Southern California Conference on Women and Drugs, which brought together women in drug treatment programs with representatives of state agencies, who then formed ongoing organizations to further their interests and concerns. (See Ruzek 1975a for discussion of CSCWD; see also "Women Air Health Care Discontent" 1975; "Women Gather for Drug Conference" 1974; "Women and Drugs Subject of Statewide Media Campaign" 1974).

Under pressure from free and community clinic proponents, the California Department of Health Bureau of Licensing established an Advisory Committee on Free and Community Clinics in 1976 to review proposed changes in licensing regulations applicable to these clinics. Two appointees to the advisory committee were known to be involved in feminist health activities,[*] and representatives from local women's health clinics in northern California attended the first public hearing on clinic regulations held in Oakland, California, in December 1976. Most recently (January 1978), the Office of Civil Rights in the Department of Health has initiated an Advisory Committee on Women's Health to consider issues involved in sterilization regulations and provision of abortion to low-income women who are no longer eligible to receive federally funded abortions. The FWHCs have had an active voice in nominating appointees to this committee. Members of the Los Angeles FWHCs also attend meetings and public hearings of the state Medical Quality Assurance Board and are increasingly called upon by state officials to serve as consultants on pending matters, such as licensing of lay midwives, rewriting community clinic regulations, and developing certification for paraprofessionals.

FWHC representatives initially found it somewhat incongruous that the same public agencies which had been harassing them with threats of arrest were now __paying__ them to fly to Sacramento to provide

---

[*]Ginny Cassidy, RN, a nurse-practitioner with the Los Angeles FWHC, and the author were both appointed.

"expert" opinions. The chief of the California State Office of Maternal and Child Health and the Director of Health have solicited input from the Coalition for the Medical Rights of Women on health matters relating to women and children. The California Medical Association has negotiated with the Coalition and sends its own lawyers and physicians to respond to petitions (Corea 1977, p. 256).

These and other developments suggest that a feminist health policy system is emerging that is similar to that which developed earlier in the larger feminist movement (Freeman 1975, pp. 228-29). Such social policy systems often take years to develop, because significant people in different institutions must become known to each other, establish meeting patterns, conferences, and mutual activities to support the informal network through which substantive issues of concern are hammered out.

As these policy systems emerge, large numbers of "woodwork feminists" in government come to serve important functions. That these supporters were waiting in the wings became clear at the Santa Cruz conference in 1977. One participant who had been involved in lay alternative services commented that community women would really be surprised to see how much potential support there was among high-level academic and government women. Conferees openly discussed the reciprocal relationships that can develop between "insiders" and "outsiders" in efforts to influence public policy ("Proceedings of the Conference on Women's Leadership and Authority in the Health Professions" 1977).

On the national level, the National Women's Health Network, the Women and Health Roundtable, and WEAL seek to develop reciprocal relationships between women in government agencies and health activists. Both WEAL and the Network recently released pamphlets outlining how to establish liaison with public bodies and outside pressure groups, listing key contact persons in Congress, the NIH, and other federal agencies (Rosenbach and King 1977; "NWHC Activists Guide: An Action Index to Your Resources in Washington" 1977).

By late 1977, representatives of the Network had participated in various government activities. Board member Doris Haire testified at the FDA advisory committee hearing on behalf of the American Foundation for Maternal and Child Health, citing and dangers of using oxytocin in childbirth. Another board member, Judy Lipschutz, represented the Network at other meetings, including those within the FDA and at the International Women's Year meeting ("Network Hotline" 1977, pp. 5-7). Belita Cowan is facilitating efforts to elect individual women as representatives of feminist consumer groups to seats on the over 60 FDA advisory committees, each of which can have one nonvoting consumer representative ("Consumer Input in FDA" 1977). The Network is considering petitioning the FDA to demand that pharmacists be informed that patients are legally entitled to receive physicians' information flyers for all prescription drugs ("Labeling: Only Your Doctor Knows" 1977). And Network committees are attempting to monitor ACOG activities ("Network Hotline" 1977).

As Gilb (1966) points out, professional organizations, such as the ACOG and the AMA, wield such power and influence over public policy that they can be regarded as "private governments." To influence public policy, health activists must take into account the role these organizations play and develop means of influencing them—that is, they must learn how to lobby, petition, and exert public pressure as if these organizations were "official" government organizations that were responsive and accountable to the public.

INSTITUTIONALIZATION, COOPTATION, AND INTERDEPENDENCE

While the medical profession's responsiveness to health movement demands is viewed positively by many women, others are fearful of cooptation. Discouraged rather than encouraged by physicians' growing willingness to treat at least their private patients in a more egalitarian fashion, one health activist fumed (in 1973): "Before you know it the doctors will be setting up their own 'women's clinics.' They'll even coopt that! Every good idea we have, they coopt it!"

Of course, every reform-movement runs a risk of cooptation. Not even the most radical program can escape this hazard. Nonetheless, as Chomsky (1971, p. 79) points out, "Those who oppose a program of social action merely on the grounds that it might be 'coopted' doom themselves to paralysis: they are opposed to everything imaginable." Thus far, health activists have not been immobilized by the radical paradox, which in the larger feminist movement paralyzed many women. Pursuing "reformist" issues, which did not alter the basic nature of the system, was repugnant to radical women, because they felt such reforms would just strengthen the system. Thus, they were immobilized for fear their activity might be counterrevolutionary (Freeman 1975, p. 241).

Health activists' fear of cooptation centers largely on the medical establishment's adopting feminist "forms"—for example, using paramedics, providing an informal atmosphere, and emphasizing education—without placing real control in the hands of women themselves. Recent moves to institutionalize highly professionalized home-style birth is a good example of the cooptation many radicals fear. Nonetheless, there are recognizable gains—even to those who despise continued medical dominance. Nurse-midwives are regarded as more suitable birth attendants than male physicians, and programs that encourage making birth a family affair offer an experience vastly different from that available in the surgical suite.

There is increasing evidence that proposed changes in birth practices will have a significant effect on the psychological development of both parents and children. Tanzer (1973), for example, reports that mothers who give birth when they are fully awake and with husbands present adjust better to motherhood, develop more self-esteem, and perceive their spouses more positively than women who are anesthetized for delivery. Both animal and human studies reveal that bonding occurs through early postpartum mother-infant contact. And behavioral differences have been observed in the quality of mother-infant interaction between women who have had even as little as one-half hour of direct skin contact followed by 12 hours of separation and mothers who did not have direct contact. The effects were still observable after one year. (See, for example, Barnett et al. 1970; Seashore et al. 1973; Klaus et al. 1972; and Kennell et al. 1974.)[*] Overall, then, most health activists view new medical options in childbirth positively, even when they are concerned over cooptation.

Fear over professional women usurping control continues to be of concern, particularly as greater emphasis is placed on organized lobbying and influencing social policy, where credentials and expertise are valued and valuable. However, more probably, increased participation of academic and professional women will result in the growth of new constituencies of similarly situated women. This actually facilitates the growth of symbiotic relationships between insiders and outside pressure groups. Activists perceive that pressure for change must come from outside, but insiders, particularly newly incorporated marginal individuals (as are most women in powerful institutions) are often effective change agents. Indeed, Freeman (1975, p. 236) argues that whole agencies can be "captured" by outside challenging groups with the cooperation of sympathetic insiders.

However, it seems unlikely that academic and professional women and agency insiders can be successful change agents without the existence of a broad-based—and generally more radical—social movement.[†] The relationship between different segments of the

---

[*]Peterson and Mehl (1977) review these studies on the effects of early maternal contact and separation and discuss various factors involved in the attachment process between parents and children.

[†]My own experience in attempting to influence social policy by presentation of social-scientific "facts" underscores my conviction that "expertise" is most effective in bringing change when the experts have strong political constituencies. When I was involved in the CSCWD, I complimented the state drug abuse staff for making the policy and program changes our committee had requested. One staff

movement is one of mutual interdependence. Differences in strategies, tactics, and priorities, as well as style, are part of the division
of labor that is essential in a movement seeking far-reaching changes
in major social institutions. The most radical flank of the movement
is essential, not only to press for change but to make other groups
appear respectable (Freeman 1975, pp. 235-36).

IMPLICATIONS FOR SOCIAL CHANGE

The women's health movement shows how incremental social
change occurs on many levels and how changes in self-conception and
self-determination can stimulate widespread social action. By studying this movement, we learn much about how organized client groups
can alter the direction of major social institutions.

While the women's health movement does not seriously challenge the structure of the society at large, or even the entire health
system (except in ideological appeals), many of the reforms achieved
have significance for quality of life. For women, control over the
means of reproduction and control over definitions of body-self are
crucial. Dismissing them as trivial or as insignificant reformism,
as do Carden (1974) and Guettel (1974), is to accept the dominant
male value system, which devalues female spheres of life.* As Bernard (1973a, p. 783) points out: "The topics that have preoccupied
sociologists have been the topics that preoccupy men: power, work,

-----

member grimly remarked that we (CSCWD professional and academic
women) had been on their backs so much that they felt they had to
respond. Besides, he added, our requests seemed quite "reasonable"
after he had been strongly attacked by several vocal community wom-
en's groups. As I had suspected, the agency representatives responded
to our suggestions not because they were convinced by our research
but because, correctly or incorrectly, we were perceived as more
moderate representatives of a growing pressure group of insurgent
women. Without such a militant and broad-based pressure group
hovering nearby, it is difficult to see how much can be accomplished.
See Ruzek 1975a.

*For discussion of how male perspectives in social science
have made women and women's concerns "invisible" until feminist
scholars began exploring "women's issues," see especially Daniels
1975b; Lorber 1975b; McCormack 1975; Oakley 1974; and Tuchman
1975.

climbing the occupational ladder, conflict." Perhaps sociologists' general inattention to the role of social movements in social change (Banks 1972; Killian 1964) is due to male domination of social science. Because most social reform movements involve large numbers of women, their role in social change may not be studied as seriously as political revolutions, which are usually organized and controlled by men.

The women's health movement also offers insight into how routine health care might be restructured in areas beyond obstetrics and gynecology and suggests how social change can be brought about, even in institutions dominated by powerful professions. Patient education, legislative and lobbying efforts, selective utilization of practitioners, judicial measures, and direct pressure can all be used to change other areas of the health care system. For example, routine pediatric care, services for the chronically ill, and care for persons suffering minor disorders could all be provided along models suggested by self-help clinics. This type of primary care improves people's health at a fraction of the cost of high-technology specialty care needed by relatively few patients.

The more general question feminists raise when they demand control over all reproductive research and training concerns the appropriateness and desirability of granting professions the right to make decisions that affect persons significantly different from themselves. The objection is grounded in the democratic principle that the governed—or otherwise controlled—should have a voice in the government. As powerful professions become more like private governments (making decisions that affect the public) (Gilb 1966), their governing power should be acknowledged—and balanced—by organized consumer participation. Organized health groups' willingness and ability to establish quality criteria and to evaluate professional practice suggests that outside accountability structures are both feasible and beneficial.

APPENDIX A

PROGRAMS AND CONFERENCES

California Commission on the Status of Women Hearings, Department of Public Health, San Francisco, December 8-9, 1972.

"The Medical Mystique," Pacific Medical Center, San Francisco, March 9-11, 1973.

Women's Weekend, Feminist Women's Health Center, Oakland, California, March 16-17, 1973.

"Women Health Workers, A Conference," John Adams Adult School, San Francisco, April 6, 1973.

San Francisco Women's Health Center Self-Help Group, April-May, 1973.

"The Childbirth Controversy—Home and Hospital," University of California, San Francisco, June 30, 1973.

Planned Parenthood Volunteer Training, Spring 1973.

Feminist Women's Health Centers, University of California, Berkeley, February 25, 1974.

"Sex Differences in Health Care," Panel, American Association for the Advancement of Science, San Francisco, March 1, 1974.

Hawaii Health Network Meeting, San Francisco, April 5-7, 1974.

Self-Help Clinic Demonstration, California State University, Northridge, April 14, 1974.

Women and Alcohol Panel, California State University, Northridge, April 14, 1974.

Menstrual Extraction Conference, sponsored by the Feminist Women's Health Centers, San Francisco, April 27, 1974.

"Healing Systems in Cross-Cultural Perspective," University of California, Berkeley, May 3-5, 1974.

"Northern California Conference on Women, Drugs and Alcohol," University of California, Davis, February 1-2, 1975.

Breast Cancer Discussion Group, San Francisco Women's Health Center, Spring 1975.

"Abortion," Film showing, Planned Parenthood of Marin, Spring 1975.

"Women and Their Health: Research Implications for a New Era," University of California, San Francisco, August 1-2, 1975.

"Self-Health," Film showing, San Francisco Women's Health Center, Summer 1975.

"Women on Trial for Taking Control of Their Bodies," Benefit for the Santa Cruz Midwives, University of California, Berkeley, August 20, 1975.

"Double Dynamics: Women's Roles in Health and Illness," Conference, Philadelphia, December 7-9, 1975.

"Self-Care Conference," Institute for the Study of Human Knowledge and the University of California, San Francisco, March 19-20, 1977.

"Women's Health: Research, Communication and Policy," University of California, San Francisco, May 20-21, 1977.

"Women's Leadership and Authority in the Health Professions," University of California, Santa Cruz, June 19-21, 1977.

APPENDIX B

FEMINIST PERIODICALS—WOMEN'S HEALTH PERIODICALS

Amazon Quarterly, Box 434, West Somerville, MA 02144.

Boston Women's Health Book Collective, Inc., Health Packets, Box 192, West Somerville, MA 02144.

Broadside, P.O. Box 4190, Berkeley, CA 94701.

Capitol Alert, P.O. Box 214982, Sacramento, CA 95821.

Chrysalis Magazine, Women's Building, 1727 N. Spring Street, Los Angeles, CA 90012.

Coalition for the Medical Rights of Women News, 4079A 24th Street, San Francisco, CA 94114.

Congressional Clearinghouse on Women's Rights, (order from your own Congressman), U.S. House of Representatives, Washington, D.C. 20515.

Everywoman, 1043 B. West Washington Blvd., Venice, CA 90291.

Family Planning Perspectives, Planned Parenthood-World Population, The Alan Guttmacher Institute, 515 Madison Avenue, New York, NY 10022.

Feminist Studies, 417 Riverside Drive, New York, NY 10025.

51%, P.O. Box 371, Lomita, CA 90717.

The Furies, Lesbian/Feminist Monthly, P.O. Box 8843, S.E. Station, Washington, D.C. 20003.

Health/Pac Bulletin, Health Policy Advisory Center, 17 Murray Street, New York, NY 10007.

HealthRight, Women's Health Forum, 175 Fifth Avenue, New York, NY 10010.

Her-Self, 225 E. Liberty, Ann Arbor, MI 48108 (ceased publication 1977).

ICEA News, International Childbirth Education Association, P.O. Box 20852, Milwaukee, WI 53220.

Journal of Female Liberation, Cell 16, 16 Lexington Avenue, Cambridge, MA 02138.

The Lesbian Tide, 373 North Western, Room 202, Los Angeles, CA 90004.

Majority Report, 74 Grove Street, New York, NY 10014.

Marin Women's News Journal, P.O. Box 1412, San Rafael, CA 94902.

Medical Self-Care Magazine, P.O. Box 718, Inverness, CA 94937.

Momma, The Newspaper for Single Mothers, P.O. Box 567, Venice, CA 90291.

The Monthly Extract, New Moon Communications, Box 3488 Ridgeway Station, Stamford, CT 06905.

Mother Lode, P. O. Box 40213, San Francisco, CA 94140.

Mountain Moving, c/o Women at Northwestern, 619 Emerson Street, Evanston, IL 60201.

Mother Lode, P. O. Box 40213, San Francisco, CA 94140.

NARAL Newsletter, 706 Seventh Street, S.E., Washington, D.C. 20003.

National Black Feminist Organization Newsletter, 285 Madison Avenue, Room 1720, New York, NY 10017.

Network News, National Women's Health Network, 1302 18th Street, N.W., Suite 203, Washington, D.C. 20024.

NOW Monthly Newsletter, 49 East 91 Street, New York, NY 10028.

Ob. Gyn. News, Physicians International Press, 4907 Cordell Ave., Washington, D.C. 20014.

Off Our Backs, 1724 20th St., N.W., Washington, D.C. 20005.

Quest, a Feminist Quarterly, 2000 P St., N.W., Washington, D.C. 20009.

Rough Times, P.O. Box 89, Somerville, MA 02144.

Roundtable Reports, Women and Health Roundtable, Federation of Professional Women, 2000 P St., N.W., Washington, D.C. 20009.

The Second Wave, A Magazine of the New Feminist, P.O. Box 344, Cambridge A, Cambridge, MA 02139.

Sister, Westside Women's Center, 218 S. Venice, Venice, CA 90291.

Skirting the Capitol, P.O. Box 4569, Sacramento, CA 94825 (discontinued 1975).

SWS Newsletter, Sociologists for Women in Society, Department of Sociology, American University, Washington, D.C. 20016.

The Spokeswoman, 5464 South Shore Drive, Chicago, IL 60615.

Up From Under, 399 Lafayette Street, New York, NY 10009.

WEAL Washington Report, 733 15th Street, N.W., Suite 200, Washington, D.C., 20005.

Women & Health, Issues in Women's Health Care, SUNY/College at Old Westbury, Old Westbury, NY 11568.

Women: A Journal of Liberation, 3028 Greenmount Avenue, Baltimore, MD 21218.

Women Today, Today Publications and News Service, National Press Building, Washington, D.C. 20045.

Women's Lobby Quarterly, Women's Lobby, 201 Massachusetts Avenue, N.E., Washington, D.C.

Women's Washington Report, 324 C Street S.E., Washington, D.C. 20003.

WONAAC Newsletter, Women's National Abortion Action Coalition, 150 Fifth Avenue, Room 315, New York, NY 10011.

APPENDIX C

WOMEN'S HEALTH RELATED ORGANIZATIONS
AND DIRECT SERVICE GROUPS

Australia

Hobart Women's Centre, 340 Elizabeth St., North Hobart, 7000
Tasmania.

Leichhardt Women's Community Health Centre, 164 Flood St.,
Leichhardt, New South Wales, 2040.

The "Body Politic," 2/46 Anderson Road, East Hawthorn 3123,
Victoria.

Austria

Gesundheitsgruppe, c/o Freda Blau, Starlfriedgasse 11/3a, 1180 Wien.

Belgium

Collectif contraception, 34 av. des Celtes, 1040 Bruxelles.

La Maison des femmes, 70 rue du Méridien, 1030 Bruxelles.

Les cahiers du Grif, 14 rue du Musée, 1000 Bruxelles.

Sabine Grau, rue Potagère, 71, 1030 Bruxelles.

Canada

Centre de santé de femmes du quartier, 5091 Delandière, Montréal.

Vancouver Birth Center, 1520 West 6th Ave., Vancouver, B.C.

Vancouver Women's Health Collective, 1520 West 6th Ave., Vancouver, B.C.

Women's Health Center, 134 Darcy St., Toronto, Ontario.

France

Collectif Notre corps, nous-même, c/o Sophie Mayoux, 4 rue Myrha, 75018 Paris.

Femmes en lutte, 70 rue Jean-Pierre Timbaud, 75011 Paris.

GIS, c/o Jeanne Weiss, 128 bd Montparnasse, 75014 Paris.

Groupe de femmes de la place des Fêtes, 9 rue du Pré Saint-Gervais, 75019 Paris.

Groupe Grenoble, c/o Nicole Duperray, 80 Galerie Arlequin (S. 55), 38100 Grenoble.

Lyba Spring, 44, rue d'Aubagne, 13100 Marseille.

Maison des femmes, 19 rue des Couteliers, 3100 Toulouse.

MLAC, La Commune, Chemin de la Pierre de Feu, Le Pey Blank, 13100 Aix-en-Próvence.

Great Britain

Association of Radical Midwives, 19 Bromfield Cres., Leeds LS 6 3DD, York.

British Our Bodies, Ourselves, c/o Angela Phillips and Jill Rakusen, 62 Albert Palace Mansions.

Essex Road Women's Health Group, 108 Essex Road, London N1.

Leeds Women's Health Group, 34 Delph Lane, Leeds 6W, York.

Spanish Women's Health Group, Box 33, 142 Drummond St., London NW1.

Women's Report Collective, 14 Aberdeen Rd., Wealdstone, Harrow, Middlesex.

Greece

Greek Women's Liberation Movement, Tsimiski 39, Atene.

Multi National Women's Liberation Group, 3 Ellanikou, Pangrati, Atene.

Italy

CED, Via Amedei 13, Milano.

Centro di medicina della donna, Via dei Mille 22, Pinerolo.

Centro per la salute della donna, Galleria Trieste 6/9, Padova.

Centro per la salute della donna, Via Montanaro 24, Barriera di Milano, Torino.

Collettivo 8 Marzo, Via Traversa Vittorio Veneto 14, Brescia.

Collettivo dell'ospedale Sant'Anna, c/o Anna Negro, Via Revello 2 Bis, Torino.

Collettivo Femminista Appio Alberone, c/o Luciana Marzilli, Via Latina 499, Roma.

Collettivo Femminista S. Lorenzo, Via dei Sabelli 100, int. 11, Roma.

Collettivo Leoncavallo, Via Leoncavallo, c/o Maria Pina Usai, Milano.

Collettivo Mercati Generali, Via Montevideo 45, Torino.

Collettivo Ospedale S. Carlo, c/o Franca Fumagalli, Via Diaz 6, Corsio Milano.

Collettivo Per Una Medicina Della Donna, Via S. Nicolo 6, Firenze.

Collettivo Pratica Consultori, c/o Vicky Franzinetti, Via Bertholet 42, Torino.

Collettivo Via Imbriani Spaziodonna, Via Imbriani 12, Trieste.

Consultorio Autogestito, Via A. Genocchi 9, Piacenza.

Consultorio Femminista, Via Antonio Genovesi 30, Salerno.

Consultorio Per i Problemi Della Donna, Via Broseta 118, Bergamo.

Graziella Rondano, Via S. Giorgio 2/2 Bologna.

Gruppo di Studio Sulla Medicina e la Donna, Via Ugo Bassi, 13/A
Ferrara.

Gruppo Femminista Per la Salute Della Donna, c/o Spina, Piazza
del Monte de Pietá 30, 00186 Roma.

Gruppo Femminista Per Una Medicina Della Donna, Via Col di Lana 8,
Milano.

Gruppo "Salario al Lavoro Domestico," Via del Governo Vecchio 39,
Roma.

Movimento di Liberazione Della Donna, Via del Governo Vecchio 39,
Roma.

Movimento Femminista Romano, Via Pompeo Magno 94, Roma.

Vittoria Uberti, Via XX Settembre 8, Brescia.

Women's Support Group, 23 Via Poggio Imperiale, Firenze.

Mexico

Colectivo "La Revuelta," Malitzin 38 Coyoacan, Citta del Messico.

Netherlands

Vrouwen gez. centr. Amst., Lidwien van der Hulst, Nikolaas Wit-
senkade 19, Amsterdam.

Norway

Helsegruppa (Women's) Huset, Radhusgata 2, Oslo.

Spain

Col. Feminista, Trav. de Bracia 272 1°, Barcelona.

Colectivo Feminista Pelvis, Rector Vives 45A, Génova, Palma de Mallorca.

Colectivo Self-Help, c/o Carmen 16, 3° Teresa Ingles, Barcelona.

Grup de Mujers Independientes, c/o Pasteur, 49 - bis, Barcelona.

La Mar, c/o Rita Prieto, Julio n. 21, Satico 2^d, Barcelona.

LA SAL, Local Feminista, c/o Riereta S. Barcelona.

Magas, c/o Felin y Codina, 45 es. A 3°3a, Barcelona.

Sweden

Gruppo 8, c/o Kjerstin Novéu, Rabyvagen 32 c, S-223 57 Lund.

Switzerland

Cassarate Dispensaire Gynéco-obstétrique, Centre des Femmes, 5 Bd St-Georges, 1205 Genève.

Movimento Femminista Tichinese, Cas. post. 29, 6906 Lugano.

United States

Alabama

Martin Luther King Clinic, Rt. 1, Box 125A, Browns, AL 36724.

Alaska

Anchorage Women's Liberation, 7801 Peck Ave., Anchorage, AK 99504.

North America Indian Women's Association, 807 River View Dr., Fairbanks, AK 99701.

Arizona

American Medical Women's Association, Professional Resources Research Center, Speedway Professional Bldg., Suite 206A, 2302 East Speedway Blvd., Tucson, AZ 85719.

Center Against Sexual Assault, P.O. Box 3786, Phoenix, AZ 85030.

Arkansas

Fayetteville Women's Health Collective, 210 Locust St., Fayetteville, AR 72701.

California

Abortion Praxis Collective, c/o Women's Studies, Kresge College, University of California, Santa Cruz, CA 95064.

Association for Childbirth at Home, 16705 Monte Cristo, Cerritos, CA 90701.

Berkeley Women's Health Collective, 2908 Ellsworth, Berkeley, CA 94705.

Black Women Organized, P.O. Box 15072, San Francisco, CA 94115.

Chicana Services Action Center, 4811 Telegraph Rd., Los Angeles, CA 90022.

Chico Feminist Women's Health Center, 330 Flume St., Chico, CA 95926.

Ching Nin Clinic, 511 Columbus Ave., San Francisco, CA 94133.

Claremont Women's Self-Help Center, 256 W. 6th St., Claremont, CA 91711.

Coalition for the Medical Rights of Women, 4079A 24th St., San Francisco, CA 94114.

Comision Feminil Mexicana Nacional, 279 S. Loma Dr., Los Angeles, CA 90803.

Common Women's Force, 572A Miles Ave., Oakland, CA 94618.

Everywoman's Clinic, 2600 Park Ave., Concord, CA 94520.

Feminist Health/Mental Health Project, American Friends Service Committee, 2160 Lake St., San Francisco, CA 94121.

Feminist Women's Health Center, 1112 Crenshaw Blvd., Los Angeles, CA 90019.

Gay Community Services Center, Women's Gynecology Clinic, 1614 Wiltshire Blvd., Los Angeles, CA 90017.

Gay Health Workers, Box 42242, San Francisco, CA 94142.

GNA West, Box 1793, San Diego, CA 94112.

Haight Ashbury Women's Clinic, 1101 Masonic, San Francisco, CA 94117.

Herself Health Clinic, 4164 Santa Monica Blvd., Los Angeles, CA 90029.

Holistic Childbirth Institute, 1627 10th Ave., San Francisco, CA 94112.

Los Angeles NOW Health Task Force, c/o Monique Harriton, 2413 Ronda Vista Dr., Los Angeles, CA 90027.

The Marin County Women's Health Collective/YWCA, 1618 Mission Ave., San Rafael, CA 94901.

Network Against Psychiatric Assault/Women Against Psychiatric Assault (NAPA/WAPA), 2150 Market St., San Francisco, CA 94114.

Nevada City Women's Health Collective, 12585 Jones Bar Rd., Nevada City, CA 94949.

Oakland Feminist Women's Health Center, 2930 McClure, Oakland, CA 94609.

Orange County Feminist Women's Health Center, 429 S. Sycamore, Santa Ana, CA 92701.

Palo Alto Self-Help Collective, 270 Grant, Palo Alto, CA 94306.

Program for Women in Health Sciences, University of California, San Francisco, 1343 Third Ave., San Francisco, CA 94143.

Religious Coalition for Abortion Rights, Box 250, Mill Valley, CA 94941.

San Francisco Women's Health Center, 3789 24th St., San Francisco, CA 94132.

Santa Cruz Birth Center, 208 Escalona St., Santa Cruz, CA 95060.

Santa Cruz Women's Health Center, 250 Locust St., Santa Cruz, CA 95060.

Society for Humane Abortion, P.O. Box 1862, San Francisco, CA 94101.

Urban Indian Health Board, Native American Health Center, 56 Julian Ave., San Francisco, CA 94103.

Westside Women's Health Care Project, 1711 Ocean Park Blvd., Santa Monica, CA 90405.

Womancare—A Feminist Women's Health Center, 424 Pennsylvania, San Diego, CA 92109.

Womankind Health Services, 250 Locust St., Santa Cruz, CA 95060.

Women Acting Together to Combat Harassment (WATCH), c/o FWHC, 1112 Crenshaw Blvd., Los Angeles, CA 90019.

Women's Community Clinic, 696 E. Santa Clara, San Jose, CA 95112.

Women's Health Collective, 250 Locust Ave., Santa Cruz, CA 95060.

Women's Health Collective, Humboldt Open Door Clinic, 10th & H Sts., Arcata, CA 95521.

Women's Need Center, Haight Ashbury Free Medical Clinic, 558 Clayton St., San Francisco, CA 94117.

Colorado

Fort Collins Self-Help Clinic for Women, 629 South Hawes, Ft. Collins, CO 80521.

Women's Health Services of Colorado Springs, 1703 North Weber, Colorado Springs, CO 80907.

Connecticut

Grace Hirsch Self-Help Clinic, 2 Hemlock Dr., Stamford, CT 06902.

Hartford Women's Health Co-op, c/o Mary Palmer, 92 Rowe Ave., Hartford, CT 06106.

Therapy Rights Committee, 215 Park St., New Haven, CT 06511.

Women's Health Services, 19 Edwards St., New Haven, CT 06511.

Delaware

Rape Crisis Center of Wilmington, P.O. Box 1507, Wilmington, DE 19889.

District of Columbia

American College of Nurse-Midwives, 100 Vermont Ave. NW, Washington, DC 20005.

American Public Health Association, Standing Committee on Women's Rights, 1015 18th St., NW, Washington, DC 20036.

American Society for Psychoprophylaxis in Obstetrics, 1523 L St. NW, Washington, DC 20005.

Catholics for a Free Choice, 201 Massachusetts Ave. NE, Washington, DC 20001.

Citizen Action Group, 133 C St. SE, Washington, DC 20003.

Feminist Alliance Against Rape, Box 21033, Washington, DC 20009.

Health Research Group, 2000 P St. NW, Washington, DC 20036.

Home Oriented Maternity Experience, 511 New York Ave., Tacoma Park, Washington, DC 20012.

Human Rights for Women, 1128 National Press Bldg., Washington, DC 20004.

National Abortion Rights Action League, 706 Seventh St. SE, Washington, DC 20003.

National Organization for Women (NOW), 425 13th St. NW, Suite 1001, Washington, DC 20004.

National Women's Health Network, 1302 18th St. NW, Washington, DC 20036.

Neighborhood Consumer Information Center, 3005 Georgia Ave. NW, Washington, DC 20001.

Religious Coalition for Abortion Rights, 100 Maryland Ave. NE, Washington, DC 20002.

Secretary's Advisory Committee on the Rights and Responsibilities of Women, Department of Health, Education and Welfare, North Bldg., 330 Independence Ave. SW, Washington, DC 20201.

Women and Health Roundtable, Federation of Organizations for Professional Women, 2000 P St. NW, Washington, DC 20005.

Women's Equity Action League (WEAL), Women and Health Committee, 733 15th St. NW, Suite 200, Washington, DC 20005.

Women's Legal Defense Fund, 1424 16th St. NW, Washington, DC 20036.

Women's Lobby, 201 Massachusetts Ave. NE, Washington, DC 20002.

Florida

Association for Breast Cancer Detection Earlier (ABCDE), 1110 S. Dixie Highway, Coral Gables, FL 33146.

Feminist Women's Health Center, 1017 Thomasville Rd., Tallahassee, FL 32303.

Gainesville Women's Health Center, 805 SE 4th St., Gainesville, FL 32601.

Mothers of the Whole Earth Revolt (MOTHER), c/o FWHC, 1017 Thomasville Rd., Tallahassee, FL 32303.

Tampa Women's Health Center, 1200 West Platt St., Tampa, FL 33606.

WATCH (Women Acting Together to Combat Harassment), c/o FWHC, 1017 Thomasville Rd., Tallahassee, FL 32303.

Women's Center Health Group, Box 1350, Tampa, FL 33601.

Georgia

Feminist Women's Health Center, 580 14th St. NW, Atlanta, GA 30318.

National Association of Abortion Facilities, Box 18774, Atlanta, GA 30326.

Hawaii

Women's Health Center, 1820 University Ave., Honolulu, HI 96822.

Idaho

Moscow Rape Crisis Center, c/o University of Idaho, Department of Psychology, Moscow, ID 83201.

Pocatello Free Clinic, 421 Memorial Dr., Pocatello, ID 83201.

Illinois

Champaign-Urbana Women's Health Collective, 612 W. Elm St., Urbana, IL 61801.

Chicago Women's Health Center, 745 West Armitage, Chicago, IL 60614.

Chicago Women's Liberation Union, 2748 North Lincoln, Chicago, IL 60614.

Coalition for the Right to Choose, Box 514, Normal, IL 61761.

DES Action Group, 407 E. Adams, Springfield, IL 62701.

Emma Goldman Women's Health Center, 1317 West Loyola, Chicago, IL 60626.

Fritzi Englestein Health Center, 2751 North Wilton, Chicago, IL 60614.

Health Evaluation and Referral Service (HERS), 3411 W. Diversy, Chicago, IL 60647.

La Leche League, 9616 Minneapolis Ave., Franklin Park, IL 60631.

Resource Center on Women and Health Care, Rockford School of Medicine, 1601 Parkview Ave., Rockford, IL 61101.

Society for the Protection of the Unborn Through Nutrition (SPUN), 17 N. Wabash Ave., Chicago, IL 60602.

Women Act to Control Health Care (WATCH), 1318 W. Newport, Chicago, IL 60657.

Women in Medicine Committee, American Medical Student Association, 1171 Tower Rd., Schaumberg, IL 60196.

Women's Health Information Center, 261 Kemberly Rd., Barrington, IL 60010.

Indiana

Indianapolis Women's Center, 5656 East 16th St., Indianapolis, IN 46218.

Women's Health Group, 507 Dodge St., West Lafayette, IN 47906.

Iowa

Cedar Rapids Clinic for Women, 86 1/2 16th Ave. SW, Cedar Rapids, IA 52404.

Emma Goldman Clinic for Women, 215 North Dodge, Iowa City, IA 52240.

Women's Community Health Center, 819 Lincoln Way, Ames IA 50010.

Kansas

Gay Women's Liberation, Box 234, Lawrence, KS 66044.

Pan American Medical Women, 1019 West 50th N, Wichita, KS 67204.

Wichita Workers and Oppressed People United, 1715 N. St. Francis, Wichita, KS 67214.

Kentucky

Appalshop, P.O. Box 743, Whitesburg, KY 41858.

Kentucky Women's Rights Organization, P.O. Box 128, Prestonburg, KY 41653.

Mountain People's Rights, Rt. 3, Box 462A, Manchester, KY 40962.

New Womankind, P.O. Box 18102, Beuchel, KY 40218.

Louisiana

Delta Women's Clinic, 1406 St. Charles Ave., New Orleans, LA 70130.

New Orleans Women's Health Collective, 1117 Decatur, New Orleans, LA 70116.

NOW Women's Health Collective, 1117 Decatur, New Orleans, LA 70116.

Maine

Maine Feminist Health Project, 105 Dresden Ave., Gardiner, ME 04345.

Maine Feminist Health Project, 183 Water St., Augusta, ME 04330.

Maine Health Collective, c/o Donna Roux, Box 472, York Beach, ME 03910.

Maryland

Birth, 1304 Ludlow Dr., Temple Hills, MD 20031.

Breast Cancer Advisory Service, Box 422, Kensington, MD 20795.

Research Group One, 2743 Maryland Ave., Baltimore, MD 21218.

Women's Crisis Hotline, University of Maryland Health Center, College Park, MD 20742.

Massachusetts

Association for Childbirth at Home, 47 Ronald Rd., Arlington, MA 02174.

Athol Women's Health Center Group, 235 Main St., Athol, MA 01331.

Birth Day, 128 Lowell Ave., Newtonville, MA 02160.

Boston Women's Health Book Collective, Box 192, Somerville, MA 02144.

Framingham Women's Health Project, 73 Union Ave., Framingham, MA 01701.

Harvard Reduced Schedule Residency Project, Harvard Medical School, 25 Shattuck St., Boston, MA 02115.

Homebirth, 89 Franklin St., Suite 200, Boston, MA 02110.

Marlborough Women's Health Services, P.O. Box 160, Marlborough, MA 01752.

New Bedford Women's Center Health Services, 15 Chestnut St., New Bedford, MA 02740.

New Bedford Women's Clinic, 347 County St., New Bedford, MA 02740.

Salem Women's Health Collective, 140 Washington St., Salem, MA 01970.

Somerville Women's Health Project, 326 Somerville Ave., Somerville, MA 02143.

Valley Women's Center, 200 Main St., Northampton, MA 01060.

Women's Community Health Center, 137 Hampshire, Cambridge, MA 02139.

Women's Health Clinic, 14 Center St., P.O. Box 1011, Provincetown, MA 02657.

Worcester Women's Liberation, Women's Health Project, Box 164, Turnpike Station, Shrewsburg, MA 01545.

Michigan

American Lesbian Medical Association (ALMA), c/o Ambitious Amazons, P.O. Box 811, East Lansing, MI 48823.

Ann Arbor Advocates for Medical Information, c/o Belita Cowan, 556 Second St., Ann Arbor, MI 48103.

Ann Arbor Health Care Collective, Room 2209, Michigan Union, University of Michigan, Ann Arbor, MI 48109.

Community Women's Clinic, c/o Women's Crisis Center, 306 North Division St., Ann Arbor, MI 48104

Detroit Women's Health Project, 18700 Woodward, Detroit, MI 48203.

Feminist Self-Help Center, 5325 South Cedar St., Lansing, MI 48910.

Feminist Women's Health Center, 2445 West Eight Mile Road, Detroit, MI 48345.

Self-Help/Women's Crisis Center, 306 N. Division St., Ann Arbor, MI 48104.

The Birth Center, c/o Kellog & Sinclair, 141 W. Margaret St., Detroit, MI 48203.

Women's Health and Information Center (WHIP), Box 110 Warriner, CMU, Mt. Pleasant, MI 48858.

Minnesota

Abortion Counseling Service of Minnesota, 549 Turnpike Rd., Golden Valley, MN 55416.

Elizabeth Blackwell Clinic, 2000 South 5th St., Minneapolis, MN 55405.

Mississippi

Jackson Women's Center, P.O. Box 3234, Jackson, MS 39207.

Lesbian Front, P.O. Box 8342, Jackson, MS 39204.

Lowell Women's Center, Rt. 1, Box 975, Ruleville, MS 38971.

Missouri

St. Louis Women's Health Collective, 6010 Kingsbury, St. Louis, MO 63112.

St. Louis Women's Health Collective, Women's Resource Center, Box 1182, St. Louis, MO 63130.

Montana

Women's Place, 1130 W. Broadway, Missoula, MT 59801.

Nebraska

Women's Communication Center, 1432 North St., Lincoln, NE 68508.

Nevada

Community Action Self-Help, 960 W. Owens St., Las Vegas, NV 89106.

Women's Center & Rape Crisis Line, P.O. Box 8448, Reno, NV 89507.

New Hampshire

Every Women's Center/YMCA, 72 Concord St., Manchester, NH 03101.

New Hampshire Feminist Health Center, 38 South Main St., Concord, NH 03301.

New Jersey

New Jersey Women's Health, 450 Hamburg Turnpike, Wayne, NJ 07470.

Woman Health, 11 Emily Court, Demarest, NJ 07627.

New Mexico

Southwest Maternity Service, 504 Luna SW, Albuquerque, NM 87102.

Women's Health Services, 700 Franklin, Santa Fe, NM 87501.

New York

Abortion Rights Mobilization, 333 E. 23 St., Suite 6, New York, NY 10010.

Abused Women's Aid in Crisis, 137 E. 2nd St., New York, NY 10009.

Action for Women in Chile, P.O. Box 530, Cathedral Station, New York, NY 10025.

American Women's Committee for Medical Aid to Indochina, 1 Union Square West, Room 408, New York, NY 10003.

American Women's Hospital Service, 255 W. 34th St., New York, NY 10001.

American Federation for Maternal and Child Health, 30 Beekman Place, New York, NY 10022.

American Foundation for Maternal and Child Health, 30 Beekman Place, New York, NY 10022.

American Medical Women's Association, 1740 Broadway, New York, NY 10019.

Association of Mothers for Educated Childbirth, 1161 Beach & 9th St., Far Rockaway, NY 11691.

Association for the Study of Abortion, 120 W. 57th St., New York, NY 10019.

Association for Voluntary Sterilization, 788 Third Ave., New York, NY 10017.

Buffalo Women's Self-Help Clinic, c/o Buffalo Women's Center, 498 Franklin St., Buffalo, NY 14212.

Catholics for a Free Choice, 515 Madison Ave., New York, NY 10022.

Center for Medical Consumers and Health Care Information, Inc., 410 E. 62 St., New York, NY 10021.

Coalition Against Sterilization Abuse, c/o TWWA, 244-48 W. 27th St., New York, NY 10011.

Committee to End Sterilization Abuse, Box 839, Cooper Station, New York, NY 10003.

DES-Watch, P.O. Box 141, Jericho, NY 11753.

DES-Watch, P.O. Box 12, Wantagh, NY 11793.

Eastern Women's Center, 14 E. 60 St., New York, NY 10022.

Feminist Health Research Committee, 9 Susan Court, White Plains, NY 10605.

Health Organization Collective of NY/Women's Health and Abortion Project, 36 W. 22nd St., New York, NY 10010.

Ithaca Women's Health Care Collective, 101 North Geneva St., Ithaca, NY 14850.

Lay Non-Medical Midwives for Natural Homebirth, 1364 E. 7th St., Brooklyn, NY 11230.

Maternity Center Association, 48 E. 92nd St., New York, NY 10028.

National Abortion Federation, 6 Lake Dr., Huguenot, NY 12746.

National Abortion Rights Action League, 250 W. 57th St., New York, NY 10019.

National Clergy Consultation Service on Abortion, 55 Washington Square South, New York, NY 10012.

National Women's Health Coalition, 222 W. 35th St., New York, NY 10016.

New Yorkers for Abortion Law Repeal, Box 240, Planetarium Station, New York, NY 10024.

Planned Parenthood-World Population, 810 Seventh Ave., New York, NY 10019.

Radicalesbians Health Collective Women's Center, 36 W. 22nd St., New York, NY 10010.

Rochester Women's Health Collective, 713 Monroe Ave., Rochester, NY 14607.

St. Marks Clinic, 44 St. Marks Place, New York, NY 10003.

Self-Help Action & Rap Experience for Post-Mastectomy (SHARE), c/o Dr. Eugene Thiessen, 933 Fifth Ave., New York, NY 10021.

Self-Help Clinic, 117 Avondale Place, Syracuse, NY 13210.

Women for Improved Group Health Services, c/o Elinor Polansky, 390 First Ave., New York, NY 10010.

Women's Abortion Action Alliance, 150 Fifth Ave., No. 315, New York, NY 10011.

Women's Agenda Health Task Force/Women's Action Alliance, 370 Lexington Ave., New York, NY 10017.

Women's Health Action Movement (WHAM), 175 Fifth Ave., Room 1319, New York, NY 10010.

Women's Health Alliance of Long Island, P. O. Box 645, Westbury, NY 11590.

Women's Health Forum and Women's Health Center, 175 Fifth Ave., New York, NY 10050.

Women's Rights Project/American Civil Liberties Union, 22 E. 40th St., New York, NY 10016.

Woodstock Women's Health Collective, P.O. Box 579, Woodstock, NY 12498.

North Carolina

Durham Women's Health Co-op, Central YWCA Room 29, 515 West Chapel Hill St., Durham, NC 27701.

Female Liberation/Women's Health & Pregnancy Counseling Service, Box 954, Chapel Hill, NC 27514.

National Association of Parents & Professionals for Safe Alternatives in Childbirth (NAPSAC), Box 1307, Chapel Hill, NC 27514.

North Dakota

Women's Information Collective, P.O. Box 324, Twainley Hall, Grand Forks, ND 58201.

Ohio

Cincinnati Women's Health Project, c/o Diane Porter, 2635 Bellevue, Cincinnati, OH 45219.

Cleveland NOW Health Care Task Force, 2648 Euclid Heights Blvd., Cleveland, OH 44106.

Free Afternoon Women's Clinic, 123rd St. & Euclid Ave., Cleveland, OH.

Self-Help Group, c/o Linda Goubeaux, 37 1/2 E. Frambes, Columbus, OH 43201.

Oklahoma

Oklahoma Women's Health Coalition, 12225 Candytuft Lane, Oklahoma City, OK 73132.

Oregon

Ashland Women's Health Center, 295 E. Main St., Ashland, OR 97520.

Birth Center Lucinia, 207 W. 10th St., Eugene, OR 97401.

Southeast Women's Health Clinic, 3537 SE Hawthorne, Portland, OR 92714.

The Women's Health Clinic, 3537 SE Hawthorne, Portland, OR 92714.

Women's Clinic, 750 E. 11th St., Eugene, OR 97405.

Women's Health Clinic, 4160 SE Division, Portland, OR 97202.

Pennsylvania

Baby Formula Abuse Action Group, P.O. Box 12913 Commerce Station, Philadelphia, PA 19108.

Booth Maternity Center, 6051 Overbrook Ave., Philadelphia, PA 19131.

Center for Women in Medicine, The Medical College of Pennsylvania, 3300 Henry Ave., Philadelphia, PA 19129.

CHOICE, 1501 Cherry St., Philadelphia, PA 19102.

Coalition for Abortion, 537 S. Franklin St., Wilkes Barre, PA 18702.

DES Action Group/University of Pennsylvania Women's Center, 112 Logan Hall, Philadelphia, PA 19174.

Elizabeth Blackwell Health Center for Women, 112 South 16th St., Philadelphia, PA 19103.

Gay Nurses Alliance, P.O. Box 5687, Philadelphia, PA 19129.

Gray Panthers, 3700 Chestnut St., Philadelphia, PA 19104.

Health Law Project, 133 S. 36th St., Room 410, Philadelphia, PA 19104.

Pennsylvania Women's Self-Help Group/Pennsylvania Women's Center, 112 Logan Hall, University of Pennsylvania, Philadelphia, PA 19174.

Philadelphia Women's Health Collective, 5030 Newhall St., Philadelphia, PA 19144.

Triple Jeopardy/Third World Women's Health Group, 1633 W. Bristol, Philadelphia, PA 19140.

Williamsport Women's Clinic, Clancy's Candleshop, South Williamsport, PA 17701.

Women's Ad Hoc Health Committee, 810 South 19th St., Philadelphia, PA 19102.

Women's Health Alliance/Women's Resource Center, 108 W. Beaver Ave., State College, PA 16801.

Women's Health Caucus, 2127 Green St., Philadelphia, PA 19130.

Women's Health Concerns Committee, 112 S. 16th St., Philadelphia, PA 19102.

Women's Health Services, 1209 Allegheny Tower, 625 Stanwix St., Pittsburgh, PA 15222.

Rhode Island

Rhode Island Women's Health Collective/YWCA, 423 Broad St., Central Falls, RI 02863.

Women's Health Conference, 120 Fourth St., Providence, RI 02906.

South Carolina

Abortion Interest Movement, 25 Country Club Dr., Greenville, SC 29605.

Columbia Women's Center, 1900 Haywood St., Columbia, SC 29205.

Self-Help Clinic, c/o Babette Walsh, 15 Riverside Dr., Charleston, SC 29403.

University of South Carolina, Attn. Women's Studies Institute/Linda Maloney, Columbia, SC 29208.

South Dakota

Wounded Knee Women's Health Collective, 807 Fairview St., Rapid City, SD 57701.

Tennessee

Health Group—YWCA, 200 Monroe Ave., Memphis, TN 38103.

Nashville Women's Center Health Group, 1112 19th Ave. South, Nashville, TN 37212.

Texas

Abortion Counseling and Services, 2921 Fairmont/Fairmont Center, Dallas, TX 75201.

Houston Women's Health Center, c/o Cloud, 1920 Richmond #2, Houston, TX 77006.

Women's Center of Dallas, 2001 McKinley #300, Dallas, TX 75201.

Utah

Feminist Women's Health Center, 363 East Sixth St., Salt Lake City, UT 84404.

Women's Resource Center, 293 Union Bldg., University of Utah, Salt Lake City, UT 84112.

Vermont

Green Mountain Health Center, 36 High St., Brattleboro, VT 05301.

Southern Vermont Women's Health Center, 187 N. Main St., Rutland, VT 05701.

Vermont Women's Health Center, P.O. Box 29, Burlington, VT 05401.

Virginia

Women's Health Collective, Box 3760 University Station, Charlottesville, VA 22903.

Washington

Alice Hamilton Women's Clinic, Box 525, Tacoma, WA 98401.

Aradia Clinic, 4224 University Way, NE, Seattle, WA 98105.

Country Doctor Women's Clinic, 402 15th Ave. East, Seattle, WA 98102.

Elizabeth Blackwell Women's Clinic, 1409 E. Maplewood, Bellingham, WA 98225.

Fremont Women's Clinic, 6810 Greenwood Ave. North, Seattle, WA 98103.

Lesbian Health Collective, 6817 Greenwood Ave. North, Seattle, WA 98103.

Open Door Women's Clinic, 5012 Roosevelt Way, NE, Bellingham, WA 98225.

Women's Health Resource Center, 203 W. Holly, Bellingham, WA 98225.

West Virginia

Kanawha Valley Women's Health Group, 1114 Quarrier St., Charleston, WV 25301.

Wisconsin

Amazon Women's Coalition, 2211 E. Kenwood Blvd., Milwaukee, WI 53211.

American Society for Colposcopy and Colpomecroscopy, 8700 W. Wisconsin Ave., Milwaukee, WI 53226.

Catholics for a Free Choice, Box 519, Milwaukee, WI 53201.

Coalition for Right to Choice, Box 579, Milwaukee, WI 53201.

Feminist Center of the University of Wisconsin, Milwaukee, Union Box 189 U.W.M., Milwaukee, WI 53201.

Health Writers, 306 N. Brook St., Madison, WI 53715.

International Childbirth Education Association, P.O. Box 20852, Milwaukee, WI 53220.

Women United for Action, 1012 North 3rd St., Room 414, Milwaukee, WI 53202.

Wyoming

AWARE, P.O. Box 505, Jackson, WY 83001.

Women's Resource Center, P.O. Box 3135, University Station, Laramie, WY 82070.

WYOPIRG, 1208 1/2 Gibbon, Laramie, WY 82070.

West Germany

Berlin FWHC, Postfach: 36 03 68, 1000 West Berlin 36.

Fachschaft Medizin, Universität Frankfurt, Frauenreferat 6000 Theodor-Stern Kai, Frankfurt.

Feministisches Selbsthilfszentrum "Schwarzer Mond," Gabelbergerstr. 66, 8000 München.

FFGZ, Kadettenweg 77, 1 Berlin 45.

Frauenzentrum, Gütlestrasse 8, 7750 Konstanz.

Information für Frauen c/o Free Clinic, Brunengasse 20-24, 69
Heidelberg.

APPENDIX D

SAMPLE PHYSICIAN EVALUATION SCHEDULES

Name of doctor(s):   Specialty:

Office address:

Telephone:

1. <u>Making the Appointment</u>
   When did you last visit?   Routine or special?

   Did you have trouble getting an appointment?

   Was it an emergency? (i.e., rape, excessive bleeding, etc.)

      If so, did they respond quickly?

2. <u>Arrival at the Office</u>
   How long did you wait?

   If long, who apologized to you?

   Who greeted you?

   Was there provision for entertaining children in the waiting
   room?

"Patient's Physician Evaluation" was prepared by the Health
and Abortion Information Collective of the Washington, D.C. Area
Women's Center. It appeared in <u>Off Our Backs</u>, 4 April 1974:11.
Reprinted with permission from <u>Off Our Backs</u>, a women's news
journal published monthly, 1724 20th St. NW, Washington, D.C.
20009.

3. Medical History
   Who took the history?

   Did they seem interested in you as a person?

   Was a complete history taken?

   Did you feel comfortable talking with this person?

   Were they willing to listen to your problem?

4. Initial Interview
   Who did it (doctor, nurse, etc.)?

   Did you feel relaxed?

   Was the interview done before physical exam?

5. Physical Exam
   Who did it (doctor, nurse, clinician, midwife, medic, etc.)?

   Who else was present?

   Did they assist?

   What was their sex?

   Did the examiner explain what she/he was doing?

   Were the explanations thorough and easy to understand?

   Did the examiner answer your questions to your satisfaction?

   Was the exam gentle?

   How did the examiner respond to any discomfort?

6. Laboratory Tests
   What tests were done?

   Did you discuss the reasons for the tests beforehand?

   Did you discuss the price of the tests beforehand?

Were you given a choice in the matter (that is, were you asked, or just told that the tests would be done)?

When were you given the results?

Were you told the meaning of each test result?

7. Discussion of Findings/Diagnosis
   Were you given a thorough explanation of the findings?

   Were you encouraged to ask questions?

   Were your questions answered thoroughly in language you could understand?

   Was discussion welcome on outside consultation?

8. Treatment   (Please indicate the person you talked with in each of the following questions)
   Were the reasons for suggested treatment explained?

   By whom?

   Were your questions answered thoroughly and in language you could understand?

   Were alternatives for treatment discussed?

   Were possible complications or side effects of treatment discussed?

   Was information on approximate cost volunteered?

   Were you encouraged to think things over or consult another source before beginning treatment?

FILL OUT SECTIONS 9, 10, 11 OR 12 ONLY IF APPLICABLE

9. Childbirth
   Do you feel that you were an active participant in the whole pregnancy/childbirth experience (i.e., with doctor, nurses, hospital staff, etc.)?

   Were your own needs or expectations met?

Were you given choices of delivery method?

10. Birth Control
Did you have any form of contraceptive fitted, prescribed or handed to you?

What kind of examination was performed?

Did the doctor discuss all the methods of contraception?

Did she/he ever favor one method over others?

Did the doctor inform you of possible risks, side effects and contraindications relative to your general physical health and functioning?

Was the final choice left to you?

Were you questioned about your marital status in connection with receiving birth control?

11. Surgery (including sterilization and abortion)
Was the procedure one of free choice?

Did it involve alteration, removal of any organ, body part or function?

Were you encouraged to think things over or consult another source before undergoing surgery?

Were you covered by insurance?

Did you ask to get forms from the doctor before mailing them to the insurance company?

How did they respond?

12. Pelvic Exam
Did you have a routine pelvic examination?

Was it performed by a gynecologist or an internist?

Did it include the following: breast exam; Pap smear; blood test for syphillis; gonorrhea culture; vaginal smear for vaginitis?

What kind of draping was provided?

Were you taught how to do breast self-examination?

Or anything else?

By whom?

13. General Impressions
Did you feel comfortable talking to the doctor and staff?

Did the doctor seem to relate well to the staff?

Did the staff or doctor address you by your first name?

Were you treated with dignity and respect for your intelligence?

In this particular case, how would you assess the doctor/patient relationship?

Do you think the fact that you are a woman made any difference in attitude or treatment?

Were all your expectations met?

Did you go home with unanswered questions?

What kind of literature was available in the waiting room?

Were you told in advance about the doctor's fees?

Do you think the bill was reasonable?

Was it itemized?

Was a satisfactory means of payment arranged?

Would you want to return?

Would you recommend this doctor to others?

Why, or why not?

OTHER COMMENTS:

HEALTH CARE PROVIDER EVALUATION

The information in this questionnaire is a very important part of our referral system. It is the only way that we and other women can know what kind of health care women are receiving in the Bay area. We encourage women to read these completed forms so they are better able to make informed decisions about the choosing of health care providers who are responsive to their needs. We also feel that this type of information can be a powerful tool in confronting the professional medical community about how women feel about the health care they are receiving. We know this form is very long and that some of the questions are personal, but we feel that all of the information is relevant in choosing what kind of health care we seek. We greatly appreciate you taking the time to answer these questions.

_____

DATE _____

your age _____   ethnic background _____

language spoken _____   sexual preference _____

health care provider/clinic _____

    if clinic, name of provider _____

address _____   phone _____

specialty _____   wheelchair accessible _____

_____

The "Health Care Provider Evaluation" was devloped by the San Francisco Women's Health Center, 3789 24th Street, San Francisco, CA 94122. Reprinted with permission.

what was your reason for seeking medical care? _____

_____

what treatment did you receive? _____

_____

was a relevant medical herstory taken? (e.g., family and personal herstories, including gyn, allergies, medications being taken, etc.)

_____

_____

what fees did you pay, if any, for services rendered? _____

_____

accepts medical _____ insurance _____ sliding scale _____

can you be seen without proof of payment? _____

how did you choose this health care provider? _____

how long did it take you to get an appointment? _____

how long did you wait in the waiting room? _____

can this health care provider be consulted by phone? _____

_____

did you feel the examination you received was thorough? _____

why? why not? _____

did this health care provider explain to your satisfaction?:
        any medical problem _____

        treatment _____

        medication prescribed (e.g., effects, side effects, drug inter-
actions with diet and other medications, such as tetracycline and
dairy products) _____

alternatives to medication _____

did you receive any preventive care information? (e.g., instruction in self-breast exam, prevention of bladder or vaginal infections, information about nutrition, exercise, etc.) _____

_____

_____

did you feel comfortable with the way you were treated? _____

please comment on the attitude of the health care provider and other staff. _____

_____

_____

WOULD YOU RECOMMEND THIS HEALTH CARE PROVIDER? ____

why? why not? _____

_____

_____

_____

THANK YOU very much for your contribution towards a more responsive health care system.

BIBLIOGRAPHY

BIBLIOGRAPHY

Abarbanel, Alice. (1972). "Redefining Motherhood." In L. Howe, ed., The Future of the Family, pp. 349-67. New York: Simon and Schuster.

"Activists Convicted." (1977). Network News (June): 1, 4.

Adamson, Elaine. (1971). "Critical Issues in the Use of Physician Associates and Physicians Assistants." American Journal of Public Health 61 (September): 1765-69.

Advocates for Women. (1973). San Francisco Women's Business Directory. San Francisco: Advocates for Women.

Agate, Carol. (1973). "Voluntary Sterilization: May a Spouse's Consent Be Required?" Mimeographed Stamford, Conn.: New Moon Communications.

"Alabama: Sterilization of Minors Leads to Controversy." (1973). Family Planning/Population Reporter 2 (August): 77-78.

The Alan Guttmacher Institute. (1975). Provisional Estimates of Abortion Need and Services in the Year Following the 1973 Supreme Court Decision: United States and Metropolitan Area. New York: Planned Parenthood Federation of America.

Aldrich, Alice, (1974). "Women's Health Clinic: New Approaches." Off Our Backs 9 (August/September): 9.

Alexander, Bonnie. (1974). "Quarantined Pregnancy." The Second Wave 3 (Spring): 36-37.

Alford, Robert. (1975). Health Care Politics: Ideological and Interest Group Barriers to Reform. Chicago: University of Chicago Press.

Alper, R., P. Hoffnung, and B. Solomon. (1972). "I Eat Your Flesh Plus I Drink Your Blood: The Double Features of the Abortion Business." Off Our Backs (October).

Alta. (1971). No Visible Means of Support. San Lorenzo, Calif.: Shameless Hussy Press.

Andersen, Ronald, Joanna Kravits, and Odin Anderson. (1975). Equity of Health Services: Some Emprical Analyses. Cambridge, Mass.: Ballinger.

Anonymous, Dr. (1972). Confessions of a Gynecologist. New York: Doubleday.

"Anti-Trust Suit: Verdict Before Trial." (1977). Feminist Women's Health Center Report 1 (April): 6.

Arms, Suzanne. (1975). Immaculate Deception: A New Look at Women and Childbirth in America. Boston: Houghton Mifflin.

Arneson, G. A., and W. L. Prickett. (1968). "Problems of Getting Patients off Psychotropic Drugs." Southern Medical Journal 61: 134-38. Cited in R. Seidenberg, "Drug Advertising and Perception of Mental Illness," Mental Hygiene 55 (January 1971): 26.

Ash, Roberta. (1972). Social Movements in America. Chicago: Markham.

"Atraumatic Termination of Pregnancy: A Medical Protocol." (1973). New York: National Women's Health Coalition, March.

"Bad-Dream House." (1972). Time 99 (March 20): 77.

Balter, Mitchell, and Jerome Levine. (1971). "Character and Extent of Psychotherapeutic Drug Usage in the United States." Paper presented at Fifth World Congress on Psychiatry, November 30, Mexico City. Cited in M. Silverman and P. Lee, Pills, Profits and Politics, p. 293. Berkeley: University of California Press, 1974.

——. (1969). "The Nature and Extent of Psychotropic Drug Usage in the U.S." Psychoparmacology Bulletin 5. Cited in J. Prather and L. Fidell, "Sex Differences in the Content and Style of Medical Advertising," Social Science and Medicine 9 (January 1975): 23-26.

Baltimore Chapter NOW. (1973). "How to Organize 'A Women's Right to Health,' A Panel Discussion." Mimeographed. Baltimore: Baltimore Chapter NOW.

Banks, J. A. (1972). The Sociology of Social Movements. London: Macmillan.

Bardwick, Judith, ed. (1972). Readings on the Psychology of Women. New York: Harper & Row.

———. (1971). Psychology of Women: A Study of Bio-Cultural Con flicts. New York: Harper & Row.

Barfoot, Julia McKinney. (1973). "Free Health Care for Women by Women: The Berkeley Women's Health Collective." In A. Rush, Getting Clear: Body Work for Women, pp. 89-101. New York/ Berkeley, Calif.: Random House/Bookworks.

Barker-Benfield, Ben. (1972). "The Spermatic Economy: A Nineteenth Century View of Sexuality." Feminist Studies 1 (Summer): 45-74.

Barker-Benfield, G. J. (1976). The Horrors of the Half-Known Life. New York: Harper & Row.

Barnett, C. R., P. Y. Leiderman, R. Grobstein, and M. Klaus. (1970). "Neonatal Separation: The Maternal Side of Interactional Deprivation." Peds 45 (February):197-205. Cited in G. H. Peterson and L. E. Mehl, "Parental/Child Psychology—Delivery Alternatives," Women & Health 2 (September/October 1977): 3-17.

Barry, Kathleen. (1972). "The Cutting Edge: A Look at Male Motivation in Gynecology." Mimeographed.

Bart, Pauline. (1977). "Seizing the Means of Reproduction: An Illegal Feminist Abortion Collective—How and Why It Worked." Unpublished paper. Chicago: University of Illinois, Abraham Lincoln School of Medicine.

———. (1974). "Ideologies and Utopias of Psychotherapy." In P. Roman and H. Trice, eds., The Sociology of Psychotherapy, pp. 9-57. New York: Jason Aronson.

———. (1973). "Sexism and Health Issues." The Hyde Parker (June): 65, 70.

———. (1971a). "Depression in Middle-Aged Women." In V. Gornick and B. Moran, eds., Woman in Sexist Society: Studies in Power and Powerlessness, pp. 99-117. New York: Signet.

———. (1971b). "The Myth of a Value Free Psychotherapy." In W. Bell and J. Mau, eds., Sociology and the Future. New York: Russell Sage Foundation.

Bazell, R. J. (1971). "Health Radicals: Crusade to Shift Medical Power to the People." Science 173 (August): 506.

Beam, Joanna. (1973). "Psychosurgery, Sexism and the Law." Issues in Radical Therapy 1 (Autumn): 6-10.

Becker, Howard S., Blanche Geer, Everett C. Hughes, and Anselm Strauss. (1961). Boys in White: Student Culture in Medical School. Chicago: University of Chicago Press.

Beers, Clifford. (1908). A Mind That Found Itself. New York: Longmans, Green.

Bell, Daniel. (1973). The Coming of the Post-Industrial Society. New York: Basic Books.

Ben-David, J. (1958). "The Professional Role of the Physician in Bureaucratized Medicine: A Study in Role Conflict." Human Relations 11 (August): 255-74.

BenDor, Jan. (1974). "Supercoil Abortion, Karman Part 4." Her-Self 2 (January): 8.

———. (1973a). "Harvey Karman: Another Vacuum Cleaner Salesman?" Her-Self 2 (November): 9, 21.

———. (1973b). "Karman as 'Hero,' Abortion Innovator Exhibits Sexism." Her-Self 2 (September): 1.

Berger, Peter, and Thomas Luckman. (1967). The Social Construction of Reality: A Treatise in the Sociology of Knowledge. New York: Anchor Books.

Berkeley Women's Health Collective. (1972). Feeding Ourselves. Berkeley, Calif.: Berkeley Women's Health Collective.

———. (n.d.). "Pelvic Examinations." Mimeographed. Berkeley, Calif.: Berkeley Women's Health Collective.

Bernard, Jessie. (1975). The Future of Motherhood. New York: Penguin Books.

——. (1973b). The Future of Marriage. New York: Bantam Books.

——. (1973a). "My Four Revolutions: An Autobiographical History of the ASA." American Journal of Sociology 78 (January): 773-91.

Bettelheim, Bruno. (1954). Symbolic Wounds: Puberty Rites and the Envious Male. New York: The Free Press.

Blake, Judith. (1971). "Abortion and Public Opinion: The 1960-1970 Decade." Science 171 (February 12): 540-49.

Bloch, Alice. (1973). "Women's Clinic—Not Fit for Women." The Lesbian Tide 2 (April): 9, 18.

Blumer, Herbert. (1951). "Social Movements." In A. M. Lee, ed., Principles of Sociology, pp. 199-220. New York: Barnes & Noble.

——. (1946). "Collective Behavior." In A. M. Lee, ed., A New Outline of the Principles of Sociology, pp. 167-219. New York: Barnes & Noble.

"The Book." (1977). FWHC Report 1 (April): 11.

Borgman, Robert. (1973). "Medication Abuse By Middle-Aged Women." Social Casework 54 (November): 526-32.

Borman, Nancy. (1974). "Harvey Karman: Savior or Charlatan?" Majority Report 3 (January): 6.

"Boston Conference." (1975). HealthRight 1 (Spring): 3-4.

The Boston Women's Health Book Collective. (1976). Our Bodies, Ourselves—A Book By and For Women. 2d ed. rev. New York: Simon and Schuster.

——. (1973). Our Bodies, Ourselves—A Book By and For Women. New York: Simon and Schuster.

The Boston Women's Health Course Collective. (1971). Our Bodies, Ourselves—A Course By and For Women. Boston: New England Free Press.

Bourne, Patricia. (1972). "The Three Faces of Day Care." In L. Howe, ed., The Future of the Family, pp. 268-82. New York: Simon and Schuster.

Brahen, Leonard S. (1973). "Housewife Drug Abuse." Journal of Drug Education 3 (Spring): 13-24.

Breggin, Peter. (1972). "The Return of Lobotomy and Psychosurgery." 118 Congressional Record 5567. Cited in R. Roth and J. Lerner, "Sex-Based Discrimination in the Mental Institutionalization of Women," California Law Review 62 (May 1974): 789-815.

"British Pill Study." (1974). Off Our Backs 4 (June): 8.

Brophy, Judith. (1976). "Letters," HealthRight 2:3: p. 2.

Broverman, K. B., D. M. Broverman, R. Clarkson, P. Rosenkrantz, and S. Vogel. (1970). "Sex Role Stereotypes and Clinical Judgments of Mental Health." Journal of Consulting and Clinical Psychology 34: 1-7.

Brown, Carol. (1976). "Roles for Women Health Workers in the United States and China." Women and Health 1 (March/April): 11-13.

———. (1975). "Women Workers in the Health Service Industry." International Journal of Health Services 5 (Spring): 173-84.

Brown, Judith. (1963). "A Cross-Cultural Study of Female Initiation Rites." American Anthropologist 65 (August): 837-53.

Brown, Laura. (1975). Personal communication, August.

———. (1974). Flier on Cathedral Hill Pregnancy Control Center. Mimeographed. Oakland, Calif.: FWHC.

———. (1973). "Presentation to the American Public Health Association Conference." Paper presented at meeting of the American Public Health Association, November, San Francisco. Mimeographed.

Brownmiller, Susan. (1975). Against Our Will: Men, Women and Rape. New York: Simon and Schuster.

Bullough, Bonnie, ed. (1975). The Law and the Expanding Nurse Role. New York: Appleton-Century-Crofts.

Bullough, Vern L. (1974). The Subordinate Sex: A History of Attitudes Toward Women. New York: Penguin Books.

Bullough, Vern, and Martha Voght. (1973). "Women, Menstruation, and Nineteenth-Century Medicine." Bulletin of the History of Medicine 47 (January/February): 66–82.

Bunker, John. (1970). "Surgical Manpower: A Comparison of Operations and Surgeons in the United States and in England and Wales." New England Journal of Medicine 282 (January): 135–44.

Burgess, Ann Wolbert, and Linda Lytle Holmstrom. (1974). Rape: Victims of Crisis. Bowie, Md: Robert J. Brady.

Burkons, D. M., and J. R. Willson. (1974). "Is the Obstetrician-Gynecologist a Specialist or a Primary Physician to Women?" Paper presented to American Association of Obstetricians and Gynecologists, September 4. Cited in H. Marieskind, "Restructuring Ob-Gyn," Social Policy 6 (September/October 1975): 48–49.

Burris, Barbara. (1973). "The Fourth World Manifesto." In A. Koedt, E. Levine, and A. Rapone, eds., Radical Feminism, pp. 322–57. New York: Quadrangle/The New York Times Book Company.

Burris, Carol. (1974). "Statement of Carol Burris, president, Women's Lobby, Inc." U.S. Congress, House Committee on Ways and Means Hearings on National Health Insurance, June 28, 1974. Mimeographed. Washington, D.C.: Women's Lobby.

Butler County NOW. (1973). "Ohio's Women Medical Specialists." Mimeographed. Oxford, Ohio: NOW.

Butler, Katy. (1974). "Women: Midwifery on Trial in Santa Cruz." San Francisco Bay Guardian, July 20-August 2, p. 7.

Cagan, Beth. (1970). "Giving Birth in Dignity." Up From Under 1 (May/June): 39–42.

Campbell, Kathy, Terry Dalsemer, and Judy Waldman. (1972). "Women's Night at the Free Clinic." Women: A Journal of Liberation 2: 37–38.

Campbell, Margaret (pseudonym for Mary Howell). (1973). "Why Would a Girl Go Into Medicine?" Medical Education in the United States: A Guide for Women. Old Westbury, N.Y.: The Feminist Press.

Carden, Maren Lockwood. (1974). The New Feminist Movement. New York: Russell Sage Foundation.

Caress, Barbara. (1975). "Sterilization: Women Fit to be Tied." Health/PAC Bulletin 62 (January-February): 1-6, 10-12.

Carlson, Rick J. (1975). The End of Medicine. New York: Wiley.

Carter, Richard. (1961). The Doctor Business. Rev. ed. New York: Dolphin Books.

Castleman, Michael. (1974). "Men Get Cured ... Women Get Drugged." Her-Self 3 (April): 12-13.

Cathedral Hill Medical Center. (1974). "Important Announcement." Mimeographed.

Chapman, Frances. (1973a). "Prostaglandins." Off Our Backs 3 (September): 8.

——. (1973b). "Supercoil Recoil: Karman Case Comes to Trial." Off Our Backs 3 (November): 2, 6.

Chesler, Phyllis. (1972). Women and Madness. Garden City, N.Y.: Doubleday.

——. (1971). "Patient and Patriarch: Women in the Psychotherapeutic Relationship." In V. Gornick and B. Moran, eds., Woman in Sexist Society: Studies in Power and Powerlessness, pp. 362-92. New York: Signet.

Chez, Ronald A. (1974). "Health Care and the Liberated Women." Contemporary Ob/Gyn 3 (February). Cited in H. Marieskind, "Gynecological Services and the Women's Movement: A Study of Self-Help Clinics and Other Modes of Delivery," pp. 157-84. Ph.D. dissertation, School of Public Health, University of California, Los Angeles, 1976.

Chicago Women with HealthRight. (1975). "A View From the Loop: The Women's Health Movement in Chicago." HealthRight 2 (Fall): 3-4.

Chomsky, Noam. (1971). Problems of Knowledge and Freedom: The Russell Lectures. New York: Vintage Books.

Christeve, Jackie. (1974). "Midwives Busted in Santa Cruz." The Second Wave 3 (Summer): 5-10.

Cisler, Lucinda. (1970). "Unfinished Business: Birth Control and Women's Liberation." In R. Morgan, ed., Sisterhood is Powerful, pp. 245-89. New York: Vintage Books.

Clelland, Virginia. (1971). "Sex Discrimination: Nursing's Most Pervasive Problem." American Journal of Nursing 71 (August): 1542-47.

Coalition for the Medical Rights of Women. (1976). Vital Signs, California newsmonthly from Health/PAC West 1 (June): 5.

"Coalition for the Medical Rights of Women." (1975). Mimeographed. San Francisco: Coalition for the Medical Rights of Women.

Coburn, Judith. (1974). "Sterilization Regulations: Debate Not Quelled by HEW Document." Science 183 (March): 935-39.

"Conferences, NOW or Later." (1975-76). HealthRight 2 (Winter): 4.

Connell, Elizabeth. (1974). "Menstrual Extraction." Medical Aspects of Human Sexuality 8 (January): 140-42.

"Consumer Input in FDA." (1977). Network News (October-November): 3.

Cooke, Willard R. (1943). Essentials of Gynecology. Philadelphia: Lippincott. Cited in D. Scully and P. Bart, "A Funny Thing Happened on the Way to the Orifice: Women in Gynecology Textbooks." American Journal of Sociology 78 (January 1973): 1046.

Cooper, Vicki. (1970). "Women as Health Workers: The Lady's Not For Burning." Health/PAC Bulletin (March): 2-7.

Cooperstock, R. (1971). "Sex Differences in the Use of Mood-Modifying Drugs: An Explanatory Model." Journal of Health and Social Behavior 12 (September): 238-44.

Cope, Oliver. (1977). The Breast and Its Troubles, Benign and Malignant. New York: Houghton Mifflin.

——. (1974). "The Physician's Comment Regarding Breast Cancer." Discussion guide accompanying film Taking Our Bodies Back, produced by Margaret Lazarus, Cambrige Documentary Films.

——. (1971). "Breast Cancer: Has the Time Come for a Less Muti-lating Treatment?" Psychiatry in Medicine 2 (October): 263-69.

Cope, Oliver, C. A. Wang, M. Schulz, C. C. Wang, and B. Castle-man. (1967). "Breast Cancer Reconsidered: The Rationale for Radiation Therapy Without Mastectomy." The Transactions of the New England Surgical Society (October).

Copsey, Diana. (1973). "Busing of 15 Women to Philadelphia for 'Super Coil' Abortions Provokes Wide Furor." Ob. Gyn. News 34 (April 1): 1, 34-37.

Cordtz, Dan. (1971). "Change Begins in the Doctor's Office." In H. P. Dreitzel, ed., The Social Organization of Health. New York: MacMillan.

Corea, Gena. (1977). The Hidden Malpractice: How American Medicine Treats Women as Patients and Professionals. New York: William Morrow.

Costanza, Mary. (1972). "Introduction." In Ellen Frankfort, Vaginal Politics, pp. xxiii-ix. New York: Quadrangle Books.

Cowan, Belita. (1978). Personal communication, March 18.

——. (1977). Women's Health Care: Resources, Writings, Bibli-ographies. Ann Arbor, Mich.: Anshen.

——. (1976a). "Feminists Testify at Congressional DES Hearings." Her-Self (February): 6.

——. (1976b). "Going to Washington, The Women's Health Lobby." HealthRight 2 no. 3: 4, 8.

——. (1975). "Your Health: Protest Letter Sent to FDA." Her-Self 3 (March): 9.

——. (1974a). "Copper 7 IUD Recalled." Her-Self 3 (August): 8.

——. (1974b). "Dalkon Shield IUD Called Dangerous." Her-Self 3 (August): 8.

——. (1974c). "DES Cancer Victim Files Lawsuit." Her-Self 3 (May): 9.

————. (1974d). "Lilly Won't Market Morning-After Pill." Her-Self 3 (June/July): 6.

————. (1974e). "Los Angeles Feminists Raid Karman Abortion Clinic." Her-Self 3 (November): 10.

————. (1974f). "The 'Mini Pill' Hits the Market." Her-Self 3 (April): 14.

————. (1974g). "The 'Morning After' Pill." Her-Self 3 (September/October): 6-7.

————. (1974h). "Planned Parenthood Recruits Females for Morning-After Pill Experiment." Her-Self 3 (August): 8.

————. (1974i). "Pregnant Women Lose Rights." Her-Self 3 (June/July): 6.

————. (1974j). "One Out of Three Hysterectomies Is Unnecessary." Her-Self 3 (August): 8.

————. (1974k). "Placidyl for Pregnant Women?" Her-Self 3 (April): 16.

Cowan, Belita, and Cheryl Peck. (1976). "Special Report: The Controversy at FEN, the City Club, and the Credit Union." Her-Self 5 (May): 8-17.

Crile, George, Jr. (1974). What Women Should Know About the Breast Cancer Controversy. New York: Pocket Books.

Curtis, Linda. (1976). "The Tallahassee M.D. Conspiracy." Mimeographed. Tallahassee, Fla.: Feminist Women's Health Center, April 3.

————. (1975). "Statement to the Press by Linda Curtis, Director of the Feminist Women's Health Center, Oct. 1, 1976." Mimeographed. Tallahassee, Fla.: FWHC.

Cushner, Irvin. (1965). "The Psychologic and Family Impact of the Diseases Peculiar to Women." In A. Barnes, ed., The Social Responsibility of Obstetrics and Gynecology. Baltimore: Johns Hopkins Press.

Dahrendorf, Ralf. (1959). Class and Class Conflict in Industrial Society. Stanford: Stanford University Press.

"Dalkon Shield Recall." (1974). Off Our Backs 4 (June): 9.

Daniels, Arlene Kaplan. (1977). "Development of Feminist Networks in Health." In "Proceedings of the Conference on Women's Leadership and Authority in the Health Professions," pp. 24-35. Mimeographed. University of California, Santa Cruz.

——. (1976). Personal communication, September 17.

——. (1975a). "A Feminist Organization: Equality for Women." In A. Daniels, K. Eriksson-Joslyn, and S. Ruzek, The Place of Volunteerism in the Lives of Women. Final Report, NIMH Grant no. MH 26294-01. Mimeographed. San Francisco: Institute for Scientific Analysis.

——. (1975b). "Feminist Perspectives in Sociological Research." In M. Millman and R. M. Kanter, eds., Another Voice: Feminist Perspectives on Social Life and Social Science, pp. 340-80. New York: Anchor Books.

——. (1973). "How Free Should Professions Be?" In E. Freidson, ed., The Professions and Their Prospects, pp. 39-57. Beverly Hills: Sage Publications.

Daniels, M. J. (1960). "Affect and Its Control in the Medical Intern." American Journal of Sociology 61 (November): 259-67.

Davis, Kingsley. (1938). "Mental Hygiene and the Class Structure." Psychiatry 1 (February): 55-65.

Dawson, Dena. (1975). "The Complete (At Present) Facts About the Pill." Her-Self 4 (June): 9, 15.

Dejanikus, Tacie. (1974). "Dalkon Shield Exposed." Off Our Backs 4 (July): 7, 25.

——. (1973a). "Childbirth: Not So Simple." Off Our Backs 3 (July/August): 7.

——. (1973b). "Super-Coil Controversy." Off Our Backs 3 (May): 2-3, 11.

——. (1972). "Menstrual Extraction." Off Our Backs 3 (December): 4-5.

de Maehl, Sharon, and Linda Thurston. (1973). "Crimes in the Clinic: A Report on Boston City Hospital." The Second Wave 2 no. 3: 17-20.

"DES Groups Plan Summer Programs." (1976). Coalition News (July): 3.

Deutsch, Albert. (1938). The Mentally Ill in America. 2d ed. New York: Columbia University Press.

Deutsch, Helene. (1945). The Psychology of Women. 2 vols. New York: Grune & Stratton.

"Device Legislation Empowers the FDA to Regulate IUDs as Well as Clips, Rings and Bands Used in Sterilization." (1976). Family Planning Perspectives 8 (May-June): 132-33.

Dodson, Betty. (1974). Liberating Masturbation: A Meditation on Self Love. New York: Bodysex Designs.

"Double Dynamics: Women's Roles in Health and Illness." (1975). Report of a conference conducted by The Center for Women in Medicine, The Medical College of Pennsylvania, December 7, 8, 9, 1975, Philadelphia, Pennsylvania. Mimeographed.

Downer, Carol. (1976). Letter to Larry Erskine and John Martinez, Department of Investigation of the Bureau of Consumer Affairs, Los Angeles, June 30.

——. (1974a). Personal communication, February 6.

——. (1974b). "What Makes the Feminist Women's Health Center Feminist." Feminist Women's Health Center Report, p. 12. Reprinted in The Monthly Extract 3 (March/April): 10-11, and Off Our Backs 4 (June): 2.

——. (1972). "Covert Discrimination Against Women as Medical Patients." Address to the American Psychological Association, September, Honolulu. Mimeographed.

Duffy, John. (1974). A History of Public Health in New York City, 1866-1966. New York: Russell Sage Foundation.

———. (1968). A History of Public Health in New York City, 1625-1866. New York: Russell Sage Foundation.

Duffy, Martha. (1972). "Books." Time (March 20): 98-99.

Dungan, Eloise. (1973). "Why the Patient Shouldn't Be Naked." San Francisco Sunday Examiner & Chronicle, Sunday Scene, December 2, p. 10.

Eagan, Andrea. (1976). "Breast Cancer: Facts a Woman Needs to Know." HealthRight 2 no. 3: 1, 6.

"Editorial: The Home Birth Movement." (1977). HealthRight 3 (Fall): 2.

"Editorials: Judge's Sentencing Cannot be Justified." (1977). Florida Flambeau, May 25, p. 4.

Edmiston, Susan. (1973). "A Gynecological Examination." Woman's Day 4 (October): 82, 148, 150.

Edmonds, Beverly. (1975). "Reversing Rape: Creating the Healthy Woman at a Self-Help Group." Unpublished paper, Department of Social and Behavioral Sciences, University of California, San Francisco.

Edwards, Margot E. (1973). "Unattended Home Birth." American Journal of Nursing 73 (August): 1332-35.

Ehrenreich, Barbara. (1975). "The Status of Women as Health Care Providers in the U.S." Paper presented at the International Conference on Women in Health, June 18-19, Washington, D.C. Reprinted in Social Policy 6 (November): 4-11.

Ehrenreich, Barbara, and John Ehrenreich. (1971). The American Health Empire, Power, Profits and Politics. New York: Vintage Books.

Ehrenreich, Barbara, and Deirdre English. (1973). Complaints and Disorders: The Sexual Politics of Sickness. Glass Mountain Pamphlet, no. 2. Old Westbury, N.Y.: The Feminist Press.

———. (1972). Witches, Midwives, and Nurses: A History of Women Healers. Glass Mountain Pamphlet, no. 1. Old Westbury, N.Y.: The Feminist Press.

Ehrlich, Howard J., and Carol Ehrlich. (1972). "Bardwick's Psychology of Women: A New Acquisition for the Archives of Academic Sexism." Insurgent Sociologist 3.

Eliade, Mircea. (1965). Rites and Symbols of Initiation: The Mysteries of Birth and Rebirth. New York: Harper Torchbooks.

Elling, Ray H. (1971). "The Shifting Power Structure in Health." Inquiry 8 (September): 119-43.

Emerson, Joan P. (1970a). "Behavior in Private Places: Sustaining Definitions of Reality in Gynecological Examinations." In H. Dreitzel, ed., Recent Sociology, No. 2, pp. 74-97. London: MacMillan.

——. (1970b). "Nothing Unusual Is Happening." In T. Shibutani, ed., Human Nature and Collective Behavior: Papers in Honor of Herbert Blumer, pp. 208-22. Englewood Cliffs, N.J.: Prentice-Hall.

——. (1963). "Social Functions of Humor in a Hospital Setting." Ph.D. dissertation, University of California, Berkeley.

Ephron, Nora. (1975). Crazy Salad. New York: Bantam Books.

Epstein, Cynthia. (1971). Woman's Place: Options and Limits in Professional Careers. Berkeley: University of California Press.

Etzionni, Amitai. (1974). "Review of the Coming of Post-Industrial Society." Contemporary Sociology 3 (March): 105-7.

Farber, Shelley. (1976). Personal communication, August 31.

——. (1973). "Presentation to the American Public Health Association Conference." Paper presented at meeting of the American Public Health Association, November, San Francisco. Mimeographed.

Farenza, Cynthia. (1976). "Helping Women Help Themselves." Mountain Moving 1 (March): 22-24.

Farrow, J. H., A. A. Fracchia, G. F. Robbins, and E. Castro. (1971). "Simple Excision or Biopsy Plus Radiation Therapy as Primary Treatment for Potentially Curable Cancer of the Breast." Cancer 28 (November): 1195-1201.

Fatt, Naomi. (1975-76). "Florida Women Sue M.D.'s." HealthRight 2 (Winter): 7.

———. (1975a). "Where Does All the Money Go?" HealthRight 1 (Spring): 4.

———. (1975b). "The Caucus." HealthRight (Summer): 1, 4.

"FDA Approves Depo-Provera." (1974). The Spokeswoman 4 (November): 1-2.

"Federal Court Rules in Favor of Pregnant Women in Unemployment Benefits Case." (1973). Women Today 3 (October): 6.

The Feminist Counseling Collective. (1975). "Feminist Psychotherapy." Social Policy 6 (September/October): 54-62.

The Feminist Mental Health Project. (n.d.). "Women's Medical Directory." San Francisco: American Friends Service Committee.

The Feminist Women's Health Center. (1973). "A Synopsis of the Activities of Harvey Karman." The Monthly Extract 2 (December/ January): 3-6.

———. (n.d.a). "Physicians Training Program." Mimeographed. Los Angeles: FWHC.

———. (n.d.b). "Synopsis of the FWHC Development." Mimeographed. Los Angeles: FWHC.

Feminist Women's Health Center Newsletter. (1976). 3 (January).

"Feminist Women's Health Center Report." (1977). Los Angeles: FWHC.

"Feminist Women's Health Center Report." (1975). Los Angeles: FWHC.

"Feminist Women's Health Center Report." (1974). Los Angeles: FWHC.

"Feminist Women's Health Center Report." (1973). Los Angeles: FWHC.

"Feminist Women's Health Centers Meet Planned Parenthood Physicians." (1975). Feminist Women's Health Center Report 1 (September): 8-9.

"Feminists' Anti-Trust Suit Rejected." (1976). Abortion Trends 16 (January): 3.

"Feminists Raid Abortion Clinic in L.A." (1974). San Francisco Chronicle, September 4, p. 7.

"Feminists to Stand Trial for Reclaiming Birth." (1977). Feminist Women's Health Center Report 1 (April): 1-3.

Fidell, Linda. (1974). Memo to DAPAC Subcommittee on Women and Drugs, June 25.

Field, Mark. (1967). Soviet Socialized Medicine. New York: The Free Press.

——. (1961). "The Doctor-Patient Relationship in the Perspective of 'Fee for Service' and 'Third Party' Medicine." Journal of Health and Human Behavior 2 (Winter): 252-61.

Fields, Rona M. (n.d.). "Psychotherapy: The Sexist Machine." Pittsburgh: KNOW.

Firestone, Shulamith. (1970). The Dialectic of Sex. New York: William Morrow.

Fishel, Elizabeth. (1973). "Women's Self-Help Movement or, Is Happiness Knowing Your Own Cervix?" Ramparts (November): 29.

Fisher, JoAnne. (1975). "For Want of Water." HealthRight 2 (Fall): 6.

Fleeson, Lucinda B. (1973). "Doctors Diagnose Nurses." Ms. 2 (August): 76-77.

Ford, James Ellsworth. (1975). "Doing Obstetrics: The Organization of Work Routines in a Maternity Service." Ph.D. dissertation, University of British Columbia.

Frankfort, Ellen. (1973a). "The Surgeon Cuts—and Cuts—and Cuts." The Village Voice, October 25, pp. 23-24.

——. (1973b). "Women Doctors." The Village Voice, July 26, p. 23.

——. (1972). Vaginal Politics. New York: Quadrangle Books.

Freeman, Jo. (1975). The Politics of Women's Liberation: A Case Study of an Emerging Social Movement and Its Relation to the Policy Process. New York: David McKay.

——. (1973). "The Tyranny of Structurelessness." In A. Koedt, E. Levine, and A. Rapone, eds., Radical Feminism, pp. 285-99. New York: Quadrangle/The New York Times Book Company.

Freidl, Ernestine. (1966). "Hospital Care in Provincial Greece." In W. R. Scott and E. H. Volkart, eds., Medical Care: Readings in the Sociology of Medical Institutions, pp. 508-16. New York: John Wiley & Sons.

Freidson, Eliot. (1975). Doctoring Together: A Study of Professional Social Control. New York: Elsevier.

——. (1973a). "Prepaid Group Practice and the New 'Demanding Patient'." Milbank Memorial Fund Quarterly/Health and Society 51 (Fall): 473-88.

——. (1973b). "Professionalisation and the Organization of Middle-Class Labor in Post-Industrial Society." In P. Halmos, ed., The Sociological Review Monograph, no. 20, Professionalisation and Social Change (University of Keele), December.

——. (1970). Profession of Medicine: A Study of the Sociology of Applied Knowledge. New York: Dodd, Mead.

——. (1969). "Client Control and Medical Practice." American Journal of Sociology 65 (January): 374-82.

——. (1968). "The Impurity of Professional Authority." In H. Becker, B. Geer, D. Riesman, and R. Weiss, eds., Institutions and the Person, pp. 25-34. Chicago: Aldine.

——. (1961). Patients Views of Medical Practice. New York: Russell Sage Foundation.

Freidson, Eliot, and Buford Rhea. (1963). "Processes of Control in a Company of Equals." Social Problems 2 (Fall): 119-31.

Freudenberger, H. J. (1974). "Staff Burn-Out." Journal of Social Issues 30 (January/March): 159-65.

Fried, John J. (1974). "Tranquilizers: Rx for the 'Woman Problem'." Playgirl (July): 53, 92, 109, 126.

Friedman, Lawrence J. (1971). "Art Versus Violence." Arts in Society 8:1: 325-31. Cited in B. Seaman, Free and Female, p. 162. New York: Fawcett Publications, 1972.

Friedman, Samuel R. (1973). "Perspectives on the American Student Movement." Social Problems 20 (Winter): 283-99.

Fruchtbaum, Harold. (1976). "A Review of the Horrors of the Half-Known Life: Male Attitudes Toward Women and Sexuality in Nineteenth-Century America by G. J. Barker-Benfield." Women and Health 1 (March/April): 30-31.

Fruchter, Rachel. (1976). "ERT: A Risky Proposition." HealthRight 2:3: 7.

———. (1970). "On Abortion." Up From Under 1 (August/September): 9-12.

Fuller, Richard C., and Richard R. Myers. (1941). "The Natural History of a Social Problem." American Sociological Review 6 (June): 320-29.

"Funeral for a Fetus." (1974). Her-Self 3 (August): 4.

"FWHC Plans Birth Control Subscriptions." (1976). Feminist Women's Health Center Newsletter 3 (January): 1.

"FWHC Response." (1974). Off Our Backs 4 (August/September): 17-21.

Gallyot, Jeanne. (1978). Personal communication, January 14.

Galper, Miriam, and Carolyn Kott Washburne. (1976). "A Women's Self-Help Program in Action." Social Policy 6 (March/April): 46-52.

Garai, Pierre R. (1964). "Advertising and Promotion of Drugs." In P. Talalay, ed., Drugs in Our Society. Baltimore: Johns Hopkins Press.

Gartner, Alan, and Frank Riessman. (1974). The Service Society and the Consumer Vanguard. New York: Harper & Row.

Geiger, Jack. (1971). "Hidden Professional Roles: The Physician as Reactionary, Reformer, Revolutionary." Social Policy 1 (March/April): 24-33.

Gendel, Evalyn S., with Dalma Heyn. (1974). "It's Your Body ... Not Your Doctor's." Redbook 142 (March): 88-89, 165-70.

Gibson, Campbell. (1976). "The U.S. Fertility Decline, 1961-1975: The Contribution of Changes in Marital Status and Marital Fertility." Family Planning Perspectives 8 (September/October): 249-52.

Gilb, Corinne Lathrop. (1966). Hidden Hierarchies: The Professions and Government. New York: Harper & Row.

Glaser, Barney G., and Anselm L. Strauss. (1967). The Discovery of Grounded Theory: Strategies for Qualitative Research. Chicago: Aldine.

——. (1965). Status Passage: A Formal Theory. New York: Aldine.

Glasscote, Raymond, James B. Raybin, Clifford B. Reifler, and Andrew W. Kane, eds. (1975). The Alternate Services: Their Role in Mental Health. Washington, D.C.: Joint Information Service of the American Psychiatric Association and the National Association for Mental Health.

Goffman, Erving. (1963). Behavior in Public Places: Notes on the Social Organization of Gatherings. New York: The Free Press.

Goldberg, Michael. (1974). "Birth Center/Midwives Busted!" Sundaz! (March 1974). Reprinted in Rough Times 4 (March/April/May 1974): 4.

Goldsmith, Sadja. (1972). "Non-Electric Methods of Vacuum Aspiration." In T. M. Hart, ed., Abortion in the Clinic and Office Setting, p. 36. San Francisco: The Society for Humane Abortion.

Goldsmith, Sadja, and Alan J. Margolis. (1971). "Aspiration Abortion Without Cervical Dilation." American Journal of Obstetrics and Gynecology 110 (June 15): 580-82.

Goodman, Robin Reba. (1974). "Diethylstilbestrol: Gynecology or Gynecide?" Her-Self 3 (April): 8.

Gornick, Vivian, and Barbara K. Moran, eds. (1971). Woman in Sexist Society: Studies in Power and Powerlessness. New York: Signet.

Gossett, Jay W. (1971). "Medical Consumerism Flexes Its Muscles." Medical Economics 48 (August 16): 29-40.

Gould, Lois. (1975). "Pornography for Women." In U. West, ed., Women in a Changing World, pp. 126-40. New York: McGraw-Hill.

Graedon, Joe. (1976). The People's Pharmacy. New York: St. Martin's Press.

Grau, Peggy. (1971). "Menstrual Extraction." Everywoman 11 (October).

Gray, Marian Johnson, and Roger W. Gray. (1971). How to Take the Worry Out of Being Close. P.O. Box 2822, Oakland, CA 94616. Distributed by authors.

Green, T. (1971). Gynecology: Essentials of Clinical Practice. Boston: Little, Brown. Cited in S. Shapiro, "The Politics of Dysmenorrhea." Unpublished paper, 1975.

Greene, Chayse. (1974). "Morning After Pill: A Cautionary Tale." Off Our Backs 4 (May): 22.

Greenwald, P., J. J. Barlow, P. C. Nasca, and M. S. Burnett. (1971). "Vaginal Cancer After Maternal Treatment with Synthetic Estrogens." New England Journal of Medicine 285 (August): 390-92.

Griffin, Susan. (1971). "Rape: The All-American Crime." Ramparts 10 (September): 26-35.

Grinker, Roy. (1974). Psychosomatic Concepts. New York: Jason Aronson.

Groesser, Antoinette. (1972). "Is Gynecology for Women?" In M. Alleyn, ed., The Witch's Os, pp. 9-19. Stamford, Conn.: New Moon Publications.

Guettel, Charnie. (1974). Marxism & Feminism. Toronto: Canadian Women's Educational Press/Hunter Rose Company.

Gustitas, Rasa. (1975). "The Herb Doctors Are Coming Back."
City of San Francisco (September 17): 20.

Haas, Charlie. (1977). "Judy Chicago's 'The Dinner Party': A
Room of Her Own." New West (August 1).

Haire, Doris. (1973). "The Cultural Warping of Childbirth." Environmental Child Health 19 (June): 171-91.

——. (1972 and 1975). "The Cultural Warping of Childbirth: Special
Report of the President of the International Childbirth Education
Association." ICEA News, Special Issue (Spring). Reissued with
Postscript, 1975.

Haire, D., and J. Haire. (1971a). Implementing Family Centered
Maternity Care with a Central Nursery. Milwaukee, Wis.: ICEA.

——. (1971b). The Nurse's Contribution to Successful Breast-Feeding. Milwaukee, Wis.: ICEA.

Halleck, Seymour. (1971). The Politics of Therapy. New York:
Science House.

Haller, John S. (1971). "Neurasthenia: The Medical Profession and
the 'New Woman' of the Late Nineteenth Century." New York State
Journal of Medicine 71 (February 15): 473-82.

Haller, John S., and Robin M. Haller. (1974). The Physician and
Sexuality in Victorian America. Urbana: University of Illinois
Press.

Hammer, Signe, ed. (1975). Women: Body and Culture—Essays on
the Sexuality of Women in a Changing Society. New York: Harper
& Row.

Handlin, Oscar. (1957). Race and Nationality in American Life.
New York: Doubleday.

Handy, Gladys. (1975). Personal communication, August.

Hansen, Lynn K., Barbara Reskin, and Diana Gray. (1972). How to Have Intercourse Without Getting Screwed: A Guide to Birth Control, Abortion, Venereal Disease. Seattle: Associated Students of University of Washington Women's Commission.

"Harassing Jane Doe." (1974). Off Our Backs 4 (June): 10.

Harding, Elizabeth, Charlene Harrington, and Gloria Jean Manor. (1973). "The Berkeley Free Clinic." Nursing Outlook 21 (January): 40-43.

Hart, Thomas M. (1970). First American Symposium on Office Abortions. The Proceedings of the Symposium of Office Abortion Procedures. San Francisco: The Society for Humane Abortion.

Haug, Marie, and Marvin Sussman (1969). "Professional Autonomy and the Revolt of the Client." Social Problems 17 (Fall): 153-61.

Hayden, Trudy. (1973). Punishing Pregnancy: Discrimination in Education, Employment, and Credit. (Women's Rights Project.) New York: American Civil Liberties Union.

Hazell, L. D. (1975). "Outcomes of 300 Elective Home Births." Birth and the Family Journal 2 (Winter): 11-23.

"Health Centers: Surviving Boston." (1977). Network News (October-November): 2.

"Health Conference." (1975). HealthRight 1 (Spring): 3.

"Health News Briefs." (1977). HealthRight 3 (Summer): 11.

Health/PAC Bulletin. (1971). 34 (October).

"HEALTH: Project Includes Service, Education and Direct Action." (1972). The Spokeswoman 2 (June 1): 1.

HealthRight. (1975a). 1 (Spring).

——. (1975b). 2 (September-October).

Heberle, Rudolf. (1951). Social Movements: An Introduction to Political Sociology. New York: Appleton-Century-Crofts.

Heide, Wilma Scott. (1973). "Nursing and Women's Liberation: A Parallel." American Journal of Nursing 73 (May): 824-27.

Heidelberg, Lynn. (1978). Personal communication, May 11.

Hendel, Samuel. (1971). The Politics of Confrontation. New York: Appleton-Century-Crofts.

Herbst, A. L., and R. E. Scully. (1970). "Adenocarcinoma of the Vagina in Adolescence: A Report of Seven Cases including Six Clear-Cell Carcinomas (So-Called Mesonephromas)." Cancer 25 (April): 745-57.

Herman, Judith. (1976). "Forced Sterilization." Sister Courage (January).

——. (1975). "Letters." HealthRight 2 (Summer): 2.

Her-Self. (1975). 3 (March).

Hibbard, Lester T. (1973). "Despite Higher Risks, Some Doctors Still Prefer Hysterectomy to Tubal Ligation." Family Planning Digest 2 (January): 9.

Higham, John. (1969). Strangers in the Land: Patterns of American Nativism. New York: Atheneum.

Hilberman, E., J. Konanc, M. Perez-Reyes, et al. (1975). "Support Groups for Women in Medical Schools: A First Year Program." (1975). Journal of Medical Education 50 (September): 867-75.

Hirsch, Jeanne. (1973). "Some Unorthodox Methods of Birth Control." The Monthly Extract 2 (May/June): 6-7.

——. (1972). "The Third Eye." In M. Alleyn, ed., The Witch's Os, pp. 31-37. Stamford, Conn.: New Moon Communications.

Hirsch, Lolly. (1977). The Breeders. New York: Simon and Schuster.

——. (1975). "Phone Interview from Stamford, Conn. to Carol Downer and Marilyn Skerbeck in Los Angeles." The Monthly Extract 4 (April/May): 16-17.

——. (1974-75). "Second Women—Controlled Women's Health Center Conference." The Monthly Extract 3 (December/January): 2-9.

——. (1972). "The Breeders." In M. Alleyn, ed., The Witch's Os. Stamford, Conn.: New Moon Communications.

Hirsch, Lolly, and Millie Alleyn. (1972). The Monthly Extract 1 (August/September): 2. Cited in M. Reynard, "Gynecological Self-Help: An Analysis of Its Impact on the Delivery and Use of Medical Care for Women," p. 110. Master's thesis, State University of New York at Stony Brook, 1973.

Hoffman, Charles A. (1972). "We Can't Save Private Practice—But Our Patients Can." Medical Economics 49 (March 13): 35-45.

Holder, Maryse. (1973). "Another Cuntree: At Last, A Mainstream Female Art Movement." Off Our Backs 3 (September): 11-17.

Hole, Judith, and Ellen Levine. (1971). Rebirth of Feminism. New York: Quadrangle Books.

Holmstrom, Lynda. (1972). The Two-Career Family. Cambridge, Mass.: Schenkman.

Hornstein, Frances. (1974a). "An Interview on Women's Health Politics, Part I." Quest 1 (Summer): 27-36.

——. (1974b). "An Interview on Women's Health Politics, Part II." Quest 1 (Fall): 75-80.

——. (1973). "Lesbian Health Care." Mimeographed. Los Angeles: Feminist Women's Health Center.

Hospital Tribune Report. (1973). "Trend to Do-It-Yourself Abortion Decried." Hospital Tribune, May 14, p. 6.

"Hospitals Bow to Couples Wanting Special Births." (1977). Medical World News 18 (October 3): 38-39.

"How to Get Hooked: Your Family Doctor as Pusher." (1972). Mother Lode 4 (Spring): 12.

Howard, Jan, Fred Davis, Clyde Pope, and Sheryl Ruzek. (1977). "Humanizing Health Care: The Implications of Technology, Centralization and Self-Care." Medical Care Supplement, 15 (May): 11-26.

Howard, John R. (1974). The Cutting Edge: Social Movements and Social Change in America. New York: J. B. Lippincott.

Howell, Mary. (1976). "Can We Be Feminist Physicians? Mirages, Dilemmas and Traps." Speech delivered to Women Medical Students Conference, February 14, University of California, Irvine. Mimeographed.

——. (1975a). Helping Ourselves: Families and the Human Network. Boston: Beacon Press.

——. (1975b). "A Women's Health School?" Social Policy 6 (September/October): 50-53.

——. (1974). "What Medical Schools Teach About Women." The New England Journal of Medicine 291 (August): 304-307.

——. (1973). Why Would a "Girl" Go Into Medicine? A Guide For Women. Old Westbury, N.Y.: The Feminist Press. Published under the pseudonym Margaret Campbell, M.D.

Huber, Joan, ed. (1973). "Changing Women in a Changing Society." American Journal of Sociology 78 (January).

Hughes, Everett. (1958). Men and Their Work. New York: The Free Press of Glencoe.

Hurvitz, Nathan. (1974). "Peer Self-Help Psychotherapy Groups: Psychotherapy Without Psychotherapists." In R. Roman and H. Trice, eds., The Sociology of Psychotherapy, pp. 84-138. New York: Jason Aronson.

Illich, Ivan. (1976). Medical Nemesis: The Expropriation of Health. New York: Pantheon Books.

"The Indians' Herbal Answer to the Pill." (1970). Mother Earth 3 (May): 8.

The Inforwomen Collective. (1974). Chicago Women's Directory. Chicago: Inforwomen.

Jackson, Leah. (1973). "Natural Birth Control." The Second Wave 2 ( ): 4-6, 24.

Jacobs, Shelley. (1978). AMSA Women in Medicine Committee Newsletter (January): 3-4.

Jeffcoate, Thomas. (1967). Principles of Gynecology. London: Butterworth. Cited in D. Scully and P. Bart, "A Funny Thing Happened on the Way to the Orifice: Women in Gynecology Textbooks." American Journal of Sociology 78 (January 1973): 1048.

Jenness, Linda, Caroline Lund, Andrea Morell, and Maxine Williams. (1973). Abortion: Women's Fight for the Right to Choose. New York: Pathfinder Press.

Johnson, Anita. (1975). "Humans: The Real Guinea Pigs." Her-Self 4 (June): 4-5.

Jones, Beverly, and Judith Brown. (1970). "Toward a Female Liberation Movement." In L. Tanner, ed., Voices From Women's Liberation. New York: Mentor.

Jones, Georgia. (1974). "DES Warning." Off Our Backs 4 (July): 7.

Jones, Vicki. (1973). "The Self-Help Clinic Movement." Paper presented at the 101st Annual Meeting of the American Public Health Association, November 5, San Francisco. Mimeographed.

Jong, Erica. (1975). Loveroot. New York: Holt, Rinehart and Winston.

———. (1973). Fear of Flying. New York: Holt, Rinehart and Winston.

———. (1971a). Fruits and Vegetables. New York: Holt, Rinehart and Winston.

———. (1971b). Half-Lives. New York: Holt, Rinehart and Winston.

Jourard, Sidney. (1971). The Transparent Self. New York: D. Van Nostrand.

Joyce, Virginia. (1972). "The Abortion: A Story." Woman Becoming 1 (December): 89-100.

Kaiser, Barbara, and Irwin Kaiser. (1974). "The Challenge of the Women's Movement to American Gynecology." American Journal of Obstetrics and Gynecology 120 (November): 652-61.

Kaiser, Irwin. (1978). Personal communication, April 8.

Kaplan, Helen Singer. (1974). The New Sex Therapy: Active Treatment of Sexual Dysfunctions. New York: Brunner/Mazel.

"Karman Found Guilty." (1974). Off Our Backs 4 (December/Janu-
ary): 13.

Karman, Harvey, and Malcolm Potts. (1972). "Very Early Abortion
Using Syringe as Vacuum Source." The Lancet 7759 (May 13):
1051-52.

Katz, Barbara. (1976). "Unnatural Childbirth ... Is the Jump in
the Cesarean Rate Too Great?" National Observer, January 17.

——. (1975). "The IUD's Unnatural Birth." National Observer,
September 8.

Kelman, Sander. (1971). "Toward the Political Economy of Medical
Care." Inquiry 8 (September): 30-38.

Kennedy, Edward M. (1972). In Critical Condition: The Crisis in
America's Health Care. New York: Simon and Schuster.

Kennell, J. H., R. Jerauld, H. Wolfe, D. Chester, N. Kerger,
W. McAlpine, M. Steffa, and M. Klaus. (1974). "Maternal Be-
havior One Year After Early and Extended Postpartum Contact."
Deviant Medical Child Neurology 16 (April): 172-79. Cited in
G. H. Peterson and L. E. Mehl, "Parental/Child Psychology—
Delivery Alternatives," Women & Health 2 (September/October
1977): 3-17.

Killian, Lewis M. (1964). "Social Movements." In R. Farls, ed.,
Handbook of Modern Sociology, pp. 426-55. Chicago: Rand
McNally.

Kinsey, Alfred C., N. Pomeroy, G. Martin, and P. Gebhard. (1953).
Sexual Behavior in the Human Female. Philadelphia: W. B. Saun-
ders.

Klaus, M. H., R. Jerauld, N. Kreger, W. McAlpine, M. Steffa,
and J. H. Kennell. (1972). "Maternal Attachment: Importance
of the First Post-Partum Days." New England Journal of Medicine
286 (March): 460-63. Cited in G. H. Peterson and L. E. Mehl,
"Parental/Child Psychology—Delivery Alternatives," Women &
Health 2 (September/October 1977): 4, 16.

Kleiber, Nancy. (1974). "Vancouver Women's Health Collective, Self-Help Clinic." Unpublished paper, School of Nursing, University of British Columbia.

Kleiber, Nancy, and Linda Light. (1978). Caring for Ourselves; An Alternative Structure for Health Care. Vancouver, B.C.: School of Nursing, University of British Columbia. National Health Research and Development Project No. 610-1020A of Health and Welfare, Canada.

Klemesrud, Judy. (1973). "Why Women Are Losing Faith in Their Doctors." McCalls 100 (June): 76-77.

Kobrin, Frances. (1966). "The American Midwife Controversy: A Crisis of Professionalization." Bulletin of the History of Medicine 40 (July/August): 350-63.

Koedt, Anne. (1973a). "Loving Another Woman." In A. Koedt, E. Levine, and A. Rapone, eds., Radical Feminism, pp. 85-93. New York: Quadrangle/The New York Times Book Company.

——. (1973b). "Women and the Radical Movement." In A. Koedt, E. Levine, and A. Rapone, eds., Radical Feminism, pp. 318-21. New York: Quadrangle/The New York Times Book Company.

Koedt, Anne, Ellen Levine, and Anita Rapone, eds. (1973). Radical Feminism. New York: Quadrangle/The New York Times Book Company.

Korsch, M. B., and V. F. Negrete. (1972). "Doctor-Patient Communication." Scientific American 227 (August): 66-74.

Kotelchuck, Ronda, and Howard Levy. (1975). "MCHR: An Organization in Search of an Identity." Health/PAC Bulletin 63 (March/April): 1-29.

Krauss, Elliott A. (1977). Power and Illness: The Political Sociology of Health and Medical Care. New York: Elsevier.

——. (1971). "Health Care and the Politics of Technology." Inquiry 8 (September): 51-59.

Kravits, Joanna. (1976). "Sex Differences in Health Care Social Survey Research Methods." In V. Olesen, ed., Women and Their Health: Research Implications for a New Era. Washington, D.C.: National Center for Health Services Research.

Kuchera, Lucile. (1971). "Postcoital Contraception with Diethylstilbestrol." Journal of the American Medical Association 218
(October 26): 562-63.

Kuhn, Thomas. (1962). The Structure of Scientific Revolutions.
Chicago: University of Chicago Press.

Kushner, Rose. (1975). Breast Cancer: A Personal History and an
Investigative Report. New York: Harcourt Brace Jovanovich.

Kushner, Trucia D. (1973). "The Nursing Profession—Condition:
Critical." Ms. 2 (August): 72-77, 99-102.

"Labeling: Only Your Doctor Knows." (1977). Network News (Octo-
ber/November): 1, 7.

Lader, Lawrence. (1973). Abortion II: Making the Revolution.
Boston: Beacon Press.

——. (1972). Foolproof Birth Control: Male and Female Sterilization. Boston: Beacon Press.

——. (1967). Abortion. Boston: Beacon Press.

——. (1955). Margaret Sanger and the Fight for Birth Control. New
York: Doubleday.

Lang, Raven. (1972). The Birth Book. Ben Lomond, Calif.: Gene-
sis Press.

Lanson, Lucienne. (1975). From Woman to Woman: A Gynecologist
Answers Questions About You and Your Body. New York: Knopf.

Lazarus, Margaret, producer. (1974). Taking Our Bodies Back.
Cambridge, Mass.: Cambridge Documentary Films.

Leach, Gerald. (1972). The Biocrats: Ethics and the New Medicine.
Rev. ed. Baltimore, Md.: Penguin Books.

Lederer, Wolfgang. (1968). The Fear of Women. New York: Harcourt Brace Jovanovich.

Lee, Nancy Howell. (1969). The Search for an Abortionist. Chicago:
University of Chicago Press.

Leinfelder, Mary. (1974). "More Abortion Stories." Her-Self 3 (August): 19.

Lembcke, Paul. (1956). "Medical Auditing by Scientific Methods, Illustrated by Major Female Pelvic Surgery." Journal of the American Medical Association 162 (October 13): 646-55.

Lennane, K. J., and R. J. Lennane. (1973). "Alleged Psychogenic Disorders in Women—A Possible Manifestation of Sexual Prejudice." New England Journal of Medicine 288 (February): 288-92.

Lennard, Henry L., and Leon J. Epstein. (1970). "Hazards Implicit in Prescribing Psychoactive Drugs." Science 169 (July 31): 438-41.

Lennard, Henry L., Leon J. Epstein, Arnold Bernstein, and Donald C. Ransom. (1971). Mystification and Drug Misuse: Hazards in Using Psychoactive Drugs. New York: Harper & Row.

Leonard, George. (1976). "The Holistic Health Revolution." New West (May): 40-49.

Lerner, Gerta. (1967). The Grimke Sisters From South Carolina: Rebels Against Slavery. Boston: Houghton-Mifflin.

"Letters—Controversy Over Controversy, OOB Replies." (1973). Off Our Backs 3 (November): 14-15.

Levin, David, Susan Devesa, David Godwin, and Debra Silverman. (1974). Cancer Rates and Risks. 2d ed. Department of Health, Education and Welfare publication, no. (NIH) 75-691. Washington, D.C.

Levin, Pamela, and Eric Berne. (1972). "Games Nurses Play." American Journal of Nursing 72 (March): 483-87.

Lewis, Deborah A. (1976). "Insuring Women's Health." Social Policy 7 (May/June): 19-25.

Lichtman, Richard. (1971). "The Political Economy of Medical Care." In H. P. Dreitzel, ed., The Social Organization of Health. New York: MacMillan.

Lieberman, Sharon. (1977). "A Hospital is Not a Home." Health-Right 3 (Fall): 3.

Light, Linda. (1974). "Vancouver Women's Health Collective, Profile of Membership." Unpublished paper, School of Nursing, University of British Columbia.

Light, Linda, and Nancy Kleiber. (1975a). "Report #1, Membership Process of the Vancouver Women's Health Collective." Unpublished paper, School of Nursing, University of British Columbia.

———. (1975b). "Report #3, State of the Research Health Education Groups of the Vancouver Women's Health Collective." Unpublished paper, School of Nursing, University of British Columbia.

———. (1975c). "Report #4, New Directions of the Vancouver Women's Health Collective." Unpublished paper, School of Nursing, University of British Columbia.

Linn, Lawrence S. (1971). "Physician Characteristics and Attitudes Toward Legitimate Use of Psychotherapeutic Drugs." Journal of Health and Social Behavior 12 (June): 132-40.

Linn, Lawrence, and Milton S. Davis. (1972). "Physicians-Orientation Toward the Legitimacy of New Drug Information." Social Science and Medicine 6 (April): 199-203.

———. (1971). "The Use of Psychotherapeutic Drugs by Middle-Aged Women." Journal of Health and Social Behavior 12 (December): 331-40.

Lipman-Blumen, Jean. (1975). "Changing Sex Roles in American Culture: Future Directions for Research." Annals of Sexual Behavior. Cited in Signs (1975) 1 (Autumn): 230.

"Liver Tumors and the Pill." (1974). Her-Self 3 (April): 3.

Lloyd, J. William. (1964). The Karezza Method. Mokelumne Hill, Calif.: Health Research.

Lomas, Peter. (1964). "Childbirth Ritual." New Society 31 (December). Cited in A. Oakley, Sex, Gender and Society. New York: Harper Colophon Books, 1972.

Lorber, Judith. (1975a). "Good Patients and Problem Patients: Conformity and Deviance in a General Hospital." Journal of Health and Social Behavior 16 (June): 213-25.

——. (1975b). "Women and Medical Sociology: Invisible Professionals and Ubiquitous Patients." In M. Millman and R. M. Kanter, eds., Another Voice: Feminist Perspectives on Social Life and Social Science, pp. 75-105. New York: Anchor Books.

Luy, Mary Lynn. (1974). "What's Behind Women's Wrath Toward Gynecologists." Modern Medicine 42 (October 14): 17-21.

McAfee, Kathy, and Myrna Wood. (1970). "Bread and Roses." In L. Tanner, ed., Voices From Women's Liberation. New York: Mentor.

McArthur, Sharon. (1973). "Childbirth in Four Non-Western Cultures." In D. Tennov and L. Hirsch, eds., Proceedings of the First International Childbirth Conference, p. 9. Stamford, Conn.: New Moon Communications.

McCarthy, Mary. (1963). The Group. New York: Harcourt, Brace and World.

McCormack, Thelma. (1975). "Toward a Nonsexist Perspective on Social and Political Change." In M. Millman and R. M. Kanter, eds., Another Voice: Feminist Perspectives on Social Life and Social Science, pp. 1-33. New York: Anchor Books.

McKinlay, John. (1977). "The Business of Good Doctoring or Doctoring as Good Business: Reflections on Freidson's View of the Medical Game." International Journal of Health Services 7 (Summer): 459-83.

——. (1975). "Who Is Really Ignorant—Physician or Patient?" Journal of Health and Social Beahvior 16 (March): 3-11.

——. (1973). "On the Professional Regulation of Change." In P. Halmos, ed., The Sociological Review Monograph, no. 20, Professionalisation and Social Change (University of Keele), December.

McLaren, Angus. (1975). "Medicine and Private Morality in France, 1800-1850." Feminist Studies 2 (Fall-Winter): 39-54.

McTigue, Joan. (1977). "Taking Our Bodies Back." HealthRight 3 (Fall): 1, 4-5.

"Machine May Cause Many Birth Defects." (1974). Her-Self 3 (April): 9.

Macintyre, Sally. (1977). Single and Pregnant. New York: Prodist.

Malinowski, Bronislaw. (1955). Sex and Repression in Savage Society. New York: Meridian Books.

Margolis, Susan. (1972). "Guides, for the New Woman." San Francisco Sunday Examiner & Chronicle, Calivornia Living, October 8.

Marguerite, Jeanne. (1973). "Birthing at Home." Broadside 1 (February 16): 7, 12-13.

Margulies, Leah. (1977). "Exporting Infant Malnutrition." Health-Right 3 (Spring): 1, 4.

Marieskind, Helen. (1976). "Gynecological Services and the Women's Movement: A Study of Self-Help Clinics and Other Modes of Delivery." Ph.D. dissertation, School of Public Health, University of California, Los Angeles.

——. (1975a). "The Women's Health Movement." International Journal of Health Services 5 (Spring): 217-23.

——. (1975b). "Restructuring Ob-Gyn." Social Policy 6 (September/October): 48-49.

Marieskind, Helen, and Barbara Ehrenreich. (1975). "Toward Socialist Medicine: The Women's Health Movement." Social Policy 6 (September/October): 34-42.

Matthews, Washington. (1902). "Myths of Gestation and Parturition." American Anthropologist 4: 737-42.

Maxtone-Graham, Katrina. (1973). Pregnant by Mistake: The Stories of Seventeen Women. New York: Liveright.

Mead, Margaret. (1972). "Forward." In H. Wortis and C. Rabinowitz, eds., The Women's Movement: Social and Psychological Perspectives. New York: Halsted Press.

——. (1949). Male and Female. New York: William Morrow.

Mead, Margaret, and Niles Newton. (1967). "Pregnancy, Childbirth and Outcome: A Review of Patterns of Culture and Future Research Needs." In S. Richardson and A. Guttmacher, eds., Childbearing: Its Social and Psychological Aspects. New York: Williams & Wilkins.

"Med Schools Prepare More Women." (1976). AWIS Newsletter (May/June): 6.

"Medical Bulletin." (1974). Majority Report 3 (January): 10.

Mehl, Lewis E. (1977). "Options in Maternity Care." Women & Health 2 (September/October): 11-23.

Mehl, L. E. (1976). "Statistical Outcomes of Homebirths in the U.S." In D. Stewart and L. Stewart, eds., Safe Alternatives in Childbirth. Chapel Hill, N.C.: NAPSAC.

Mehl, L. E., G. H. Peterson, N. S. Shaw, and D. C. Creevy. (1975). "Complications of Home Birth: An Analysis of a Series of 287 Home Births from Santa Cruz County, California," Birth and the Family Journal 2 (Winter): 123-35.

Mellinger, G. D., M. B. Balter, and D. I. Manheimer. (1971). "Patterns of Psychotherapeutic Drug Use Among Adults in San Francisco." Archives of General Psychiatry 25 (November): 385-94.

Mendelsohn, Everett, Judith P. Swazey, and Irene Taviss, eds. (1971). Human Aspects of Biomedical Innovation. Cambridge, Mass.: Harvard University Press.

"Mercurial Jelly." (1973). Off Our Backs 3 (September): 4.

Meyer, Adolph. (1935). "The Birth and Development of the Mental Hygiene Movement." Mental Hygiene 19 (January): 29-37.

Meyer, Lawrence. (1977). "Physicians and the Making of Money." The Washington Post, June 12.

Meyer, Wendy Haskell. (1974). "The Hidden Killer: Rare Cancer Hits Girls Whose Mothers Took DES." The National Observer (November 2): 1, 20.

Miles, Stephanie. (n.d.a). "Birth." Shameless Hussy Review, p. 3. San Lorenzo, Calif.: Shameless Hussy Press.

———. (n.d.b). "Labor." Shameless Hussy Review, p. 2. San Lorenzo, Calif.: Shameless Hussy Press.

Miller, John Seiden. (1962). Childbirth. New York: Atheneum.

Miller, Lindsay. (1973). "Lib Women Look at Having Babies." New York Post, June 4. Reprinted in Proceedings of the First International Childbirth Conference, p. 31. Stamford, Conn.: New Moon Communications.

Miller, N. F. (1947). "The Abuse of Pelvic Surgery in the Female." The Pennsylvania Medical Journal 50 (June): 939-44.

Millet, Kate. (1970). Sexual Politics. New York: Avon Books.

Millman, Marcia. (1977). The Unkindest Cut: Life in the Backrooms of Medicine. New York: William Morrow.

Millman, Marcia, and Rosabeth Moss Kanter. (1975). Another Voice: Feminist Perspectives on Social Life and Social Science. New York: Anchor Books.

Mintz, Morton. (1967). By Prescription Only. Boston: Beacon Press.

Mishell, Dahlia. (1974). "The CU-7 IUD." Her-Self 3 (April): 15.

Mitchell, Juliet. (1975). Psychoanalysis and Feminism. New York: Vintage Books.

——. (1973). Woman's Estate. New York: Vintage Books.

"A Modern Miracle of Organized Medicine—A Verdict Before the Trial." (1976). Mimeographed. Los Angeles: Feminist Women's Health Center, December.

Modlin, Herbert C. (1963). "Psychodynamics and Management of Paranoid States in Women." Archives of General Psychiatry 8 (March): 263-68. Cited in R. Roth and J. Lerner, "Sex-Based Discrimination in the Mental Institutionalization of Women." California Law Review 62 (May 1974): 802.

The Monthly Extract. (1974). 3 (March-April).

——. (1973). 2 (May-June).

Monty, Barbara. (1973). "Personal Action." The Second Wave 2 no. 3, p. 27.

Moorhead, Ann. (1975). Personal communication, June 30.

Morantz, Regina Markell. (1974). "The Perils of Feminist History." Journal of Interdisciplinary History 4 (Spring): 649-60.

Morehead, Mildred, and Ray Trussell. (1962). The Quantity, Quality and Costs of Medical Care Secured by a Sample of Teamster Families in the New York Area. New York: Columbia University School of Public Health and Administrative Medicine. Cited in H. Marieskind and B. Ehrenreich, "Toward Socialist Medicine: The Women's Health Movement." Social Policy 6 (September/October 1975): 42.

Morgan, Kenneth R. (1976). "Must You Coax Her into Lithotomy Position?" Medical Economics (December 13): 200-204.

Morgan, Robin, ed. (1970). Sisterhood is Powerful. New York: Vintage Books.

Morgan, Suzanne. (1976). "The Hysterectomy Experience." Unpublished paper, Sociology, College I, University of Massachusetts, Boston.

Mother Lode Collective. (1972). Mother Lode, Medical issue (Spring): 4.

Muller, Charlotte, and Frederick Jaffe. (1972). "Financing Fertility-Related Health Services in the United States, 1972-1978: A Preliminary Projection." Family Planning Perspectives 4 (January): 6-19.

Muller, Charlotte, Melvin Krasner, and Frederick Jaffe. (1975). "An Index of Insurance Adequacy for Fertility-Related Health Care." Medical Care 13 (January): 25-36.

Muller, Gretchen. (1972). "Drug Ads and the Big Lie." Rough Times 3 (December): 4-5.

Mumford, Emily. (1970). Interns: From Students to Physicians. Cambridge, Mass.: Harvard University Press.

Nader, Ralph, Peter Petkas, and Kate Blackwell, eds. (1972). Whistle-Blowing: The Report of the Conference on Professional Responsibility. New York: Bantam Books.

Naismith, Grace. (1973). "How Safe Is Do-It-Yourself Gynecology?" Family Health 5 (February): 24-25.

"NAPSAC Meeting Held, Home Birth Advocated, Decried." (1977). ACOG Newsletter (May).

National Abortion Rights Action League. (1976). "Legislative Alert!!!" NARAL Newsletter (July 23): 1.

———. (1975). NARAL Newsletter (March).

National Women's Health Coalition. (1974). "NWHC Women's Health Program." Mimeographed. (March 13). New York: National Women's Health Coalition.

———. (n.d.). "Early Atraumatic Termination of Pregnancy." Mimeographed. New York: National Women's Health Coalition.

National Women's Health Network. (1976). "Minutes May 22, 23, 1976 and Task Force Reports." Mimeographed. Washington, D.C.: National Women's Health Network.

Navarro, Vicente. (1975). "Women in Health Care." New England Journal of Medicine 292 (February 20): 398-402.

———. (1976). Medicine Under Capitalism. New York: Prodist.

Nelson, Cynthia, and Virginia Olesen. (1977). "Veil of Illusion: A Critique of the Concept of Equality in Western Thought." Catalyst 10-11 (Summer): 8-36.

"Network Hotline." (1977). Network News (October/November): 5-7.

"The New Sex Therapy: Active Treatment of Sexual Dysfunctions by Helen Singer Kaplan, M.D., Ph.D." (1976). Psychotherapy and Social Science Review 10 (October 15): 3-9.

Nochlin, Linda. (1971). "Why Are There No Great Women Artists?" In V. Gornick and B. K. Moran, eds., Women in Sexist Society: Studies in Power and Powerlessness, pp. 480-510. New York: Basic Books.

Nolan, William A. (1972). The Making of a Surgeon. New York: Pocketbooks.

Norsigian, Judy. (1976). "Women's Health Lobby Holds Demonstration in Washington, D.C." Her-Self (February): 7.

——. (1975-76). "Training the Docs." HealthRight 2 (Winter): 6.

North, Sandie. (1972). "Why all the Fuss About Gynecologists?" Family Circle (October). Cited in H. Marieskind, "Gynecological Services and the Women's Movement: A Study of Self-Help Clinics and Other Modes of Delivery." Ph.D. dissertation, School of Public Health, University of California, Los Angeles.

Novak, Edmund R., Georgeanna Seegar Jones, and Howard W. Jones. (1970). Novak's Textbook of Gynecology. Baltimore: Williams & Wilkins. Cited in D. Scully and P. Bart, "A Funny Thing Happened on the Way to the Orifice: Women in Gynecology Textbooks," American Journal of Sociology 78 (January 1973): 1048.

"NWHN Activist's Guide: An Action Index to Your Resources in Washington." (1977). Washington, D.C.: National Women's Health Network, June.

Oakley, Ann. (1974). The Sociology of Housework. New York: Pantheon Books.

Olds, Sally Wendkos. (1973). "Woman's Body, Woman's Mind: In Praise of Breast-Feeding." Ms. 1 (April): 10-13.

Olesen, Virginia, ed. (1977a). "Researchers Working in the Area of Women's Health." Roster prepared for the National Center for Health Services Research. Mimeographed. San Francisco: Department of Social and Behavioral Sciences, University of California.

——. (1977b). Women and Their Health: Research Implications for a New Era. Proceedings of a conference held at the University of California, San Francisco, August 1-2, 1975. Department of Health, Education and Welfare publication no. (HRA) 77-3138. Washington, D.C.: National Center for Health Services Research.

"$1-Million Sterilization Suit Filed." (1973). The Spokeswoman 4 (September 15): 1.

Ostrander, Sheila, and L. Schroeder. (1972). Astrological Birth Control. Englewood Cliffs, N.J.: Prentice-Hall.

Ostrum, Andrea. (1975). "Childbirth in America." In S. Hammer, ed., Women: Body and Culture—Essays on the Sexuality of Women in a Changing Society, pp. 277-92. New York: Perennial Library.

"The Overmedicated Woman." (1971). McCalls (September).

Ozonoff, Victoria Vespe, and David Ozonoff. (1975). "Steps Toward a Radical Analysis of Health Care: Problems and Prospects." International Journal of Health Services 5 (Spring): 239-314.

Page, Irvine H. (1975). "Our Critics Don't Know About Being a Doctor." Modern Medicine (January 15): 9, 13.

Palmer, Beverly. (1976). "Women's Self-Care Health Movement." Unpublished paper, Department of Psychology, California State College, Dominguez Hills.

——. (1974). "A Model for a Community-Based Women's Clinic." American Journal of Public Health 64 (July): 13-14.

Parachini, Alan. (1977). "Liberating the Delivery Room," New York Post, May 13.

Payne, Carol Williams. (1973). "Consciousness Raising: A Dead End?" In A. Koedt, E. Levine, and A. Rapone, eds., Radical Feminism, pp. 282-84. New York: Quadrangle/The New York Times Book Company.

Pearse, Warren H. (1977). "Home Birth Crisis." ACOG Newsletter (July).

Pearson, Jack W. (1975). "The Obstetrician and Gynecologist, Primary Physician for Women." Journal of the American Medical Association 231 (February 24): 815-16.

Pennell, Maryland, and Shirlene Showell, eds. (1975). Women in Health Careers: Status of Women in Health Careers in the United States and Other Selected Countries. Department of Health, Education and Welfare publication, no. (HRA) 75-55. Washington, D.C.: Department of Health, Education and Welfare, Public Health Service, Health Resources Administration.

Peskin, Ellen. (1976). Personal communication, December 6.

Peterson, Gail H., and Lewis E. Mehl. (1977). "Parental/Child Psychology—Delivery Alternatives." Women & Health 2 (September/October): 3-17.

Peterson, Karen Jean. (1976). "Creating Divisions of Labor: A Case Study of Nonprofessionals Professing Self-Help." Ph.D. dissertation, Northwestern University, Evanston, Ill.

The Philadelphia Women's Health Collective. (1973a). "Letters: Controversy Over Controversy." Off Our Backs 3 (November): 14.

——. (1973b). "The Philadelphia Story: Another Experiment on Women." Mimeographed. Philadelphia: Philadelphia Women's Health Collective.

"Physicians and Feminist Patients: Conflict Grows." (1973). Medical Tribune (November 7).

Pixa, Bea. (1975). "A Pair of Unorthodox Doctors." San Francisco Examiner & Chronicle, Sunday Scene, February 16, p. 4.

Planned Parenthood Association of Marin. (1973). "Tubal Ligation Referral Guide." Mimeographed. San Rafael, Calif.: Planned Parenthood Association of Marin.

Plath, Sylvia. (1971). Crossing the Water: Transitional Poems. New York: Harper & Row.

——. (1963). The Bell Jar. London: Heinemann. Published in the United States—New York: Harper & Row, 1971.

——. (1961). Ariel. New York: Harper & Row.

——. (1960). Colussus. London: Heinemann.

Polgar, Steven, and Ellen S. Fried. (1976). "The Bad Old Days: Clandestine Abortions Among the Poor in New York City Before Liberalization of the Abortion Law." Family Planning Perspectives 8 (May/June): 125-27.

Pollard, Vicki. (1969). "Producing Society's Babies." Women: A Journal of Liberation 1 (Fall): 18-21.

Pollner, Fran. (1975). "Feminist Movement's Impact on Ob. Gyn. Care Is Not Debatable." OB-Gyn News (June 15).

——. (1973). "NWRO Convention: Health Care." Off Our Backs 3 (July/August): 8.

"Population Report." (April 1973). Series F, no. 2. Washington, D.C.: Department of Medical and Public Affairs, The George Washington University Medical Center.

Prather, Jane, and Linda Fidell. (1975). "Sex Differences in the Content and Style of Medical Advertisements." Social Science and Medicine 9 (January): 23-26.

———. (1973). "Medical Advertising—Pressures for Prescribing Psychoactive Drugs to Women." Paper presented at the 68th Annual Meeting of the American Sociological Association, September, New York. Mimeographed.

Pratt, L. A., W. Seligman, and G. Reader. (1957). "Physicians' View on the Level of Medical Information Among Patients." American Journal of Public Health 47 (October): 1277-83. Cited in J. McKinlay, "Who Is Really Ignorant—Physician or Patient?," Journal of Health and Social Behavior 16 (March 1975): 3-11.

"Pregnancy Ruled a Disability." (1974). Off Our Backs 4 (June): 9.

Prensky, Joyce. (1975). Healing Yourself. Seattle, Wash.: The Country Doctor Clinic.

Prescott, Helen. (1976a). "A Cautious Investigation of the Hole." Her-Self 5 (July): 9.

———. (1976b). "Women's Herbal Folk Medicine—Part 1." Her-Self 5 (July): 12-13.

Price, Collette. (1972). "The Self-Help Clinic." Woman's World 1 (March/May). Reprinted by the Feminist Women's Health Centers.

"Proceedings of the Conference on Women and Health, June 27, 28, 29, 1974, Philadelphia, Pa." (1974). Commonwealth of Pennsylvania. Mimeographed.

"Proceedings of the Conference on Women's Health: Research, Policy and Communication." (1977). May 20-21, University of California, San Francisco. Program in Health Sciences. Mimeographed.

"Proceedings of the Conference on Women's Leadership and Authority in the Health Professions." (1977). June 19-21, held at the

University of California, Santa Cruz. Sponsored by the Program for Women in Health Sciences, University of California, San Francisco. Mimeographed.

Proceedings of the First International Childbirth Conference. (1973). Stamford, Conn.: New Moon Publications.

"Proceedings for the 1975 Conference on Women and Health." (1975). April 4-7, Boston. Available from Health Conference, c/o Box 192, West Somerville, Mass. 02141.

Quint, Jeanne C. (1972). "Institutionalized Practices of Information Control." In E. Freidson and J. Lorber, eds., Medical Men and Their Work. Chicago: Aldine Atherton.

——. (1965). "Institutionalized Practices of Information Control." Psychiatry 28 (May): 119-32.

Radicalesbians. (1970). "The Woman Identified Woman." In A. Koedt, E. Levine, and A. Rapone, eds., Radical Feminism, pp. 240-45. New York: Quadrangle/The New York Times Book Company, 1973.

Radicalesbians Health Collective. (n.d.). "Lesbians and the Health-Care System." Cited in P. Bart, "Sexism and Health Issues," The Hyde Parker (June 1973): 65, 70.

Rainone, Nanette, Martha Shelley, and Lois Hart. (1970). "Lesbians Are Sisters." In L. Tanner, ed., Voices from Women's Liberation. New York: New American Library.

Ramsey, Judith. (1973). "The Modern Woman's Health Guide to Her Own Body." Family Circle (July): 113-20.

Rapone, Anita. (1973). "The Body Is the Role: Sylvia Plath." In A. Koedt, E. Levine, and A. Rapone, eds., Radical Feminism, pp. 407-12. New York: Quadrangle/The New York Times Book Company.

Rau, Karen. (1974). "And Now, the 'Liberated' Woman Patient." American Medical News (October 7).

Record, Jane Cassels. (1974). "Leveling the Chinese Physician: 'Permanent Revolution' and the Medical Profession in the People's Republic of China." Paper presented at the American Sociological Association, August, Montreal. Mimeographed.

Regal, S. (1972). "My First Period." Women Becoming 1 (December): 7-8.

"Regional Reports." (1977). HealthRight 3 (Summer): 7.

"Regional Reports, New York City." (1976a). HealthRight 2 (Summer): 7.

"Regional Reports, New York City." (1976b). HealthRight 2 (Summer): 4.

"Regional Reports, New York, N.Y." (1976). HealthRight 2 (Spring): 7.

"Regional Reports, Washington, D.C." (1976). HealthRight 2 (Summer): 5.

Rennie, Susan, and Kirsten Grimsted. (1973). The New Woman's Survival Catalog. New York: Coward, McCann and Geoghegan.

Rennie, Susan, and Anna Rubin. (1977). "Catalog of Resources on Healing." Chrysalis Magazine 1: 1.

Reverby, Susan. (1975). "Alive and Well in Somerville, Mass." HealthRight 1 (Winter): 1.

———. (1972a). "Health: Women's Work." Health/PAC Bulletin 40 (April): 15-20.

———. (1972b). "The Sorcerer's Apprentice." Health/PAC Bulletin 46 (November): 10-16.

Reynard, Muriel J. (1973). "Gynecological Self-Help: An Analysis on Its Impact on the Delivery and Use of Medical Care For Women." Master's thesis, State University of New York, Stony Brook.

Rich, Adrienne. (1975). "The Theft of Childbirth." New York Review of Books (October 2): 25-30.

Richardson, Brian. (1976). "Medical Clinic Suit Dismissed." Tallahassee Democrat, December 1.

Ridenour, Nina. (1961). Mental Health in the United States. Cambridge, Mass.: Harvard University Press.

Rivers, Caryl. (1975). "The New Anxiety of Motherhood." In U. West, ed., Women in a Changing World, pp. 141-52. New York: McGraw-Hill.

Roberts, Barbara. (1972). "Psychosurgery: The 'Final Solution' to the 'Woman Problem'?" The Second Wave 2: 13-15, 43.

Roberts, Ron E., and Robert Marsh Kloss. (1974). Social Movements: Between the Balcony and the Barricade. Saint Louis: C. V. Mosby.

Robins, Joan. (1970). Handbook of Women's Liberation. North Hollywood, Calif.: Now Library Press. Cited in M. L. Carden, The New Feminist Movement, p. 64. New York: Russell Sage Foundation.

Roby, Pamela. (1975). "Sociology and Women in Working-Class Jobs." In M. Millman and R. M. Kanter, eds., Another Voice: Feminist Perspectives on Social Life and Social Science, pp. 203-39. New York: Anchor Books.

———. (1973). Childcare, Who Cares? New York: Basic Books.

Rodgers, Joann. (1975). "Rush to Surgery." New York Times Magazine, September 21, pp. 34-36.

Rogers, J. M. (1971). "Drug Abuse by Prescription." Psychology Today 5 (September): 16-20.

Rollin, Betty. (1972). "Motherhood: Who Needs It?" In L. Howe, ed., The Future of the Family, pp. 69-82. New York: Simon and Schuster.

Rosenbach, Margo, and Joan King. (1977). "Woman & Health." Washington, D.C.: WEAL.

Rosengren, William R., and Spencer DeVault. (1963). "The Sociology of Time and Space in an Obstetrical Hospital." In E. Freidson, ed., The Hospital in Modern Society. New York: The Free Press of Glencoe.

Rosoff, Jeanie. (n.d.). "Memorandum: DHEW Proposed Regulations on Sterilization." Washington, D.C.: Planned Parenthood-World Population.

——. (1973). "Sterilization: The Montgomery Case—And Its After-math." The Hastings Center Report 3 (September): 6.

Rossi, Alice. (1977). "A Biosocial Perspective on Parenting." Daedalus 106: 1-31.

Rossi, Alice, and Anne Calderwood, eds. (1973). Academic Women on the Move. New York: Russell Sage Foundation.

Roth, Julius. (1978). Personal communication, January 14.

——. (1977a). "A Yank in the NHS." In A. Davis and G. Horobin, eds., Medical Encounters, pp. 191-205. London: Croom-Helm.

——, with the collaboration of Richard R. Hanson. (1977b). Health Purifiers and Their Enemies: A Study of the Natural Health Move-ment in the United States with a Comparison to Its Counterpart in Germany. New York: Prodist.

——. (1973). "Care of the Sick: Professionalism vs. Love." Science, Medicine and Man 1 (July): 173-80.

——. (1972). "Some Contingencies of the Moral Evaluation and Con-trol of Clients." American Journal of Sociology 77 (March): 839-56.

——. (1963a). "Information and the Control of Treatment in Tuber-culosis Hospitals." In E. Freidson, ed., The Hospital in Modern Society. New York: The Free Press of Glencoe.

——. (1963b). " 'Management Bias' in Social Science Study of Medi-cal Treatment." Human Organization 21 (Spring): 47-50.

Roth, Robert T. (1973). "Break Through the Looking Glass—Sexism in Psychiatry." Issues in Radical Therapy 1 (Autumn): 11-13.

Roth, Robert T., and Judith Lerner. (1974). "Sex-Based Discrimi-nation in the Mental Institutionalization of Women." California Law Review 62 (May): 789-815.

Rothman, Barbara Katz. (1976). "Woman's Body, Woman's Mind: In Which a Sensible Woman Persuades Her Doctor, Her Family and Her Friends to Help Her Give Birth at Home." Ms. (Decem-ber): 27-32.

Rothman, Lorraine. (1972). "Self-Help Clinic: Paramedic Politics." In M. Alleyn, ed., The Witch's Os, pp. 27-30. Stamford, Conn.: New Moon Communications.

Roundtable Report. (1977). 3 (March 30). Washington, D.C.: Women and Health Roundtable.

Rush, Anne Kent. (1973). Getting Clear: Body Work for Women. New York/Berkeley, Calif.: Random House/Bookworks.

Rush, Anne Kent, and Anica Mander. (1974). Feminism as Therapy. New York/Berkeley, Calif.: Random House/Bookworks.

Rushing, William. (1971). "Public Policy, Community Constraints, and the Distribution of Medical Resources." Social Problems 19 (Summer): 21-36.

Russell, Diana E. H. (1975). Politics of Rape: The Victim's Perspective. New York: Stein and Day.

Ruzek, Sheryl. (1977a). "Emergent Modes of Utilization: Gynecological Self-Help." In V. Olesen, ed., Women and Their Health: Research Implications for a New Era. Department of Health, Education and Welfare publication, no. (HRA) 77-3138. Washington, D.C.: National Center for Health Services Research.

———. (1977b). "Where Do We Go From Here? Strategies for Change." In "Proceedings of the Conference on Women's Leadership and Authority in the Health Professions," June 19-21, University of California, Santa Cruz, pp. 265-75. Mimeographed.

———. (1975a). "Social Science and Pressure Groups: Policy Making on Women and Drugs." Paper presented to the Society for the Study of Social Problems, August 23, San Francisco. Mimeographed.

———. (1975b). Women and Health Care: A Bibliography with Selected Annotation. Occasional Papers, no. 1. Evanston, Ill.: Program on Women, Northwestern University.

———. (1974). "The Women's Health Movement from a Feminist Perspective." Paper presented at the Annual Meeting of American Association for the Advancement of Science, March 1, San Francisco. Mimeographed.

——. (1973). "Making Social Work Accountable." In E. Freidson, ed., The Professions and Their Prospects, pp. 217-43. Beverly Hills, Calif.: Sage Publications.

Ryder, N. B., and C. F. Westoff. (1965). "National Fertility Study." In C. F. Westoff, E. C. Moore, and N. B. Ryder, Milbank Memorial Fund Quarterly 47 (1969): 11. Cited in J. Blake, "Abortion and Public Opinion: The 1960-1970 Decade," Science 171 (February 1971): 540.

Sablosky, Ann. (1976). "The Power of the Forceps: A Comparative Analysis of the Midwife, Historically and Today." Women & Health 1 (January/February): 10-13.

Sabol, Blair. (1972). "Menstrual Extraction: The at Home Abortion." Village Voice, August 3, p. 11.

Sade, Robert M. (1971). "Medical Care as a Right: A Refutation." New England Journal of Medicine 285 (December): 406-12.

Sadler, Alfred M., B. Sadler, and A. Bliss. (1972). The Physician's Assistant: Today and Tomorrow. New Haven, Conn.: Yale University Press.

Salmon, Thomas W. (1913). "Immigration and the Mixture of Races in Relation to the Mental Health of the Nation." In W. A. White, ed., Medical Treatment of Nervous and Mental Disease, pp. 241-86. New York: Lea and Febiger.

Salomon, Mathilde. (1974). "Taking Our Bodies to the Body Shop." Majority Report 3 (January): 7, 10.

Samuels, Mike, and Hal Bennett. (1973). The Well Body Book. New York/Berkeley, Calif.: Random House/Bookworks.

Sandmaier, Marian. (1976). "Fighting for Our Lives: Women and U.S. Health Care." AAUW Journal (April).

Sanger, Margaret. (1938). Margaret Sanger: An Autobiography. New York: Dover Publications. Reissued 1971.

——. (1920). Woman and the New Race. New York: Truth Publishing.

"Santa Cruz Center Victory." (1976). Her-Self 5 (July): 4.

Sartwell, P. E. (1974). "Iatrogenic Disease: An Epidemiological Perspective." International Journal of Health Services 4 (Winter): 89-93.

Sarvis, Betty, and Hyman Rodman. (1973). The Abortion Controversy. New York: Columbia University Press.

Scheff, Thomas, ed. (1967). Mental Illness and Social Processes. New York: Harper & Row.

———. (1966). Being Mentally Ill: A Sociological Theory. Chicago: Aldine.

Schutz, Alfred. (1964). "The Well Informed Citizen: An Essay on the Social Distribution of Knowledge." In A. Schutz, Collected Papers II: Studies in Social Theory. The Hague: Martinez Nijhoff.

Scully, Diana, and Pauline Bart. (1973). "A Funny Thing Happened on the Way to the Orifice: Women in Gynecology Textbooks." American Journal of Sociology 78 (January): 1045-50.

Seaman, Barbara. (1975). "Pelvic Autonomy: Four Proposals." Social Policy 6 (September/October): 43-47.

———. (1972). Free and Female. New York: Fawcett.

———. (1969). The Doctors' Case Against the Pill. New York: Avon.

Seaman, Barbara, and Gideon Seaman. (1977). Women and the Crisis in Sex Hormones. New York: Rawson Associates.

Seashore, M. J., A. D. Leifer, C. R. Barnett, and P. H. Lederman. (1973). "The Effects of Denial of Early Mother-Infant Interaction on Maternal Self-Confidence." Journal of Personality and Social Psychology 26: 369-78. Cited in G. H. Peterson and L. E. Mehl, "Parental/Child Psychology—Delivery Alternatives," Women & Health 2 (September/October 1977): 3-17.

Seidenberg, Robert. (1971). "Drug Advertising and Perception of Mental Illness." Mental Hygiene 55 (January): 21-31.

———. (1960). "Interpersonal Determinants of Reality-Testing Capacity." Archives of General Psychiatry 3 (October): 368-72.

Seligmann, Jean, with Mariana Gosnell and Dan Shapiro. (1976). "New Science of Birth." Newsweek (November 15): 55-60.

Service, Elman R. (1963). Profiles in Ethnology. New York: Harper & Row.

Shandall, Ahmed Abu-El-Futuh. (1967). "Circumcision and Infibulation of Females." Sudan Medical Journal 5 (December): 178-212.

Shapiro, Eileen. (1977). "Some Thoughts on Counseling Women Who Perceive Themselves to be Victims of Nonactionable Sex Discrimination: A Survival Guide." In "Proceedings of the Conference on Women's Leadership and Authority in the Health Professions," June 19-21, 1977, University of California, Santa Cruz. Mimeographed.

Shapiro, Eileen, and Shirley G. Driscoll. (1977a). "Reduced-Schedule Graduate Medical Education: A Status Report." In "Proceedings of the Conference on Women's Leadership and Authority in the Health Professions," June 19-21, 1977, University of California, Santa Cruz. Mimeographed.

——. (1977b). "Reduced Schedule Residencies: Innovations in Medical Education." Journal of the American Medical Women's Association 32 (August): 291-92.

Shapiro, Susan E. (1975). "The Politics of Dysmenorrhea." Unpublished paper.

Shaw, Nancy. (1974). Forced Labor: Maternity Care in the United States. New York: Pergamon Press.

——. (1972). "So You're Going to Have a Baby: Institutional Treatment of Maternity Patients." Ph.D. dissertation, Brandeis University.

Shinder, Dorothy. (1972). Mayhem on Women. San Rafael, Calif.: Ombudswoman.

Shostak, Arthur B. (1974). Modern Social Problems: Solving Today's Social Problems. New York: Macmillan.

Showalter, Elaine. (1973). "Women Writers and the Female Experience." In A. Koedt, E. Levine, and A. Rapone, eds., Radical Feminism, pp. 391-406. New York: Quadrangle/The New York Times Book Company.

Shryock, Richard H. (1966). Medicine in America: Historical Essays. Baltimore, Md.: Johns Hopkins Press.

Sidel, Ruth. (1975). "New Roles for Women in Health Care Delivery in the People's Republic of China." Paper presented at the International Conference on Women in Health, June 16-18, Washington, D.C. Mimeographed.

Sidel, Victor, and Ruth Sidel. (1974). "The Delivery of Medical Care in China." Scientific American 230 (April): 19-27.

Silverman, Arlene. (1976). "Women Watching Out for Women." San Francisco Sunday Examiner & Chronicle, California Living, August 29, pp. 14-16.

Silverman, Milton, and Philip R. Lee. (1974). Pills, Profits and Politics. Berkeley: University of California Press.

Skipper, James K. (1965). "Communication and the Hospitalized Patient." In J. Skipper and R. Leonard, eds., Social Interaction and Patient Care. Philadelphia: J. B. Lippincott.

Skipper, J. K., D. L. Tagliacozzo, and H. O. Mauksch. (1964). "Some Possible Consequences of Limited Communication Between Patients and Hospital Functionaries." Journal of Health and Human Behavior 5 (Spring): 34-40. Cited in J. McKinlay, "Who Is Really Ignorant—Physician or Patient?," Journal of Health and Social Behavior 16 (March 1975): 3-11.

Smith, Dorothy, and Sara David, eds. (1975). Women Look at Psychiatry. Vancouver, B.C.: Press Gang Publishers.

Smith, Margot. (1973). "A Preliminary Paper on Menstrual Extraction." Unpublished paper, School of Public Health, University of California, Berkeley.

Smith, Page. (1970). Daughters of the Promised Land: Women in American History. Boston: Little, Brown.

Smith-Rosenberg, Carroll. (1975). "The Female World of Love and Ritual: Relations Between Women in Nineteenth-Century America." Signs 1 (Autumn): 1-29.

——. (1973). "Puberty to Menopause: The Cycle of Feminity in Nineteenth-Century America." Feminist Studies 1 (Winter-Spring): 58.

——. (1972). "The Hysterical Woman: Sex Roles in 19th Century America." Social Research 39 (Winter): 652-78.

Snow, Eleanor. (1975). "Overview, International Women's Year Conference and Tribunal." Feminist Women's Health Center Report 1 (April): 1-2.

Social Problems. (1975). 22 (April).

Sociologists for Women in Society. (1977). SWS Newsletter 7 (October).

Spake, Amanda. (1978). "The Pushers." In Claudia Dreifus, ed., Seizing Our Bodies: The Politics of Women's Health. New York: Vintage Books.

The Spokeswoman. (1975). 3 (November 1).

Stacey, Margaret, ed. (1976). The Sociology of the N.H.S. The Sociological Review monograph, no. 22 (University of Keele).

Stafford, William. (1976). "Order Denying Preliminary Injunction, Feminist Women's Health Center, Inc. vs. Mahmood Mohammad, M.D., et al." U.S. District Court, Tallahassee Division, June 9, 1976.

Stamm, Karen, and Suzanne Williamson. (1978). "The Sterilization Con-nection." HealthRight 4 (Winter): 3.

Stannard, Una. (1970). "Adam's Rib, Or the Woman Within." Trans-Action 8 (November/December): 24-35.

"State of California Goes Fishing Without a License." (1977). Feminist Women's Health Center Report (April): 12.

"Statement of Chicago Women." (1974). Majority Report 3 (January): 6.

Steele, Darlene. (1974). "A Study of Women Using a Self-Help Clinic." Master's thesis, School of Nursing, University of British Columbia. Cited in N. Kleiber, "Vancouver Women's Health Collective Self-Help Clinic." Unpublished paper, School of Nursing, University of British Columbia.

Stephen, Beverly. (1975). "The IUD Controversy." San Francisco Chronicle, January 30, p. 17.

———. (1974). "U.S. Input into World Lib." San Francisco Chronicle, September 16, p. 17.

———. (1973a). "Perinatal Care at Home." San Francisco Chronicle, October 4, p. 21.

———. (1973b). "What Women Want From Their Doctors." San Francisco Chronicle, July 20, p. 20.

"Sterilization Abuse of Women: The Facts." (1975). Mimeographed. New York: Committee to End Sterilization Abuse.

"Sterilization Guidelines Criticized by ACLU." (1973). The Spokeswoman 4 (November): 2.

Stim, Edward M. (1973). "Minisuction: An Office Abortion Procedure." Paper presented at the American Association of Planned Parenthood Physicians, April 13, Houston, Texas. Mimeographed. Reprinted by National Women's Health Coalition, New York.

Stimson, Gerry, and Barbara Webb. (1975). Going to See the Doctor. London: Routledge and Kegan Paul.

"Supercoil Suit." (1973). Off Our Backs 3 (July/August): 6.

"Support, Information by Ob. Gyn. 'Best Response' to Women's Lib." (1975). OB-Gyn News (March 1).

Sweeney, William J., with Barbara Lang Stern. (1973). Woman's Doctor: A Year in the Life of an Obstetrician-Gynecologist. New York: William Morrow.

Switzer, Ellen. (1976). "New and Better Breast Cancer Treatments." Woman's Day 40 (November): 92-98, 164.

Szasz, Thomas. (1970). The Manufacture of Madness: A Comparative Study of the Inquisition and the Mental Health Movement. New York: Harper & Row.

———. (1963). Law, Liberty and Psychiatry. New York: Macmillan.

———. (1961). The Myth of Mental Illness. New York: Harper & Row.

Szasz, Thomas, and M. H. Hollender. (1956). "A Contribution of the Philosophy of Medicine: The Basic Models of the Doctor-Patient."

American Medical Association Archives of Internal Medicine 97 (May): 585-92.

"Tallahassee FWHC Fights Back." (1976). *Network News* (December): 1, 4.

"Tallahassee FWHC Update." (1976). *Feminist Women's Health Center Newsletter* 3 (January): 2.

Tanner, Leslie B. (1970). *Voices From Women's Liberation*. New York: Mentor.

Tanzer, Deborah. (1973). "Natural Childbirth: Pain or Peak Experience?" In Carol Tavris and the editors of *Psychology Today*, eds., *The Female Experience*, pp. 26-32. Del Mar, Calif.: C/R/M.

Teixeira, Linda. (1976). "Health Highlights of the 94th Congress." *Network News* (October): 2-3.

Tennov, Dorothy. (1975). *Psychotherapy: The Hazardous Cure*. New York: Abelard-Schuman.

———. (1973). "Feminism and Psychotherapy and Professionalism." *Journal of Contemporary Psychotherapy* 5 (Summer): 107-11.

"Testimony Heard on IUD, Pap Smears." (1976). *Coalition News* (July): 5.

Theodore, Athena, ed. (1971). *The Professional Woman*. Cambridge, Mass.: Schenkman.

Thompson, Kathleen, and Andra Medea. (1974). *Against Rape*. New York: Farrar, Straus & Giroux.

Thomsen, Russel J. (1975). "Viewpoints Supporting the Classification of Intrauterine Devices as Drugs." Statement prepared for a Hearing of the Department of Health, State of California, San Francisco, March 5. Mimeographed. San Francisco: Coalition for the Medical Rights of Women.

Thorne, Barrie. (1975). "Protest and the Problem of Credibility: Uses of Knowledge and Risk-Taking in the Draft Resistance Movement of the 1960's." *Social Problems* 23 (December): 111-23.

Tietze, Christopher. (1968). "Statistical Assessment of Adverse Experiences Associated with the Use of Oral Contraceptives." Clinical Obstetrics and Gynecology 11 (September): 698–715. Cited in B. Seaman, Free and Female, p. 181. New York: Fawcett, 1972.

Tietze, Christopher, and Sara Lewit. (1973). "Early Medical Complications of Abortion by Saline: Joint Program for the Study of Abortion." Studies in Family Planning 4 (June): 133–38.

"Tinidazole: Another Carcinogen for Women." (1974). Off Our Backs 4 (August/September): 9.

Treseder, A. (1970). "Obstetrics in the Wrong Hands." Everywoman 1 (October): 13.

Tuchman, Gaye. (1975). "Women and the Creation of Culture." In M. Millman and R. M. Kanter, eds., Another Voice: Feminist Perspectives on Social Life and Social Science, pp. 171–202. New York: Anchor Books.

Turner, Castellano, and William A. Darity. (1973). "Fears of Genocide Among Black Americans as Related to Age, Sex and Region." American Journal of Public Health 63 (December): 1029–34.

Turner, Ralph. (1969). "The Theme of Contemporary Social Movements." British Journal of Sociology 20 (December): 390–405.

U.S. Department of Labor. (1975). 1975 Handbook on Women Workers. Bulletin 297. Washington, D.C.: Department of Labor, Women's Bureau.

"Vaginal Sprays." (1973). Her-Self 2 (July/August): 4.

Vancouver Women's Health Collective. (n.d.). "Doctor Questionnaire." Mimeographed. Vancouver, B.C.: Vancouver Women's Health Collective.

Verbrugge, Martha H. (1975). "Historical Complaints and Political Disorders: A Review of Ehrenreich and English's Study of Medical Ideas About Women." International Journal of Health Services 5 (Spring): 323–34.

"Vitamin C Abortion." (1974). Off Our Backs 4 (December/January): 14.

"Vitamin C Abortion." (1973). Monthly Extract 2 (December/January): 14-15.

Von B, Marge. (1974). "A New Cause—Midwifery." Watsonville Register-Pajaronia, March 8, p. 1.

Walsh, Mary Roth (1977). "Doctors Wanted: No Women Need Apply." In Sexual Barriers in the Medical Profession 1835-1975. New Haven, Conn.: Yale University Press.

———. (1975). "Feminism: A Support System for Women Physicians." Journal of the American Medical Women's Association 31 (June): 247-50.

Walstedt, Joyce Jennings. (1971). "The Anatomy of Oppression: A Feminist Analysis of Psychotherapy." Mimeographed. Pittsburgh: KNOW.

Weber, Max. (1958). From Max Weber: Essays in Sociology. H. H. Gerth and C. W. Mills, eds., trans. New York: Oxford University Press.

———. (1947). Max Weber: The Theory of Social and Economic Organization. A. M. Henderson and T. Parsons, trans. New York: The Free Press.

Weinerman, E. Richard. (1969). Social Medicine in Eastern Europe. Cambridge, Mass.: Harvard University Press.

Weiss, Kay. (1975a). "Epidemiology of Vaginal Adenocarcinoma and Adenosis: Current Status." American Medical Women's Association 30 (February): 59-63.

———. (1975b). "What Medical Students Learn About Women." Off Our Backs 5 (April/May): 24-25.

———. (1974a). "Vaginal Cancer." The Monthly Extract 3 (May/June): 10-11.

———. (1973). "Afterthoughts on the Morning-After Pill." Ms. (November): 22, 24-26.

———. (1972, 1974b). "Fact Sheet on DES." Mimeographed. Pittsburgh: KNOW.

——. (n.d.). "Epidemiology of Vaginal Adenocarcinoma and Adenosis: A Literature Review." Mimeographed. Pittsburgh: KNOW.

Weisstein, Naomi. (1971). Psychology Constructs the Female, or the Fantasy Life of the Male Psychologist. Boston: New England Free Press.

"Well Women Clinics Are Wave of Future." (1973). The Spokeswoman 3 (April 15): 1-2.

Wellford, Harrison. (1972). Sowing the Wind: Nader Study Group Report on Food Safety and the Chemical Harvest. New York: Bantam Books.

The West Coast Sisters. (1971). "Self-Help Clinics." Mimeographed. Los Angeles: Feminist Women's Health Center.

"WHAM Will Demonstrate on Women's Health Issues at Democratic Convention." (1976). Women Today (July 5): 96.

"What Is 'Feminist Health'?" (1974). Off Our Backs 4 (June): 2-5.

Wheeler, Robinetta. (1975). "Tools for Change: WIN Program." Unpublished paper, Department of Social and Behavioral Sciences, University of California, San Francisco.

Whiting, J. W. M., R. Kluckhohn, and A. Anthony. (1958). "The Function of Male Initiation Ceremonies at Puberty." In E. Maccoby, T. Newcomb, and E. Hartley, eds., Readings in Social Psychology, 3d ed. New York: Holt Rinehart & Winston.

"Who Speaks for Women in Washington?" (n.d.). Mimeographed. Washington, D.C.: Women's Lobby.

Wilson, Angela. (1976-77). "Black Women's Health." HealthRight 3 (Winter): 1, 6.

Wilson, John. (1973). Introduction to Social Movements. New York: Basic Books.

Wilson, J. R. (1970). "Health Care for Women: Present Deficiencies and Future Needs." Obstetrics and Gynecology 36 (August): 178-86.

Wolfe, Sidney M. (1977). Letter to HEW Secretary Joseph Califano, December 12. Mimeographed. Washington, D.C.: Health Research Group.

———. (1973). "Statement of Sidney M. Wolfe, M.D., Health Research Group, Washington, D.C." Presented at the "Quality of Health Care—Human Experimentation" Hearings before the U.S. Congress, Senate, Subcommittee on Health of the Committee on Labor and Public Welfare, 93rd Cong., 1st sess., March 7, 8, 1973, pt. 3: 809-13.

———. (1971). "Consumerism and Health Care." Public Administration Review 31 (September/October): 528-36.

Wolfson, Alice. (1970). "Caution: Health Care May Be Hazardous to Your Health." Up From Under 1 (May/June): 5-10.

Womanpower Project. (1973). The New York Woman's Directory. New York: Workman.

A Woman's Place. (1972). A Vancouver Women's Health Booklet. Vancouver, B.C.: Press Gang Publishers.

"Women Air Health Care Discontent." (1975). California Aggie 87 (February 3): 1.

"Women and Drugs Subject of Statewide Media Campaign." (1974). Joint Newsletter State Department of Health, State Office of Narcotics and Drug Abuse 1 (December): 6.

Women & Health. (1976). 1 (January-February).

"Women Gather for Drug Conference." (1974). Joint Newsletter State Department of Health, State Office of Narcotics and Drug Abuse 1 (December): 1.

"Women's Clinics." (1971). Health/PAC Bulletin 34 (October): 14-16.

Women's Community Health Center. (1976). "Letter." HealthRight 2: 2.

———. (1976). "Experiences of a Pelvic Teaching Group." Women & Health 1 (July-August).

Women's Equity Action League. (1976). "National Legislative Program, Unanimously Adopted at Philadelphia Convention, May 1976." Mimeographed. Washington, D.C.: WEAL.

Women's Health and Abortion Collective. (1973). "D.C. Abortion Clinic Evaluation." Off Our Backs 3 (September): 5-7.

Women's Health Consumers Union. (July 7, 1973). Letter. Duplicated and mailed to women's health groups.

"Women's Liberation and the Practice of Medicine." (1973). Medical World News 14 (June 22): 33-38.

Women's Work Project of the Union for Radical Political Economics. (1976). "USA—Women Health Workers." Women & Health 1 (May/June): 14-23.

Wood, Ann Douglas. (1973). "The Fashionable Diseases: Women's Complaints and Their Treatment in Nineteenth-Century America." Journal of Interdisciplinary History 4 (Summer): 25-52.

Woodside, Nina. (1975). "Women in Health Care Decision Making." Philadelphia Medicine (October): 431-41.

Yost, Kaye. (1974). "At Home or in the Hospital?" San Francisco Sunday Examiner & Chronicle, California Living, November 6, pp. 6-11.

Young, Frank. (1965). Initiation Ceremonies: A Cross-Cultural Study of Status Dramatization. New York: Bobbs-Merrill.

——. (1962). "The Function of Male Initiation Ceremonies: A Cross-Cultural Test on an Alternative Hypothesis." American Journal of Sociology 67 (January): 379-96.

Young, Frank W., and Albert A. Bacdayan. (1965). "Menstrual Taboos and Social Rigidity." Ethnology 4 (April): 225-40.

Zahler, Leah. (1973-74). "Abortion." Aphra 5 (Winter): 46-47.

Zald, Mayer N., and Roberta Ash. (1966). "Social Movement Organizations." Social Forces 44 (March): 327-41.

Ziegler, Vicki, and Elizabeth L. Campbell. (1973). Circle One: Self Health Handbook. Pittsburgh: KNOW.

Zola, Irving Kenneth. (1972). "Medicine as an Institution of Social Control." _The Sociological Review_ 20 (November): 487–504.

Zola, Irving Kenneth, and Stephen J. Miller. (1973). "The Erosion of Medicine from Within." In E. Freidson, ed., _The Professions and Their Prospects_, pp. 155–72. Beverly Hills, Calif.: Sage Publications, 1976.

NAME INDEX

SUBJECT INDEX

ABOUT THE AUTHOR

SHERYL BURT RUZEK is Community Coordinator, Program for Women in Health Sciences, University of California, San Francisco. She is also Research Associate and Member of the Advisory Board, Center for the Study of Women, Institute for Scientific Analysis, San Francisco.

Previous publications include <u>Women and Health Care: A Bibliography With Selected Annotation</u>, available from the Program on Women, Northwestern University. She has also published in the areas of medical self-help and client-professional relations.

Dr. Ruzek holds a B.A. from San Francisco State University and received an M.A. and Ph.D. from the University of California, Davis.

RELATED TITLES
Published by
Praeger Special Studies

THE HIGHER EDUCATION OF WOMEN:
Essays in Honor of Rosemary Parks

> edited by
> Helen S. Astin
> Werner Z. Hirsch

*WOMEN'S RIGHTS AND THE LAW:
The Impact of the ERA on State Laws

> Barbara A. Brown
> Ann E. Freedman
> Harriet N. Katz
> Alice M. Price
> with Hazel Greenberg

WOMEN AND MEN: Changing Roles,
Relationships and Perceptions

> Libby A. Cater
> Ann Firor Scott
> with Wendy Martyna

IMPACT OF FAMILY PLANNING PROGRAMS
ON FERTILITY: The U.S. Experience

> Phillips Cutright
> Frederick S. Jaffe

PASSAGE THROUGH ABORTION: The Personal
and Social Reality of Women's Experience

> Mary K. Zimmerman

*Also available in paperback.